ALLERGIC DISEASES OF THE EYE

July 2001

To Stevie

Your insight + focus have made a difference Hope to see you back in Ophthalmic Pharma Industry soon Fond Regards

THARK

ALLERGIC DISEASES OF THE EYE

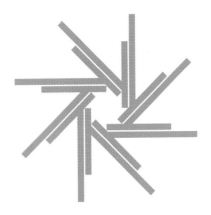

MARK B. ABELSON, M.D., C.M., F.R.C.S. (C)

Clinical Associate Professor of Ophthalmology
Harvard Medical School

Senior Clinical Scientist
Schepens Eye Research Institute
Boston
Ophthalmic Research Associates
North Andover, Massachusetts

Illustrated by David Anders Tilden, A.M.I.

W.B. SAUNDERS COMPANY
A Harcourt Health Sciences Company
Philadelphia ■ London ■ New York ■ St. Louis ■ Sydney ■ Toronto

W.B. SAUNDERS COMPANY
A Harcourt Health Sciences Company

The Curtis Center
Independence Square West
Philadelphia, Pennsylvania 19106

Library of Congress Cataloging-in-Publication Data

Allergic diseases of the eye / [edited by] Mark B. Abelson; illustrated by David Anders Tilden.

p.   cm.

ISBN 0–7216–8679–6

1. Eye—Diseases—Immunological aspects.   2. Allergy.   3. Eye—Inflammation.   I. Abelson, Mark B.   [DNLM: 1. Eye Diseases—immunology.   2. Hypersensitivity.   3. Eye Diseases—therapy.   WW 160 A434 2000]

RE68.A44 2000   617.7'1—dc21
DNLM/DLC
                                                            99–23446

Editor-in-Chief: Lisette Bralow
Acquisitions Editor: Richard Lampert
Project Manager: Mary Anne Folcher
Production Manager: Linda Garber
Illustration Specialist: Francis Moriarty
Book Designer: Steven Stave
Indexer: Angela Holt

ALLERGIC DISEASES OF THE EYE   0–7216–8679–6

Printed in the United States of America

Last digit is the print number: 9   8   7   6   5   4   3   2   1

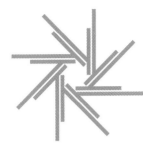

CONTRIBUTORS

Mark B. Abelson, M.D., C.M., F.R.C.S. (C)
Clinical Associate Professor of
  Ophthalmology
Harvard Medical School

Senior Clinical Scientist
Schepens Eye Research Institute
Boston

Ophthalmic Research Associates
North Andover, Massachusetts

Gregg J. Berdy, M.D., F.A.C.S.
Clinical Instructor
Department of Ophthalmology
Washington University School of
  Medicine
St. Louis, Missouri

Susan Schukar Berdy, M.D.
Assistant Professor
Clinical Medicine
Washington University School of
  Medicine
St. Louis, Missouri

Sergio Bonini, M.D.
Ophthalmology
University of Rome Tor Vergata
Rome, Italy

Stefano Bonini, M.D.
Ophthalmology
University of Rome Tor Vergata
Rome, Italy

Salim Butrus, M.D.
Assistant Clinical Professor
Department of Ophthalmology
George Washington University
  School of Medicine

Associate Clinical Professor
Department of Ophthalmology
Georgetown University School of
  Medicine
Washington, D.C.

Richard Casey, M.D.
Assistant Professor
Charles R. Drew University of
  Medicine and Science
Associate Professor
Jules Stein Eye Institute
Interim Chairman
Department of Ophthalmology
King/Drew Medical Center
Cornea, Faculty
University of California, Los
  Angeles, Medical Center
Los Angeles, California

Matthew J. Chapin, B.S.
Ophthalmic Research Associates
North Andover, Massachusetts

**Louis M. T. Collum, F.R.C.S.,
  F.R.C.S.I., F.R.C.ophth., E.B.O.D.**
Professor of Ophthalmology
Royal College of Surgeons in
  Ireland
Consultant Ophthalmic Surgeon
Royal Victoria Eye and Ear Hospital
Dublin, Ireland

Denise De Freitas, M.D.
Assistant Professor
Federal University of São Paulo
Paulista School of Medicine
Head, External Eye Disease and
  Cornea Service
São Paulo Hospital

Federal University of São Paulo
Paulista School of Medicine
São Paulo, Brazil

Kristine Erickson, O.D., Ph.D.
Associate Professor
Departments of Ophthalmology and
  Pharmacology
Boston University School of Medicine
Associate Professor of Optometry
New England College of Optometry
Boston, Massachusetts

Michelle George, B.S.
Ophthalmic Research Associates
North Andover, Massachusetts

Anne Giovanoni, B.S.
Ophthalmic Research Associates
North Andover, Massachusetts

Paulo J. Gomes, M.S.
Ophthalmic Research Associates
North Andover, Massachusetts

Kelly K. Grant, B.S.
Ophthalmic Research Associates
North Andover, Massachusetts

**Jack V. Greiner, O.D., D.O., Ph.D.,
  F.A.A.O.S.**
Clinical Instructor
Department of Ophthalmology
Harvard Medical School
Clinical Associate Scientist
Schepens Eye Research Institute
Harvard Medical School
Boston, Massachusetts

Thomas John, M.D.
Clinical Associate Professor
Loyola University of Chicago Stritch
  School of Medicine
Maywood, Illinois

Connie Katelaris
Department of Clinical Terminology
  and Allergy
Westmead Hospital
Westmead, Sydney, Australia

**Dara J. Kilmartin, M.Med.Sc.,
  F.R.C.S.I., F.R.C.ophth., E.B.O.D.**
Clinical Research Fellow in
  Ophthalmology
University of Aberdeen Medical
  School
Specialist Registrar in
  Ophthalmology
Aberdeen Royal Infirmary
Grampian University Hospitals
  NHS Trust
Aberdeen, Scotland

Alessandra Lambiase, M.D.
Ophthalmology
University of Rome Tor Vergata
Rome, Italy

Andrea Leonardi, M.D.
Professor
Institute of Ophthalmology
University of Padova
Allergy and Immunology Service
Department of Laboratory Medicine
Padova Hospital
Padova, Italy

Jaqueline M. Nevius, B.S.
Ophthalmic Research Associates
North Andover, Massachusetts

Jin Pyun, B.S.
Ophthalmic Research Associates
North Andover, Massachusetts

Kevin P. Richard, B.S.
Ophthalmic Research Associates
North Andover, Massachusetts

Luiz Rizzo, M.D.
São Paulo University
São Paulo, Brazil

Elizabeth R. Sandman, B.S.
Ophthalmic Research Associates
North Andover, Massachusetts

Elcio H. Sato, M.D.
Assistant Professor
Federal University of São Paulo

Paulista School of Medicine
Medical Director
São Paulo Hospital Eye Bank
Federal University of São Paulo
Paulista School of Medicine
São Paulo, Brazil

Kendyl Schaefer, B.S.
Ophthalmic Research Associates
North Andover, Massachusetts

Clyde Schultz, Ph.D.
Schepens Eye Research Institute
Harvard Medical School
Boston, Massachusetts

Erika Schwartz, B.S.
Ophthalmic Research Associates
North Andover, Massachusetts

Antonio G. Secchi, M.D.
Professor of Physiopathological
  Optics
Institute of Ophthalmology
School of Medicine
University of Padua
Regional Center for Inflammatory
  Diseases of the Eye
Padua, Italy

Jennifer Sloan, B.S.
Ophthalmic Research Associates
North Andover, Massachusetts

Andrew P. Slugg, B.S.
Ophthalmic Research Associates
North Andover, Massachusetts

Lisa M. Smith, B.S.
Professor
Department of Medicine
School of Laboratory Technology
University of Padova
Editorial Services in Science and
  Medicine
Padova, Italy

Donna Welch, R.N.
Ophthalmic Research Associates
North Andover, Massachusetts

Paula J. Wun, B.S.
Ophthalmic Research Associates
North Andover, Massachusetts

Betsey Zbyszynski, B.S.
Ophthalmic Research Associates
North Andover, Massachusetts

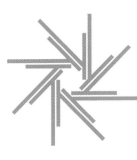

PREFACE

Diseases of the ocular surface are an important and frequent group of ophthalmic disorders. By their general nature, they affect most individuals at some point in their lives. External ocular diseases are therefore a component of the human condition. To truly understand external ocular diseases, in terms of the clinical aspects of differential diagnosis and appropriate therapeutic selection, it is necessary to first understand the pathophysiology of these diseases. Practitioners must have a deep understanding of ocular allergic diseases, which are perhaps the most frequent manifestations of external ocular diseases.

Numerous advances have been made in the understanding of the nature of inflammatory cellular involvement and mediators, cytokines, adhesion molecules, and receptors. Clinical management of ocular allergic disease is no more and no less than the management of the sum total of the effects produced by the "cocktail" of mediators released into and onto the ocular surface. The more we understand ocular allergy, the more we see the similarities to and differences from general inflammatory disease. The "external disease expert" must be able to recognize, understand, and treat all the manifestations of ocular allergies, which can exist by themselves or in conjunction with other inflammatory diseases.

Allergic Diseases of the Eye addresses the relevant new developments in the field of ocular allergy. This text presents a foundation for an understanding of the clinical manifestations and appreciation of the multitude of therapeutic interventions currently available and those available in the near future. The incidence of ocular allergy cases has been increasing. Ocular allergy is estimated to affect 20% of the general population annually. With the advent of more effective agents, the opportunity to treat patients with related symptoms has improved dramatically.

The contributors we have assembled, to present information in their specific areas of expertise, represent a group of clinical scientists with an interest in clinical practice and an interest in basic science. These individuals have played an important role in driving forward our understanding of ocular allergy and aiding in the availability of new therapeutic agents. We express our deep appreciation to the clinical scientists who straddle the divide: the clinicians with an appreciation for and interest in external disease and the researchers with an interest in providing further understanding of the underlying pathophysiology of ocular allergic disease. They must be recognized as they continue to play an important role in the advancement of this exciting area.

The clinician will not be disappointed by the information contained in *Allergic Diseases of the Eye*. The basic researcher will have a greater appreciation for the current problems that we all must solve.

Mark B. Abelson, M.D.

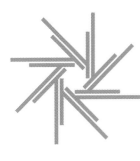

CONTENTS

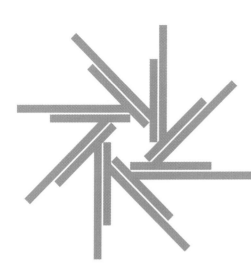

CHAPTER 1

Genetic and Environmental Factors in Ocular Allergy

STEFANO BONINI ■ **ALESSANDRO LAMBIASE** ■ **SERGIO BONINI**

The genetics of ocular allergy is a complex and largely unexplored puzzle. Many different clinical entities are grouped together under the term "allergic eye disease," and the nomenclature is confusing. Despite these variations, predisposition to atopy is the common denominator for all these diseases. Much more is known about the genetics and environmental factors of other atopic conditions such as asthma, eczema, and rhinitis. It is to our advantage that most of this knowledge can also be applied to ocular allergic diseases.

In this chapter, we analyze the clinical and epidemiological features of each form of allergic conjunctivitis. We focus on pathophysiological, constitutional, and environmental factors contributing to this complex and multifactorial genetic process.

CLASSIFICATION

Allergic diseases of the eye are mostly confined to the conjunctiva and are classified as acute allergic conjunctivitis, seasonal hay fever, perennial allergic conjunctivitis, vernal conjunctivitis, and atopic conjunctivitis.[1-4] Giant

1

papillary conjunctivitis (GPC), which is frequently associated with the use of contact lenses, is also discussed with allergic disease, although it does not seem to have a true allergic origin.[5]

Acute allergic conjunctivitis is an acute hypersensitivity reaction caused by an exposure to allergens or chemicals. It is characterized by hyperemia and chemosis of the conjunctiva, edema of the lid, and tearing, itching, and burning sensations.

Seasonal hay fever is a relatively mild form of allergic conjunctivitis, often associated with rhinitis, that occurs every year during spring and late summer or early autumn. This ocular reaction follows exposure to pollen allergens in sensitized persons. The precise onset and duration of seasonal hay fever depend on the allergen and on the regional pollination season. Perennial allergic conjunctivitis is a mild, chronic form of allergic conjunctivitis related to exposure to allergens such as house dust mites.

Vernal keratoconjunctivitis (VKC) is a severe, bilateral, and chronic disease, primarily of young boys, with seasonal exacerbations in early spring. Corneal involvement in the form of superficial punctate keratitis or shield-shaped corneal ulcers is common. Itching, photophobia, a thick, cord-like mucus discharge, and the presence of giant cobbles on the upper tarsal conjunctiva are the main features of this disease.

Atopic keratoconjunctivitis is a severe, bilateral inflammation affecting the conjunctiva and cornea. This entity predominantly affects patients older than 40 years of age. A diffuse periocular eczema is frequently associated with atopic conjunctivitis. Severe itching and foreign body sensation are the most common symptoms. Blepharitis is almost always present, and ocular complications such as anterior polar cataract, keratoconus, or retinal detachment may also occur.

GPC is a syndrome generally seen in contact lens wearers. It is characterized by hyperemia, mucus discharge, feeling of a foreign body in the presence of contact lenses, and eruption of giant papillae in the upper conjunctiva. This reaction is probably due to lid movement over the lens edge or adherence of foreign material to the contact lens.

EPIDEMIOLOGY

The clinical entities of allergic conjunctival disease have different prevalence rates and are influenced by different developmental factors. The seasonal or perennial forms are usually grouped as "allergic conjunctivitis" and represent the most common ocular allergic disease. These forms accounted for 66% of all ocular allergic diseases observed in a large series of patients attending an outpatient allergy clinic.[6, 7] The prevalence of hay fever and perennial rhinitis in population studies varies from 5 to 22%, with clear evidence that the prevalence of the disease has increased considerably in recent years. The reason for this increase is not known, but it seems to correlate with an increase in allergic disease as a whole.

VKC is a rare disease: its prevalence is less than 1% of all eye diseases.[8] The disease has a worldwide distribution; it is more common in the Mediterranean area, in Central and South America, and in the Balkans, but it is rare in Northern Europe and North America. The incidence of the disease differs from country to country and may change considerably within a single region from year to year. In our clinic, VKC represents 8% of all cases of allergic conjunctivitis.

Atopic keratoconjunctivitis is a severe conjunctival and corneal disorder that is the ocular manifestation of atopic dermatitis. The reported incidence of ocular involvement in atopic disorders is between 25 and 40%.[9–11]

FACTORS INFLUENCING THE DEVELOPMENT OF ALLERGIC DISEASES

Age

Although we often consider allergic conjunctivitis as a homogeneous group of diseases, the mean age of those affected and the age at onset of disease vary considerably for each of the three major clinical entities.[6]

Allergic conjunctivitis is a disease of young adults (mean age of 27 ± 10 years) with a mean age at the onset of symptoms of 20 years. In contrast, VKC is a disease of childhood (mean age, 12 ± 5 years). The mean age at onset is 7 years. Atopic keratoconjunctivitis is a disease of adults that generally occurs after age 40 years.

GPC associated with contact lens wear follows the same age patterns as contact lens wear; thus, it is rare in the elderly and in children. GPC can also be associated with postsurgical sources of mechanical ocular trauma or irritation (i.e., exposed sutures), which are more prevalent in an older population.

Gender

Before the age of 15 years, allergic disease is more prevalent in males. After age 15, it becomes more prevalent in females.[8, 12, 13] For example, the ratio of males to females with VKC is 3:1. However, evidence indicates that, with advancing age, the ratio changes in favor of the female sex.[14] The explanation for this change is not clear, but it is seems possible that sex hormones may influence the progression of the disease. Similarly, a slightly higher prevalence of males has been observed for hay fever conjunctivitis[7, 15] and atopic keratoconjunctivitis.[16] A retrospective study of patients with GPC did not reveal any association with gender.[9]

Race

The question of racial predisposition to ocular allergy is controversial. Most investigators who studied large, multiracial groups of patients with VKC could not find any differences in prevalence associated with race. However, several reports indicate a preponderance of the limbal form of VKC in blacks. No marked racial predisposition has been observed in patients with hay fever, atopic keratoconjunctivitis, or GPC.

Family History

Atopic conditions frequently occur within families, and children of allergic parents have a greater chance to develop an atopic condition. In a survey of 148 patients with VKC, we found that 45% had a family history of atopic diseases. A similar familial predisposition has also been observed in patients with hay fever conjunctivitis and atopic keratoconjunctivitis. Perhaps genetic factors permit, rather than cause, the development of atopic conditions including ocular allergic disease.[17]

Natural Course of Allergic Conjunctivitis

Although no data from long-term follow-up studies are available, clinical observation suggests a different evolution for each clinical entity. Patients with VKC generally have a spontaneous resolution of the disease after puberty without any further symptoms or visual complications. VKC is rarely seen after age 30 years. Similarly, seasonal allergic conjunctivitis and, to a lesser extent, perennial conjunctivitis show a marked reduction or disappearance of signs and symptoms with advancing age. In contrast, atopic keratoconjunctivitis has a more prolonged course, probably because of the severity of the disease, the late appearance in life, and associated ocular complications. Because cases of GPC largely depend on a source of mechanical trauma, they often resolve rapidly following removal of the offending source.

PATHOPHYSIOLOGICAL VARIABLES INFLUENCING PHENOTYPIC EXPRESSION AND HETEROGENEITY OF OCULAR ALLERGY

We have described allergic eye diseases as a heterogeneous group of conditions primarily affecting the conjunctiva. These diseases are usually defined as "allergic," based on a putative prominent role of an IgE-mediated hypersensitivity mechanism. This mechanism is referred to as a type I reaction (Coombs and Gell).[18] This type I or immediate hypersensitivity mechanism may well explain the typical form of seasonal allergic conjunctivitis (hay fever conjunctivitis). For other ocular allergies, such as atopic keratoconjunctivitis or VKC, the pathogenesis is likely to be much more complex and multifactorial. We do not intend to give a definitive answer to the question: "What is ocular allergy?" However, we try to give a practical interpretation of the different forms of ocular allergy by suggesting that allergic eye diseases result from a combination of the following abnormalities:

- An aptitude for allergen recognition and an amplified specific response.
- Increased polyclonal IgE and IgG4 production.
- Up-regulation of inflammatory cells, particularly mast cells and eosinophils.
- Hyperresponsiveness of ocular tissues.

The ability to respond to substances (such as pollen or dust allergens) that do not elicit a clinically relevant immune response in the majority of persons is a typical feature of allergic patients. The molecular mechanism for antigen recognition and response at the level of the T-cell receptor/major histocompatibility complex is currently unknown.[19] Allergic patients are high IgE and IgG4 responders. Increased levels of both immunoglobulins are present in serum and tears of patients with various forms of allergic conjunctivitis.[20] This increased polyclonal IgE activation seems to be, at least in part, independent from a specific IgE response to common allergens. In fact, high total serum and tear IgE have been reported in forms of atopic keratoconjunctivitis or VKC without clinical evidence of sensitization.[21, 22] Ongoing research should soon provide a better understanding of relevant epitopes involved in antigen recognition with reference to different allergens and HLA specificity.[23, 24]

Increased number, altered distribution, and exaggerated degranulation of tissue mast cells are factors known to play a central role in type I hypersensitivity mechanisms. However, investigators have clearly shown that several other cells also take part in the immune network leading to allergic inflammation and symptoms.[25] A significant contribution to our understanding of the events leading from mast cell degranulation to allergic inflammation has been derived from studies of late-phase reactions following allergen challenge. We have been able to show that conjunctival allergen challenge in human patients causes persisting inflammatory changes within ocular tissues similar to those previously described in rats.[26] In the eye, the late-phase reaction is characterized by redness, mild itching and tearing, and a foreign body sensation persisting long after allergen exposure.[27] Analysis of conjunctival scrapings or cells in tears shows an early accumulation of neutrophils, followed by a prevalent recruitment of eosinophils 6 to 10 hours after provocation and a later infiltration of lymphocytes and monocytes. Inflammatory changes are noted up to 24 hours after challenge.[27] The recruitment of inflammatory cells during the ocular late-phase reaction is associated with the detection in tears of mediators released by primary and secondary effector cells.[28] For instance, we were able to detect significant amounts of leukotriene C_4, eosinophil peroxidase, eosinophil cationic protein, and histamine during ocular late-phase reactions.[28] Tryptase was not detected. This last finding is in agreement with the hypothesis of the Baltimore group (Naclerio and co-workers) that, based on the pattern of mediators found in nasal washings at different times after allergen challenge, basophils have a role in the late-phase reaction, but mast cells do not.[29]

Clinical and cytological changes associated with the conjunctival late-phase reaction appear to be due to a continuous, dose-dependent process.[27] When low allergen doses are used for challenge, or when the sensitivity of the patients is low, only cytological changes that are not associated with clinical symptoms are observed during the early phase of conjunctival reaction. Increasing the dose of allergen results in a more intense cellular reaction and a typical immediate clinical response of the conjunctiva. When the dose of allergen is further increased, or when patients with higher sensitivity are challenged, a more intense and prolonged cell recruitment is induced, including a clinically manifest late-phase reaction.

In summary, data derived from studies of conjunctival allergen challenge and late-phase ocular reaction clearly indicate that up-regulation of inflammatory cells, particularly mast cells and eosinophils, occurs in allergic disease of the eye, just as in allergic diseases involving other organs. Studies of the allergic conjunctiva reveal the presence of several inflammatory cell types and mediators as a constant finding in allergic eye diseases,[30] as well as a close a relationship between these findings and the severity of clinical symptoms.[31, 32]

Extensive studies in target organs other than the eye indicate that allergic patients are hyperreactive to various nonspecific substances in addition to the sensitizing allergen. Although close relationships exist between reactivity to allergens and reactivity to nonallergic substances, specific and nonspecific hyperreactivity responses represent distinct concurrent mechanisms in the pathogenesis of allergic diseases.

We compared conjunctival responsiveness to histamine diphosphate (0.1–1.0 mg/mL) in patients with VKC and in healthy controls.[33] Both patients and controls reacted to histamine with a dose-dependent conjunctival redness 2 to 5 minutes after allergen challenge. However, at low histamine doses (0.01–0.5 mg/mL), patients with VKC had a significantly ($P <$ .05) more intense reaction than controls. Moreover, the concentration of histamine diphosphate causing a threshold conjunctival redness, termed the provoking concentration, was significantly lower ($P <$ .02) in patients with VKC than in controls.

The existence of conjunctival hyperresponsiveness to histamine in VKC, and possibly in other allergic external eye diseases, may be relevant to the pathogenesis and some of the clinical features of this disease. Abelson and Leonardi[70] have postulated that histamine deficiencies in a subgroup of patients, based on high levels of histamine found in active vernal conjunctivitis, are unlike those in patients with active vernal conjunctivitis. For instance, nonspecific conjunctival hyperreactivity may play a role in variations observed in the course of VKC that are not related to environmental changes of the sensitizing allergen. Sun, wind, dust, or other natural agents may represent triggers for a nonspecific abnormal reactivity of the conjunctiva. We can also speculate that nonspecific conjunctival hyperreactivity has a primary pathogenic role in other forms of "allergic" conjunctivitis in which no clinical evidence of sensitization is detectable.

The CD4 T-cell phenotype T_H2 plays a role in influencing allergen recognition and an amplified response through the production of cytokines, such as interleukin-3 (IL-3), IL-4, IL-5, and granulocyte-macrophage–colony-stimulating factor (GM-CSF).[34] Neural influences appear to be important in the development of the inflammatory component of allergic diseases and the hyperresponsiveness of ocular tissues. Moreover, bi-directional influences occur among all these reported abnormalities.

The relative role of the four abnormalities identified may vary in different forms of allergic eye disease, as in vernal conjunctivitis versus inactive vernal conjunctivitis. In grass-sensitive persons with hay fever conjunctivitis, the specific IgE response to grass allergens appears to be the major pathophysiological abnormality. In other cases of seasonal allergic conjunctivitis, the classic type I hypersensitivity mechanism represents the basic pathophysiological abnormality. In subjects with high sensitivity to allergens or in patients sensitized to perennial allergens, late-phase inflammatory events contribute to a distinct pathogenic mechanism, clinical picture, and response to therapy. In most cases of VKC and atopic keratoconjunctivitis, IgE antibodies and inflammation can be well documented. However, in other cases, specific IgE antibodies are not found, and eosinophilic inflammation and conjunctival hyperresponsiveness appear to be the prevalent abnormalities.

Finally, patients with GPC often have no sign of atopy,[5] but inflammation and abnormal nonspecific reactivity to foreign substances seem to represent the most important pathophysiological features. If this heterogeneous pathophysiology of "allergic conjunctivitis" is correct, the classic nosography of allergic eye disease may need revision.

GENETIC AND ENVIRONMENTAL INFLUENCES ON ALLERGIC EYE DISEASES

Although several studies have considered the role of genetic and environmental factors in allergic diseases,[35] the problem has not received adequate attention in allergic eye disease. Genetic influences probably do exist, as suggested by well-recognized clustering of allergic diseases in twins and families.[36] Studies assessing twins indicate that genetic influences are not consistently the dominant factor when considering allergic disease and sensitization in general, whether relating to a specific sensitization or a particular disease. In these cases, several concomitant genetic or environmental factors can be assumed. Thus, if allergic diseases are polyfactorial, a better understanding of the genetic and environmental influences can only come from studying each factor involved in the pathogenesis of these disorders.

Based on the role of HLA class II antigens in the interaction between specific antigen epitopes and T-cell receptors during antigen presentation, several studies have indicated that allergen recognition and antibody response are influenced by Ia HLA-linked genes.[37] Most of these studies used allergens from *Ambrosia artemisiaefolia* and *Lolium perenne*. Marsh found that increased responsiveness to Amb a V (Ra5) was associated with DNA sequences HLA-DR2/DW2, whereas a response to Lol pI and Lol pII was associated with HLA-DR23 and DR5. The increased responsiveness to purified antigens was not isotope specific, but it involved both IgE and IgG.

In these studies, purified simple allergens were used, thus avoiding the masking effect of other genetic influences, such as those acting on total IgE levels. In contrast, results from population studies employing crude allergens are contradictory and of limited value. For example, we failed to show any association between HLA antigens and allergic disease in studies on twins[38] or in population studies of allergic patients.[39] Therefore, despite evidence indicating that the IgE and IgG response to purified antigens is controlled by HLA-associated genes, genetic influences appear to be less pronounced than environmental influences. Thus, the atopic condition should be regarded as uncommitted susceptibility to allergic diseases in general. Environmental factors such as the quality, intensity, route, and duration of allergen exposure may be more relevant than genetic factors in determining an effective response to allergens.

Several studies of populations, families, and twins have indicated that total serum IgE is subject to strong isotypic genetic control.[40] Environmental influences, such as smoking, may also be relevant for modulating serum IgE levels.[41] The mechanism of inheritance is still unknown, and autosomal dominant, autosomal recessive, and polygenic models have been proposed.[40] Cookson et al. assigned a gene for the IgE response with maternal inheritance to chromosome 11q.[42] However, their data, which have been confirmed by some groups but disproved by others, are based on a definition of atopy that includes both a higher than normal concentration of total serum IgE and positive skin prick or radioallergosorbent tests.

The most interesting genetic finding is the identification of genes for IL-3, IL-4, IL-5, and GM-CSF on chromosome 5.[43] This cluster of cytokine genes may have a fundamental role in the genetics of allergy. The expressed cytokines have regulatory effects on IgE and IgG4 isotype switching and production (effected by IL-4), as well as on the growth, activation, priming, mediator release, and survival of mast cells and eosinophils (effected by IL-3, IL-5, and GM-CSF).[44] Because the polyclonal activation of total IgE and IgG4 and the up-regulation of inflammatory cells are common features of all allergic diseases, it may be speculated that a genetically or environmentally induced overexpression of the cytokine gene cluster represents the basic abnormality of allergic diseases. This genetic overexpression may also represent the basis for uncommitted predisposition to both IgE-mediated and non–IgE-mediated allergy (Fig. 1.1).

One may also speculate that polyclonal IgE up-regulation is capable of influencing the appearance of a specific IgE response to various allergens. However, persons with the "right" HLA-linked Ia genes can develop a monospecific sensitization, even in the absence of an up-regulation of the total IgE response. Our studies in twins indicate that strong genetic influences regulate total serum IgE and IgG4 levels, and variables of secondary inflammatory effector mechanisms, such as basophil releasability, independent from factors regulating the specific allergen response.[45] The release of mediators from mast cells and basophils is a crucial pathogenic event in allergic diseases, representing the final factor responsible for pathophysiological changes and symptoms of allergy. Conroy et al.[46] and MacGlashan[47] have shown that histamine release from human basophils in response to anti-IgE

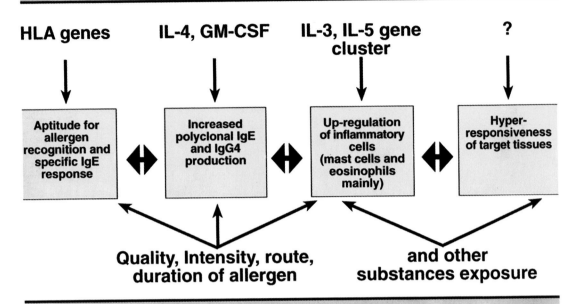

FIGURE 1.1 Environmental factors may influence the individual genetic predisposition to develop ocular allergic disease. The cluster of interleukin (IL)-3, IL-4, IL-5, and granulocyte-macrophage–colony-stimulating factor (GM-CSF) genes is located on chromosome 5. It may have a main role in the genetics of allergy, in view of the regulatory role of the expressed cytokines on immunoglobulin E (IgE) and IgG4 switching and production, as well as on the growth, activation, priming, mediator release, and survival of mast cells and eosinophils.

is not related to serum IgE levels, but to the absolute quantity of IgE antibody present on these cells when stimulated with anti-IgE or a specific allergen. Thus, two or more persons with an identical IgE response may show a different basophil mediator release depending on this intrinsic cellular property defined as "releasability" by Lichtenstein and Conroy.[48] It is conceivable that the concept of releasability can also apply to other inflammatory cells, such as eosinophils.[49, 50] Despite the central regulatory role of inflammatory cell releasability in the pathogenesis of atopic diseases, few data are available on the environmental factors affecting this mechanism, and no extensive studies have been carried out to investigate whether eosinophilic inflammation is under genetic control.

We investigated IgE-mediated (anti-IgE) and non–IgE-mediated (f-methyl-leucyl-phenylalanine: calcium ionophore, A23187) basophil releasability in 14 monozygotic twin pairs aged 25.7 ± 2.5 years and 12 dizygotic twin pairs aged 17.8 ± 0.7 years.[51, 52] A significant intrapair correlation coefficient in anti-IgE–induced histamine release was found in monozygotic twin pairs ($r = 0.84$), but not in dizygotic twin pairs. No correlation was found between serum IgE levels and basophil anti-IgE histamine release. These data indicate that basophil releasability is under genetic control and is a relevant feature of an atopic constitution. Genetic and environmental influences on basophil releasability are probably different from those affecting IgE antibody response.

The response of target tissues to mediators released following IgE-mediated phenomena is a fundamental factor in determining the final clinical outcome in sensitized subjects exposed to specific allergens. Data on this subject are limited and deal predominantly with genetic and environmental influences on bronchial responsiveness,[53] whereas factors governing the response of other tissues, such as skin, nasal tissues, and the eye, are as yet largely unexplored. Similarities between the features of ocular allergy and allergy in other body systems allow for some extrapolation with respect to influencing factors.

GENETIC AND ENVIRONMENTAL INFLUENCES ON THE EYE

Evidence indicates that environmental factors may influence the individual genetic predisposition to develop ocular allergic disease (see Fig. 1.1).[54, 55] Allergen exposure is integral to allergic conjunctivitis, whereas endocrine, neural, and physiological factors seem to have a role both in VKC and in atopic keratoconjunctivitis. These observations, once confirmed, could contribute to further differentiation between ocular allergic diseases.[56]

HLA Antigens

Specific HLA gene responses have been associated with specific antigens. Although a possible association between HLA antigens and ocular allergies has been suspected, no definite relationship has been established.[51] The variability of each clinical condition severely limits the ability to identify and study a homogeneous group of patients.

Allergen Exposure

Allergen exposure has been shown to have a particularly strong influence on those patients with a high genetic propensity for development of both seasonal and perennial allergic conjunctivitis.[17] The geographical distribution, quality of life, and the intensity and time of exposure do not allow generalizations. Pollen is the most common allergen causing allergic conjunctivitis, and pollen calendars are useful in establishing the peak recurrences in each country.

Endocrine Influence

The influence of the endocrine system on ocular allergies has long been postulated.[12] Speculations on the role of hormones in VKC date to the beginning of the 20th century, but these theories were disregarded for a long time. More recently, the evidence of bi-directional communication between the endocrine and the immune system has prompted consideration of a possible relationship between hormones and ocular allergic diseases.[57] In experimental conditions, hormones have been shown to influence the outcome and severity of allergic conjunctivitis. In particular, sex hormones (e.g., estrogens) have a greater bearing on sex differences in the development of allergic conjunctivitis.[58–63]

These studies, together with the recognition that estrogens stimulate uterine eosinophilia and edema by increasing vascular permeability in the uterus, prompted similar investigations in the eye.[64] Our group demonstrated by immunohistochemical techniques that functionally active receptors for both estrogens and progesterone are present in the conjunctiva of patients with VKC[65] and atopic keratoconjunctivitis (unpublished observations). Whether these hormone receptors could be involved in the pathogenesis of these ocular diseases should be studied further. Speculations regarding possible hormonal regulation of inflammatory cells in the conjunctiva are pertinent for future investigations.

Neural Influence

The existence of an interrelationship between the central nervous system and the eye is easily established with respect to anatomical and embryogenic origin. This interactive communications system is also strictly related to the immune system and is documented by nerve and mast cell interactions.[66] We have focused our attention on nerve growth factor, the best characterized member of a neurotrophin family, which profoundly affects several cells of the immune system. Identification of high plasma levels of nerve growth factor and the presence of a nerve growth factor high-affinity receptor in conjunctival tissues of patients with VKC indicate that neural influences may have a role in the pathogenesis of allergic diseases.[67]

Psychological Factors and Stress-Induced Symptoms

Psychological factors are known to worsen symptoms in asthmatic patients.[68] No clear or well-defined investigations of the effects of psychological factors have been reported in ocular allergies. Clinical observations and a few case reports in the literature suggest that further studies investigating the role of psychological factors in atopic and VKC should be conducted.[9]

Psychoneurotic behaviors associated with remarkable mood swings and passive-aggressive relationships with family members have been reported in patients with atopic keratoconjunctivitis. This finding indicates that psychological disturbances such as stress may affect the function of a complex system in which immune, neural, endocrine, and psychological factors interact.

SUMMARY

At present, the role of genetic influences in ocular allergic diseases remains ill defined. It is likely, as seen in other atopic conditions, that genetic and polyfunctional environmental factors influence the origin, progression, and severity of each clinical ocular allergic disease. We have sufficient evidence to prompt further investigation into the roles of genetic, constitutional, hormonal, neural, and psychological factors in ocular allergies. However, we should always keep in mind the remark of Sir Duke-Elder[8] in 1965: "We are on a safe ground only if we admit that these factors, about which after all we know very little, and that vaguely and undefinitely, form a suitable soil where disease may readily flourish."

REFERENCES

1. Abelson MB, Schaefer K. Conjunctivitis of allergic origin: immunologic mechanisms and current approaches to therapy. Surv Ophthalmol 38 Suppl:115, 1993.
2. Friedlander MH. Conjunctivitis of allergic origin: clinical presentation and differential diagnosis. Surv Ophthalmol 38 Suppl:105, 1993.
3. Allansmith MR. The eye in immunology. St. Louis, CV Mosby, 1982, p 111.
4. Donshik PC, Ehlers WH. Clinical immunologic diseases: ocular allergy. In: The cornea: scientific foundation and clinical practice. 3rd ed. Smolin G, Thoft RA, eds. Boston, Little, Brown, 1994, p 347.
5. Allansmith MR, Korb DR, Greiner JV, et al. Giant papillary conjunctivitis in contact lens wearers. Am J Ophthalmol 83:697, 1977.
6. Bonini S, Bonini S. Allergic conjunctivitis. Chibret Int J Ophthamol 5:12, 1987.
7. Weeke ER. Epidemiology of hay fever and perennial allergic rhinitis. Monogr Allergy 21:1, 1987.
8. Duke-Elder S. Diseases of the outer eye. Vol. 8, Part 1. London, Henry Kimpton, 1965, p 475.
9. Foster S, Calonge M. Atopic keratoconjunctivitis. Ophthalmology 97:992, 1990.
10. Rich LF, Hanifin JM. Ocular complications of atopic dermatitis and other eczemas. Int Ophthalmol Clin 25:61, 1985.
11. Garrity JA, Liesegang TJ. Ocular complications of atopic dermatitis. Can J Ophthalmol 19: 21,1984.
12. Wormald PJ. Age-sex incidence in symptomatic allergies: an excess of females in the childbearing years. J Hyg (Camb) 79:39, 1977.
13. Schuurs AHWM, Verheul HAM. Effects of gender and sex steroids on the immune response. J Steroid Biochem 35:157, 1990.
14. Beigelman MN. Vernal keratoconjunctivitis. Los Angeles, University of Southern California Press, 1950.
15. Montgomery Smith J. Epidemiology and natural history of asthma, allergic rhinitis and atopic dermatitis (eczema). In: Allergy: principles and practice. Middleton E, Reed CC, Ellis EF, et al., eds. St. Louis, CV Mosby, 1988, p 891.
16. Hanifin JM. Epidemiology of atopic dermatitis. Allergy 21:116, 1987.
17. Tuft SJ, Kemeny DM, Dart JKG, et al. Clinical features of atopic keratoconjunctivitis. Ophthalmology 98:150, 1991.
18. Coombs RRA, Gell PGH. Classification of allergic reactions responsible for clinical hypersensitivity and disease. In: Clinical aspects of immunology. 3rd ed. Gell PGH, Coombs RRA, Lachmann PJ, eds. Oxford, Blackwell Scientific Publications, 1975, p 761.
19. Babbitt BP, Allen PM, Matsuda G, et al. Binding of immunogenic peptides to the histocompatibility molecules. Nature 317:359, 1985.
20. Tuft SJ, Dart JKG. The measurement of IgE in the tear fluid: a comparison of collection by sponge or capillary. Acta Ophthalmol 67:301, 1989.
21. Aalders-Deestra V, Kok PTM, Bruynzeel PLB. Measurements of total IgE antibody levels in lacrimal fluid of patients suffering from atopic and non-atopic eye disorders: evidence for local production in atopic eye disorders. Br J Ophthalmol 69:385, 1985.
22. Ballow M, Mendelson L. Specific immunoglobulin E antibodies in tear secretions of patients with vernal conjunctivitis. J Allergy Clin Immunol 66: 112, 1980.
23. Bonini SE, Bonini ST, Lambiase A, et al. Vernal keratoconjunctivitis: a model of 5q cytokine gene cluster disease. Int Arch Allergy Immunol 107: 95, 1995.
24. Hoyne GF, Bourne T, Krestensen NM, et al. Peptide handling by the immune system. In: Progress in allergy and clinical immunology. Vol. 3. Johansson S, ed. Stockholm, Hogrefe & Huber, 1995, p 215.
25. Kay AB. Asthma and inflammation. J Allergy Clin Immunol 87:893, 1991.
26. Bonini S, Bonini S, Vecchione A, et al. Inflammatory changes in conjunctival scrapings after allergen challenge provocations in humans. J Allergy Clin Immunol 82:462, 1988.
27. Bonini S, Bonini S, Bucci MG, et al. Allergen dose response and late symptoms in a human model of ocular allergy. J Allergy Clin Immunol 86:869, 1990.
28. Bonini S, Bonini ST, Berruto A, et al. Conjunctival provocation test as a model for the study of allergy and inflammation in humans. Int Arch Allergy Appl Immunol 88:144, 1989.
29. Naclerio RM, Proud D, Toglas AG, et al. Inflammatory mediators in late antigen-induced rhinitis. New Engl J Med 313:6, 1985.
30. Allansmith MR, Baird RS, Greiner JV. Vernal conjunctivitis and contact lens–associated giant papillary conjunctivitis compared and contrasted. Am J Ophthalmol 87:544, 1979.
31. Irani AA, Butrus SI, Tabbara KF, et al. Human conjunctival mast cells: distribution of MCt and MCtc in vernal conjunctivitis and giant papillary conjunctivitis. J Allergy Clin Immunol 86:34, 1990.
32. Trocme SD, Aldave AJ. The eye and the eosinophil. Surv Ophthalmol 39:241, 1994.
33. Bonini ST, Bonini S, Schiavone M, et al. Conjunctival hyperresponsiveness to ocular histamine challenge in patients with vernal conjunctivitis. J Allergy Clin Immunol 89:103, 1992.
34. Ricci M, Rossi O, Bertoni M, et al. The importance of Th2-like cells in the pathogenesis of airway allergic inflammation. Clin Exp Allergy 23: 360, 1991.
35. Schlumberger HD. Epidemiology of allergic diseases. Monogr Allergy 21:1, 1987.
36. Blumenthal M, Bonini S. Immunogenetics of specific immunoresponses to allergens in twins and families. In: Genetic and environmental factors in clinical allergy. Marsh DG, Blumenthal M, eds. Minneapolis, University of Minnesota Press, 1990, p 132.
37. Marsh DG, Huang SK. Molecular genetics of human immune responsiveness to pollen allergens. Clin Exp Allergy 21 Suppl:1469, 1991.
38. Marsh DG. Immunogenetic and immunochemical factors determining immune responsiveness to allergens: studies in unrelated subjects. In: Ge-

netic and environmental factors in clinical allergy. Marsh DG, Blumenthal M, eds. Minneapolis, University of Minnesota Press, 1990, p 97.

39. Bonini S, Adorno D, Piazza M, et al. Allergic diseases and HLA antigens. In: Advances in allergology and clinical immunology. Oehling A, ed. Oxford, Pergamon Press, 1980, p 778.

40. Meyers DA. Family analysis and genetic counseling for allergic diseases. In: Genetic and environmental factors in clinical allergy. Marsh DG, Blumenthal M, eds. Minneapolis, University of Minnesota Press, 1990, p 161.

41. Bonini S. Smoking, IgE, and occupational allergy. BMJ 284:512, 1982.

42. Cookson WOCM, Sharp PA, Faux JA, et al. Linkage between immunoglobulin E responses underlying asthma and rhinitis and chromosome 11q. Lancet 1:1292, 1989.

43. Van Lee Uwen BH, Martinson ME, Webb GC, et al. Molecular organization of the cytokine gene cluster, involving the human IL-3, IL-4, IL-5, and GM-CSF genes on human chromosome 5. Blood 73:1142, 1989.

44. Arai K, Yokota T, Watanabe S, et al. The regulation of allergic response by cytokine receptors networks. ACI News 4:113, 1992.

45. Serafini U, Errigo E, eds. Proceedings of the XII Congress of the European Academy of Allergy and Clinical Immunology. Florence, OIC Medical Press, 1983, p 109.

46. Conroy MC, Adkinson NF Jr, Lichtenstein LM. Measurement of IgE on human basophil relation to serum IgE and anti-IgE induced histamine release. J Immunol 118:1317, 1977.

47. MacGlashan DW Jr. Releasability of human basophils: cellular sensitivity and maximal histamine release are independent variables. J Allergy Clin Immunol 91:605, 1993.

48. Lichtenstein LM, Conroy MC. The "releasability" of mediators from human basophils and granulocytes. In: Proceedings of the XI Congress of Allergology. Mathov E, ed. Amsterdam, Excerpta Medica, 1977, p 109.

49. Bonini S, Tomassini M, Adriani E, et al. Markers of eosinophilic inflammation in allergic diseases. Allergy 98:133, 1993.

50. Bonini SE, Tomassini M, Bonini ST, et al. The eosinophil has a pivotal role in allergic inflammation of the eye. Int Arch Allergy Appl Immunol 99:354, 1992.

51. Marone G, Casolaro V, Celestino D, et al. The role of genetic and environmental factors in the control of basophil and mast cell releasability. In: Genetic and environmental factors in clinical allergy. Marsh DG, Blumenthal M, eds. Minneapolis, University of Minnesota Press, 1990, p 153.

52. Marone G, Poto S, Celestino D, et al. Human basophil releasability. III. Genetic control of human basophil releasability. J Immunol 137:3588, 1986.

53. Hopp RJ, Nair NM, Bewtra AK, et al. Genetic bronchial hyperreactivity. In: Genetic and environmental factors in clinical allergy. Marsh DG, Blumenthal M, eds. Minneapolis, University of Minnesota Press, 1990, p 143.

54. Easty DL, Birkenshaw M, Merrett T, et al. Immunological investigations in vernal eye disease. Trans Ophthalmol Soc UK 100:98, 1980.

55. Barney NP, Foster CS. Atopic ocular disease. Int Ophthalmol Clin 33:87, 1993.

56. Cohen C. Genetic predisposition to allergic disorders: a review. In: Immunology of the eye. Workshop I. Immunogenetics and transplantation immunity. Steinberg GM, Gery I, Nussemblatt RB, eds. Sp Supp Immunology Abstracts, 1980, p 73.

57. Bonini S, Bonini S, Lambiase A, et al. Immune, endocrine and neural aspects of allergic inflammation. In: Proceedings of the XVI European Congress of Allergology and Clinical Immunology. Basomba A, Sastre J, eds. Bologna, Monduzzi, 1995, p 475.

58. Tabibzadeh S. Human endometrium: an active site of cytokine production and action. Endocr Rev 12:272, 1991.

59. Yokochi K, Sugano T. Studies on allergic conjunctivitis. 12. Effect of adrenalectomy on experimental allergic conjunctivitis. Nippon Ganka Gakkai Zasshi 75:1351, 1971.

60. Kawashima T. Studies on allergic conjunctivitis. 15. Effect of L-thyroxine on experimental allergic conjunctivitis in newborn rabbits. Nippon Ganka Gakkai Zasshi 76:581, 1972.

61. Horiuchi T. Studies on allergic conjunctivitis. 13. Effects of neonatally injected androgen on experimental allergic conjunctivitis. Nippon Ganka Gakkai Zasshi 75:1524, 1971.

62. Saruya S. Studies on allergic conjunctivitis. 5. Effects of castration and sex on hormone administration on experimental allergic conjunctivitis. Nippon Ganka Gakkai Zasshi 72:833, 1968.

63. Horiuchi T. Studies on allergic conjunctivitis. 10. Effects of neonatally injected estrogen on experimental allergic conjunctivitis. Nippon Ganka Gakkai Zasshi 74:803, 1970.

64. Tchernitchin A, Tchernitchin X, Galand P. New concepts on the action of oestrogens in the uterus and the role of eosinophils receptor system. Differentiation 5:145, 1976.

65. Bonini S, Lambiase A, Schiavone M, et al. Estrogen and progesterone receptors in vernal keratoconjunctivitis. Ophthalmology 102:1374, 1995.

66. Marshall JS, Waserman S. Mast cells and the nerve-potential interactions in the context of chronic disease. Clin Exp Allergy 25:102, 1995.

67. Lambiase A, Bonini S, Bonini S, et al. Increased plasma levels of nerve growth factor in vernal keratoconjunctivitis and relationship to conjunctival mast cells. Invest Ophthalmol Vis Sci 36: 2127, 1995.

68. Horton DJ, Suda WL, Kinsman RA, et al. Bronchoconstrictive suggestion in asthma: a role for airways hyperreactivity and emotions. Am Rev Respir Dis 117:1029, 1978.

69. Hart DE, Schkolnick JA, Bernstein S, et al. Contact lens–induced giant papillary conjunctivitis: a retrospective study. J Am Optom Assoc 60:195, 1989.

70. Abelson MB, Leonardi AA, Smith LM, et al. Histaminase activity with vernal keratoconjunctivitis. Ophthalmology 102:1958, 1995.

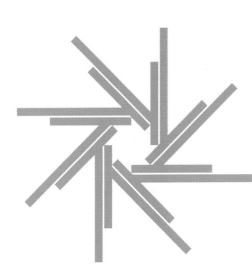

CHAPTER 2

Functional Anatomy of the Human Conjunctiva and Cornea

MARK B. ABELSON ■ **KENDYL SCHAEFER**

STRUCTURE OF THE CONJUNCTIVA

The conjunctiva is a modified integumental mucous membrane that lines the posterior surface of the lids and proceeds forward onto the globe of the eye, eventually merging with the corneal epithelium at the limbus. The conjunctiva is divided into two layers, the epithelium and the substantia propria. The epithelium is continuous with the skin at the lid margins and is composed of several upper layers of nonkeratinized squamous cells, middle layers of polyhedral cells, and a basal layer of cuboidal and columnar cells. The surface epithelial cells contain numerous microvilli, and surface crypts have been noted in the tarsal conjunctiva.[1] Investigators have postulated that the surface epithelium may contribute to the mucous layer of the tear film by secreting mucin-like glycoproteins.[2, 3]

The substantia propria is located beneath the basement membrane of the epithelial layer. The substantia propria can be divided into the superficial layer and a deeper fibrous layer. The superficial layer, which is composed of adenoid tissue, is a fine, fibrous network containing many inflammatory cells. The fibrous layer of the substantia propria is a thick meshwork of collagenous and elastic fibers, which is present in the bulbar conjunctiva and fornices and contains most of the vessels and nerves that supply the conjunctiva.

Although the conjunctiva is a continuous membrane, it is generally divided into three regions: the palpebral conjunctiva, the fornix, and the bulbar conjunctiva. The palpebral conjunctiva lines the upper and lower lids and is further divided into marginal, tarsal, and orbital sections. The marginal conjunctiva is a transition zone between the skin and the conjunctiva proper, whereas the tarsal conjunctiva is closely adherent and immovably fixed to the tarsal plates. The latter region is thin, transparent, and highly vascularized, giving it a pinkish to reddish color. Because of the transparency of the tissue, the tarsal glands are visible as yellowish streaks or lines running vertically parallel to each other. The upper conjunctiva is tightly adherent to the superior lid but is less so in the lower lid. Beyond the region of the tarsal plates is the thin, loose, orbital conjunctiva, which is thrown into horizontal folds during lid movements. The area of the superior tarsal plate has a series of shallow grooves that divide it into a mosaic of low elevations, which may appear as true papillae when inflamed.

The fornical conjunctiva is a fold lining the cul-de-sac formed by the transition of conjunctiva from the lid to the globe. It is thicker and more loosely connected than other areas of the conjunctiva, thus allowing movement of the globe independent of the lids. The space lying between the conjunctiva and the underlying fascial tissue is well supplied with visible blood vessels and is continuous with the orbital fat, a feature that accounts for the spreading of hemorrhage from the orbit into the subconjunctival tissues and possibly the cornea after trauma.

The bulbar conjunctiva covers the anterior portion of the eyeball and is so transparent that the surface vessels and white sclera are easily discernible. It is loosely attached to the underlying tissue and is freely movable. As one moves posteriorly from the cornea, the conjunctiva assumes a loose areolar structure, where the subconjunctival arteries are located. Below this area, in the anterior portion of Tenon's space, are the anterior ciliary arteries, which rise through the conjunctiva to form the pericorneal plexus. At the limbus, the deep layers of the conjunctival membrane end and the epithelial layer becomes continuous with the corneal epithelium (Fig. 2.1).

GOBLET CELLS

Mucus-secreting goblet cells are modified columnar cells that have become swollen from the accumulation of mucin droplets that displace the nucleus to the base or the side of the cell. They appear to be formed in the deeper layers of the epithelium,[4] moving toward the surface as they increase in size. Once goblet cells reach the surface, they discharge their mucin contents and degenerate. Goblet cells are present in most parts of the conjunctiva, but they are most numerous in the caruncle, the plica semilunaris, and around the area of Krause's glands in the superior fornix.[5, 6] They may occur singly in the fornices or in clusters forming crypts.

Goblet cells are true, unicellular mucous glands that moisten and protect the conjunctiva and cornea. The mucin product is essential to the proper distribution and continuity of the tear film over the ocular surface. Xerosis of the conjunctiva results in desiccation of goblet cells and drying of the ocular surface even in the presence of copious aqueous production of the lacrimal gland.[7]

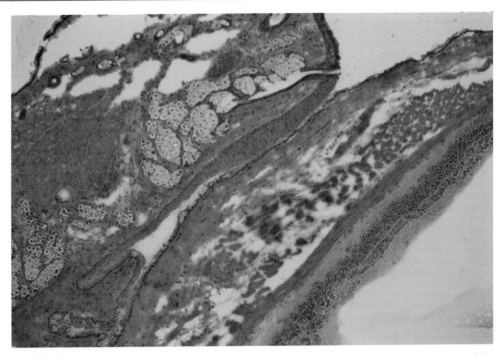

FIGURE 2.1 The conjunctiva is a modified integumental mucous membrane that lines the posterior surface of the lids and proceeds forward onto the globe of the eye, eventually merging with the corneal epithelium at the limbus. It is divided into two layers, the epithelium and the substantia propria.

LANGERHANS' CELLS

Langerhans' cells (CD1+) are present within the epithelium and the substantia propria.[8] These cells have several of the same properties as macrophages and perform a similar antigen-presenting function, although they are stationary within the tissue. Langerhans' cells have Fc and complement receptors and can express Ia (class II) histocompatibility antigens.[9] A significant increase in the number of Langerhans' cells in both the epithelium and the substantia propria has been demonstrated in patients with vernal conjunctivitis, ocular pemphigoid, and atopic keratoconjunctivitis.[10, 11]

MAST CELLS

Mast cells mediate type I (immediate) hypersensitivity reactions. Approximately 50 million mast cells can be found in the ocular and adnexal tissue of the human eye. In healthy individuals, the distribution of mast cells is limited to the substantia propria of the conjunctiva. In patients with vernal conjunctivitis or atopic keratoconjunctivitis, mast cells are also found in the conjunctival epithelium.

Each mast cell contains several hundred vesicles containing inflammatory mediators such as histamine, eosinophil chemotactic factor, platelet-activating factor, and other less well defined substances. Each mast cell also contains as many as 500,000 immunoglobulin E (IgE) receptors. Mast cell degranulation, with the resultant release of inflammatory mediators, may be initiated by the binding of allergen-IgE antibody complexes to these receptors.[12]

ROLE OF CONJUNCTIVA IN INFLAMMATION

The conjunctiva contains numerous inflammatory cells, including neutrophils, lymphocytes, plasma cells, and mast cells. Allansmith et al.[13] noted three distinct categories of inflammatory cells based on location: cells that are normally found in both the epithelium and the substantia propria (i.e., neutrophils and lymphocytes); cells that are normally located in the substantia propria (i.e., mast cells and plasma cells); and cells that are not normally found in the conjunctiva (i.e., eosinophils and basophils). The identification within the conjunctiva of even one cell in the last category would be abnormal.

Conjunctivitis can be triggered by a number of stimuli, including airborne pollens, bacteria (including normal flora), and other pathogens. The response of the conjunctiva to topical irritants may include hyperemia, tearing, chemosis, necrosis, a decrease in the number of goblet cells, and increased mucus secretion.

The study of allergic conjunctival inflammation has evolved with the advances in the study of general immunology, from the early efforts (1) to identify the inflammatory cells involved and the elaboration of their migratory time course, (2) to the isolation of their principal pre-formed and newly formed mediators, and (3) to the latest developments into what exactly, initially, calls them to the tissue. Studies now are of chemokines and cell adhesion molecules (CAMs) and their differential expression under various inflammatory conditions, which provoke the preferential adhesion of different populations of cells. Thus, a unique clinical picture is evolving for each allergic disease.[14]

Researchers have succeeded in culturing human conjunctival mast cells and epithelial cells in suspension from human cadaveric tissue.[15] This fascinating series of experiments has shown that cultured mast cells contain the cytokine—tissue necrosis factor-alpha (TNFα)—in storage granules in varying quantities, probably reflecting the immune status of specific donor cell populations. This finding is in accordance with findings from asthmatic lung tissue that was shown to have sevenfold the staining for TNFα than control lung tissue.[16] The profound effects of cytokines, such as TNFα among cells in tissues, are just lately being realized. The presence of preformed TNFα in mast cells suggests that these cells are the first source of this inflammatory cytokine to be released in response to allergen challenge. TNFα has a wide range of effects including fibroblast proliferation at low concentrations and inhibition at high concentrations.[17] It has also been shown to stimulate eotaxin, the specific eosinophil chemokine, in a human epithelial cell line.[18] Furthermore, TNFα, in this same study, upregulated intercellular adhesion molecule-1 (ICAM-1), a member of the immunoglobulin superfamily, on conjunctival epithelial cells.[15] In turn, these cells may recruit inflammatory cells to the site. This has been shown to be an important marker for inflammation in the conjunctiva.

In a similar histological study of conjunctival biopsy samples from patients with various allergic diseases, such as seasonal allergic conjunctivitis (SAC) and perennial allergic conjunctivitis (PAC), vernal keratoconjunctivitis (VKC), atopic keratoconjunctivitis (AKC), and atopic blepharoconjunctivitis (ABC), increased levels of ICAM-1, E-selectin, and vascular cell adhesion molecule-1 (VCAM-1) were found on the conjunctival microvasculature.[14] Factors that regulate these adhesion molecules are likely to be responsible for the cellular infiltration and the perpetuation of the more chronic forms of allergic eye disease (VKC, AKC, ABC) in which they were found to be particularly increased. These findings suggest that mast cell–derived cytokines prime the conjunctival epithelial cells, signalling changes in cellular adhesion and recruiting and activating other cells, such as fibroblasts, eosinophils, corneal epithelial cells, and keratinocytes. As such, cytokines surely play a fundamental role in the overall remodulation of conjunctival and corneal tissues in chronic inflammation.

STRUCTURE OF THE CORNEA[19, 20]

Between its anterior surface epithelium and posterior endothelium, the cornea is stratified in four distinct layers: epithelial basement membrane, Bowman's layer, stroma, and Descemet's membrane.

The corneal epithelium is a five to seven cell–layer stratified squamous epithelium, comprised of three to four layers of squamous cells, one to three layers of wing cells, and one layer of columnar basal cells. In addition to epithelial cells, the corneal epithelium has a vast collection of unmyelinated sensory nerve endings that penetrate from the stroma and terminate within the suprabasal and squamous cells. The study of cell-cell and cell-matrix adhesion of the corneal epithelium has led to the classification of these types of junctions that form between epithelial cells and between epithelial cells and their substrates. Morphologically, hemidesmosomes are visibly lined up along the basal epithelial surface, which during wound healing undergoes physical changes. The study of the molecular mechanisms behind these junctions has exploded with the discovery of adhesion molecules and their active, rather than passive, role in morphology and physiology.

Bowman's layer is synthesized by both epithelial cells and stromal keratocytes. It is composed of collagen fibrils arranged randomly and attached to the epithelial basement membrane and to anchoring plaques of basement membrane–like material in the fibrillar stroma, thereby creating a series of anchoring roots anteriorly and posteriorly that stabilize the cornea's various strata.

The stroma is comprised of very narrow, 20- to 30-nm diameter fibrils of primarily type I collagen in stacked lamellae. These are arranged in tightly packed parallel arrays in such a way as to minimize the scattering of light, thus resulting in a transparent tissue. This lamellar arrangement also allows for a consistent distribution of tensile strength within the whole tissue. Any stress or insult that leads to a greater diameter of the collagen fibril itself or to a distancing of the tightly grouped lamellae results in a loss of transparency of the corneal stroma. The exact nature of the interfibrillar matrix and its role in the maintenance of corneal transparency have been extensively studied. Type V collagen in the interior of the fibrils appears to play a regulatory role in their diameter. Proteoglycans containing keratan sulfate and dermatan sulfate abound within the fibrils and are thought to exert a swelling pressure by binding cations and water, thus limiting movement. A counterforce to this interior swelling pressure is thought to be created by type XII collagen bridges that hold the distance between neighboring fibrils.

Descemet's membrane is a thick basement membrane of collagen secreted by the corneal endothelium. The anterior layer is primarily composed of an elastic, hexagonal latticework of type VIII collagen. Its posterior layer provides a solid yet stretchable substrate for the endothelium. The corneal endothelium, in turn, is a single layer of confluent cells located at the posterior of the cornea, facing Descemet's membrane anteriorly and the aqueous humor posteriorly.

ROLE OF CORNEA IN INFLAMMATION

The epithelium is certainly the most critical structure regarding the cornea's potential response to external allergic stimuli. As discussed with the role of the conjunctival epithelium in inflammation, researchers no longer think that the epithelium is a passive platform on which immunologically responsive cells act in allergic reactions, but that it is a more active participant in inflammation. Histamine and cytokines released upon mast cell degranulation result in an enhanced permeability across the spaces between epithelial cells, thus increasing antigen absorption. Eosinophil major basic protein and eosinophil peroxidase were found to be potent inductors of RANTES release, a powerful eosinophil chemoattractant, from the conjunctival epithelium in vitro.[21] In the same cell line, interferon-γ was shown to upregulate ICAM-1 expression, demonstrating further promotion of eosinophil migration and attachment.[22] The extent of these effects in corneal epithelium is unknown, but they are expected to be similar. The formation of central corneal ulcers, limbal infiltrates, and epithelial defects in AKC and VKC are all thought to be the result of eosinophil-released products, such as eosinophil major basic protein[23] and eosinophil cationic protein,[24] due to the greatly increased expression of adhesion molecules in these diseases compared with SAC and PAC and normal individuals.

REFERENCES

1. Greiner JV, Covington HI, Allansmith MR. Surface morphology of the human upper tarsal conjunctiva. Am J Ophthalmol 83:892, 1997.
2. Gipson IK, Yankauckus M, Spurr-Michaud, et al. Characteristics of a glycoprotein in the ocular surface glycocalyx. Invest Ophthal Vis Sci 33:218, 1992.
3. Greiner JV, Weidman TA, Korb DR, et al. Histochemical analysis of secretory vesicles in nongoblet conjunctival epithelial cells. Acta Ophthalmol 63:89, 1985.
4. Duke-Elder WS, ed. In: System of ophthalmology: the anatomy of the visual system. Vol II. London, Henry Kimpton, 1961, p. 546.
5. Breitbach R, Spitznas M. Ultrastructure of the paralimbal and juxtacaruncular human conjunctiva. Graefes Arch Clin Exp Ophthalmol 226:567, 1988.
6. Kesing SV. Investigations of the conjunctival mucin. Acta Ophthalmol 44:439, 1966.
7. Parsons JH. The pathology of the eye. Vol. 1. London, 1904.
8. Sugiura S, Matsuda H. Jpn J Ophthalmol 13:197, 1969.
9. Tagawa Y, Takeuchi T, Saga T, et al. Langerhan's cells. In: Advances in immunology and immunopathology of the eye. O'Connor GR, Chandler JW, eds. New York, Masson, 1985.
10. Fujikawa LS, Bhan AK, Foster CS. T-cell subsets and Langerhan's cells in conjunctival lesions. In: Advances in immunology and immunopathology of the eye. O'Connor GR, Chandler JW, eds. New York, Masson, 1985.
11. Soukiasian SH, Rice B, Foster CS, et al. The T-cell receptor in normal and inflamed conjunctiva. Invest Ophthalmol Vis Sci 33:453, 1992.
12. Allansmith MR. Immunology of the eye. In: The Eye and immunology. St. Louis, CV Mosby, 1982.
13. Allansmith MR, Greiner JV, Baird RS. Number of inflammatory cells in the normal conjunctiva. Am J Ophthalmol 86:250, 1978.
14. Bacon AS, McGill JI, Anderson DF, et al. Adhesion molecules and relationship to leukocyte levels in allergic eye disease. Invest Ophthalmol Vis Sci 39:322–330, 1998.
15. Cook EB, Stahl JL, Gern JE, et al. Isolation of human conjunctival mast cells and epithelial cells: tumor necrosis factor-alpha from mast cells affects intercellular adhesion molecule-1 expression on epithelial cells. Invest Ophthalmol Vis Sci 39:336–343, 1998.
16. Bradding P, Roberts JA, Britten KM, et al. Interleukin-4, -5, and -6 and tumor necrosis factor-α in normal and asthmatic airways: evidence for the human mast cell as a source of these cyto-

kines. Am J Respir Cell Mol Biol 10:471–480, 1994.

17. Thorton SC, Por SB, Walsh BJ, et al. Interaction of immune and connective tissue cells. I. The effect of lymphokines and monokines on fibroblast growth. J Leukoc Biol 47:312–320, 1990.

18. Garcia-Zepeda E, Rothenberg M, Ownby R, et al. Human eotaxin is a specific chemoattractant for eosinophil cells and provides a new mechanism to explain tissue eosinophilia. Nat Med 2:449–456, 1996.

19. Gipson IK, Sugrue SP. Cell biology of the corneal epithelium. *In:* Principles and practices of ophthalmology. Albert DA, Jakobiec FA, eds. Philadelphia, WB Saunders, 1994, pp 17–37.

20. Olsen BR, McCarthy MT. Molecular structure of the sclera, cornea, and vitreous body. *In:* Principles and practices of ophthalmology. Albert DA, Jakobiec FA, eds. Philadelphia, WB Saunders, 1994, pp 38–63.

21. Trocme SD, Hallberg CK, Gill KS, et al. Effects of eosinophil granule proteins on human corneal epithelial cell viability and morphology. Invest Ophthalmol Visual Sci 38:593–599, 1997.

22. Yannariello-Brown J, Hallberg CK, Haberle H, et al. Cytokine modulation of human corneal epithelial cell ICAM-1 (CD54) expression. Exp Eye Res 67:383–393, 1998.

23. Trocme SD, Kephart GM, Allansmith MR, et al. Conjunctival deposition of eosinophil granule major basic protein in vernal keratoconjunctivitis and contact lens–associated giant papillary conjunctivitis. Am J Ophthalmol 108:57–63, 1989.

24. Leonardi A, Borghesan F, Faggian D, et al. Eosinophil cationic protein in tears of normal subjects and patients affected by vernal keratoconjunctivitis. Allergy 50:610–613, 1995.

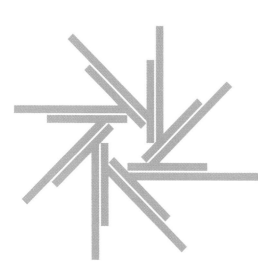

CHAPTER **3**

Ocular Immunology

MARK B. ABELSON ■ **CONNIE KATELARIS** ■ **ANDREW P. SLUGG** ■
ELIZABETH R. SANDMAN

An effective immune response depends upon the recognition of antigens and the communication between immune cells. The eye is particularly susceptible to foreign antigens due to its unique structure. The adaptive immune system, which protects the eye from foreign antigen invasion, performs three main tasks. First, it responds to a broad assortment of antigens that range from large bacteria to the smallest of viral capsid protein fragments. Second is the ability to distinguish between 'self' and 'other.' Without the ability to make this distinction, an individual can become immunocompromised. Third, the adaptive immune system has a memory in which a second antigen exposure induces a faster and more severe immune response than a primary exposure. These three characteristics combine to form the adaptive immune system composed of cellular and humoral immunity, which play roles in both nonspecific and specific immunity, respectively.

Immunological defense in the eye is mainly limited to the outer eye where pathogen invasion is a constant threat. The inner eye is characterized by immune privilege and possesses very few immunological defenses. Like the rest of the body, the eye has both specific and nonspecific defenses, which prevent or inhibit pathogenic invasion. Nonspecific defenses include the eyelids, tears, and tear components, such as IgA, lactoferrin, betalysin, lysozyme, and complement, and the normal flora of the eye. Specific defenses in the eye vary between areas of the outer eye (the cornea and conjunctiva), but generally include antigen-presenting cells, mucosa-associated lymphoid tissue (MALT), secretory IgA (S-IgA), antibodies, and cytokines. These components vary in function and presence in the cornea and conjunctiva.

NONSPECIFIC DEFENSES OF THE EYE

Apart from the physical barriers of the eye, such as the eyelids, lashes, and brows, the tears possess several important nonspecific defenses. Tears are continually produced at a rate of about 0.75 to 1.0 grams over a 24-hour period.[1] They lubricate, aid in transport, and clean and rinse the ocular surface. There are several components in tears, specifically in the aqueous layer that play roles in nonspecific defense. Secretory IgA, lactoferrin, betalysin, lysozyme, and complement all aid in prevention of infection and allergic reaction.

Secretory IgA is the main immunoglobulin component of tears. It is a dimer, composed of the Ig, the J chain, and the secretory chain, made locally in the plasma cells. Plasma cells located under the lacrimal glands produce IgA and then dimerize it with the J chain, which is bound to the secretory component. The secretory component is produced by the acinar cells in the lacrimal glands. Upon dimerization, the S-IgA is endocytosed, brought across the cytoplasm, and secreted into the tears. IgA has several immunological functions. It can prevent antigen adherence and absorption as well as neutralize cellular toxins and viruses. IgA also has the ability to eliminate plasmids.[1] It is resistant to breakdown because of its secretory component, but some bacteria do have the ability to break it down into Fab monomers.[2]

Lactoferrin, lysozyme, and betalysin are substances that prevent bacterial growth by depriving them of nutrients or by disrupting growth. Lactoferrin, which is 25% of tear protein,[2] reduces the amount of free iron in the tears needed by bacteria for reproduction. Aside from this main function, it can also be bacteriostatic. In some cases, it is bactericidal against bacteria such as *Bacillus subtilis, Staphylococcus aureus,* and *Pseudomonas aeruginosa.* Lactoferrin also plays a secondary role in primary immune response, lymphocyte production, cytokine production, natural killer cell activity, and regulation of complement activity.[2] It may also play a role in inflammatory response on the ocular surface.[2]

Lysozyme and betalysin work in conjunction by attacking the bacterial cell wall and cell membrane, respectively. Lysozyme is a low molecular weight protein with bacteriostatic and bactericidal properties[2] that makes up 40% of tear protein.[1] It destroys bacterial cell walls by enzymatically cleaving the beta $(1-4)$ glycosidic[1] linkage of muramic acid residue.[2] It cuts between *N*-acetylmuramic acid and *N*-acetylglucosamine, the same site of action as penicillin.[1] When lysozyme makes holes in the cell wall, it allows betalysin access to the cell membrane. Betalysin enzymatically attacks bacterial cell walls and is especially effective against gram-negative bacteria.[2] While this is thought to be the mode of action of this substance, its existence in tears has not yet been determined.[1]

SPECIFIC DEFENSES OF THE EYE

While the nonspecific immune response is often sufficient to ward off invading pathogens, in some cases, when a pathogen is able to surmount these defenses, a more specific response is needed. There are four main components of specific immunity that are applicable to all specific immune response. First, this type of reaction is antigen specific; it is tailored for a certain antigen using antibodies generated precisely for a particular pathogen. Second, specific immune response has a 'memory.' In other words, after the first antigen exposure, the immune system is primed for the next attack by the same antigen. The immune system retains a small number of antibodies that are produced against a pathogen, which allows these antibodies to proliferate more rapidly upon a subsequent exposure than at the primary exposure. The third characteristic of specific immune response is the immune system's ability to increase or decrease its response according to need. It does so using both cellular and humoral components and positive and negative feedback mechanisms. Fourth, specific immunity interacts with the nonspecific immune response. These two reactions do not work independently of each other and do share many of the same components. Within the ocular system, there are specific immune components in both the conjunctiva and the cornea, including antigen-presenting cells and immunoglobulins as well as distinct components.

CONJUNCTIVA

The specific immune response of the conjunctiva utilizes the antigen-presenting cells (APCs) of the eye, Langerhans' cells, macrophages, MALT system, and immunoglobulins. Antigens in the conjunctiva can stimulate cytokine production by macrophages and lymphocytes, which can attract monocytes and granulocytes. Cytokines play an important role in the up and down regulation of immunocompetent cells and in chemotaxis and cytotoxicity.[2]

The antigen-presenting cells (APCs) of the eye are mainly the Langerhans' cells, which are dendritic in origin[3] but also include macrophages. Upon antigen detection, these cells gather from the mucosal epithelium, engulf the antigen, and present the antigen proteins on their surface. These cells may carry major histocompatibility complex (MHCs), which are important in T- and B-cell activation. Langerhans' cells are considered very 'capable' cells because they can process antigen for recognition by both S-IgA and T cell–mediated response. The Langerhans' cells bind antigen to their surface and carry them to the lymph node via the lymph system. This transport may stimulate T-cell production, which can cause a hypersensitivity response or T- and B-lymphocyte production. Upon sensitization, the T cells leave the lymph nodes and travel through the bloodstream to the substantia propria in the conjunctiva; the B cells travel to the lacrimal gland to induce specific antibody response.[1]

After the Langerhans' cells have processed the antigen, S-IgA is capable of recognizing the antigen. There are also low levels of IgG, IgE, and IgM, which are made in the lacrimal gland, the conjunctiva, and accessory glands. Tears contain a wide variety of immunoglobulins, both natural and induced as a result of previous exposure to organisms such as *Staphylococcus epidermidis, Streptococcus mutans, Corynebacterium,* and several species of virus-like herpes and varicella. During an active infection, antibodies against these and similar pathogens increase. This accumulation results from a direct immune response in the conjunctiva, but can also occur in the lacrimal tissue when other mucosal tissues are stimulated by antigen. Local immunity is probably stimulated when antigen is admitted to the lacrimal ducts and when lymphoid tissue associated with the gut is stimulated.[2]

Lymphoid tissue is distributed in several areas of the body where mucoid tissue is located. This system of tissue is known as MALT. It is found in the conjunctiva-associated lymphoid tissue (CALT), intestinal and respiratory tracts. The epithelium that covers the CALT has elongated microvilli where antigens are taken up. CALT contains mainly small and medium lymphocytes, although there may be larger lymphocytes, which are undergoing mitosis. There are no plasma cells. After antigen uptake and lymphocyte sensitization, the lymphocytes travel from the CALT to local lymph nodes, then on to the thoracic duct via the bloodstream and to the specific mucosal site where they are needed. T lymphocytes travel to the substantia propria in the conjunctiva, and the B lymphocytes travel to the lacrimal and accessory lacrimal glands,[2] where they mature into plasma cells and produce S-IgA. This IgA then travels to the acinar cells in the lumen of the lacrimal ductules, where it combines with the secretory component.[1] The S-IgA travels to the conjunctiva for use. CALT may be part of a larger general secretory immune system that can use antigen sensitization in the conjunctiva to stimulate a humoral response at other mucosal sites.

CORNEA

Like the conjunctiva, the cornea's specific defenses include APCs and antibodies. Defenses also involve complement and cytokines. The antigen-presenting cells, mainly Langerhans' cells, are not distributed evenly across the cornea;[1] instead, they are compartmentalized in certain regions. The highest concentration is in the peripheral cornea, and the lowest (often no Langerhans' cells) is at the center of the cornea. Langerhans' cells can be stimulated to travel to the central cornea as a response to IL-1 and tumor necrosis factor-alpha (TNF-α)[3] secretion by corneal epithelial cells. As in the conjunctiva, the Langerhans' cells phagocytose antigens and present the proteins on their surface for Ig recognition.

Antibodies in the cornea generally reside in the stroma. Their residence in the cornea reflects previous antigenic stimulation. Antibodies usually originate from the fenestrated limbic vessels by diffusion, which suggests that immunoglobulin presence in the cornea is determined by molecular weight. For example, IgM, a high molecular weight molecule, is probably relegated to the peripheral cornea due to its size and is too large to diffuse into the central stroma. Because of this fact, and that IgM is the most effective immunoglobulin in terms of agglutination and cytolytic ability, the peripheral cornea may have more protection from pathogens.[1]

The classic pathway of the complement system is composed of a high weight protein and, like IgM, is restricted to the periphery of the cornea. Also present in the cornea are inhibitory molecules such as C1 inhibitor, C3b and decay accelerating factor in the central cornea and after injury, complement and SC5b-9, the membrane attack complex of the complement system. These complement proteins are synthesized in the plasma, although they may also be made locally.[2]

ALLERGIC REACTION: A SPECIAL CASE OF IMMUNE RESPONSE

The allergic reaction in the eye is the result of an extremely complex series of cellular and extracellular events coordinated by a number of mediators. At the center of the allergic reaction is the mast cell, which releases these mediators. Mast cells are present in loose connective tissue and contain granules, which upon mechanical or chemical disturbance (degranulation) are released. These granules contain a variety of mediators, which play important roles in the allergic reaction, and are often targets of antiallergic drugs. Mast cells can be degranulated mechanically (eye rubbing) or chemically (primarily by the binding of antigen to the IgE molecule at the membrane of the mast cell). This binding causes the linkage of IgE molecules, which results in the extrusion of the granules within the mast cell.[4] Upon degranulation, a myriad of mediators is released and causes the signs and symptoms of an allergic reaction. These signs and symptoms are increased permeability of blood vessels, contraction of smooth muscle in the bronchial tubes, and increased mucus production.[4]

The various mediators released by mast cells are as follows:

Mediators	Functions	Results
Histamine	Vasoconstriction, smooth muscle constriction	Itching, redness
Heparin	Prevents blood coagulation	Anti-inflammatory
Tryptase	Potentiates histamine, activates eosinophils and mast cells, attracts eosinophils and basophils	Bronchial hyperresponsiveness and asthma
ECF-α	Attracts eosinophils	
PAF	Platelet aggregation, neutrophil chemotaxis	Bronchoconstriction/hypotension, hyperemia, chemosis
Prostaglandins and leukotrienes	Capillary leakage, smooth muscle contraction, increased granulocyte action, platelet aggregation	Airway hyperresponsiveness, asthma

ECF-α, eosinophil chemotactic factor-alpha; PAF, platelet activating factor

The overall result of mast cell degranulation is an acute inflammatory response with local leakage of fluid from the blood vessels, which results in redness and swelling of the eyelids and nasal passages and in increased tear and mucus production. There are several antiallergic drug targets that include the prevention of mast cell degranulation, counteracting the effects of histamine and histamine blocking.[4]

Mast cells release a variety of mediators as outlined, but some of the most essential of these mediators are immunoglobulins. Immunoglobulins (Ig) are a class of glycoproteins that recognize the presence of antigen and facilitate its removal from the surrounding tissue. They are involved as messengers and effectors in both the early and the late phases of hypersensitivity reactions.

Immunoglobulins are present in two forms, secreted and membrane bound. The secreted antibodies are primarily involved in the activation of the complement cascade and the presentation of antigen to inflammatory cells such as mast cells or basophils.[5] Membrane-bound immunoglobulins (IgM) differ from secretory immunoglobulins in their structure and function.[7] Physically, membrane-bound immunoglobulins have a hydrophobic transmembrane sequence at the carboxyl end and have a short cytoplasmic tail that helps "anchor" the immunoglobulin into the membrane.

STRUCTURE

The basic structure of the Ig molecule is four polypeptide chains, two identical heavy (50,000 MW each) and two identical light (25,000 MW each).[7] The heavy chains are covalently joined together by two disulfide bonds, each with an associated light chain noncovalently joined by a single covalent bond.[6] The union of these polypeptide chains forms a Y-shaped molecule where the light chains are joined to the arms of the Y created by the bend in the heavy chains.

At one end of the immunoglobulin is the amino terminus where the antibody binds antigen at the epitope in a lock-and-key fashion.[6, 7] The other end of the immunoglobulin is the carboxyl terminus, which is involved in a variety of biological activities including immunoglobulin binding to cell surface receptors, complement fixation, and isotype determination.[5, 7]

Each immunoglobulin is composed of two regions, the variable region and the constant region. The variable region is made of the terminal 100–110 amino acids in each heavy and light chain and is where antigen binding occurs.[5] The constant region consists of the remaining portions of the polypeptide light and heavy chains. Although the variable regions of both the heavy and light chains are involved in the antigen binding, it is the arrangement of the amino acids in the constant region of the heavy chains that determines the isotype of the immunoglobulin.

The amino acid sequence consists of the heavy and light chains of the variable and constant regions as described and define the antibody's primary structure. The overall structure of the immunoglobulin molecule is defined by the composition of its primary, secondary, tertiary, and quaternary protein structures.

Immunoglobulin's secondary structure is formed as the polypeptide chain is folded back and forth in an antiparallel configuration creating a β-pleated sheet.[7] The sheets of polypeptide chains are then folded into more compact globular domains connected to neighboring domains.[7] The globular domains of the heavy and light chains then commingle to form the functional domains used in antigen binding and other biological functions.[7]

IMMUNOGLOBULIN CLASSES

To provide the diversity necessary for the binding and recognition of innumerable types of antigen epitopes, immunoglobulins have an array of light and heavy classes. Morphologically, there are two types of light chains (λ and κ) and five types of heavy chains (γ, α, μ, δ, and ε) with IgG (γ) and IgA (α) having further subclasses (four and two, respectively). This creates a total of 15 possible configurations of immunoglobulins in any individual.[5] In all, there are five forms of immunoglobulins (IgA, IgD, IgE, IgG, and IgM), which differ in structure, abundance, and function.

IgG

IgG is the most abundant immunoglobulin in serum, representing about 80% of serum antibodies.[5] The abundance of IgG is most likely due to its multiple subtypes and long half-life.[8] Produced in the conjunctiva, IgG is found in nearly all ocular tissues including the cornea, sclera, and tear film.[8, 9] IgG molecules primarily bind to the Fc receptors on a multitude of inflammatory cells and are involved in complement activation.[8]

IgA

IgA, found in 10 to 15% of serum, is the body's primary secretory immunoglobulin responsible for protecting the body's mucosal surfaces from infection.[8, 9] IgA is most abundant in tear film where it is found mostly in its dimeric form—two IgA monomers are joined at the constant region by a secretory component and J chain (a polypeptide chain that joins immunoglobulin monomers).[8] IgA is also found in the lens, cornea, and anterior chamber.

IgM

IgM is the largest immunoglobulin isotype. IgM exists in serum both in monomeric and secretory pentameric forms. Like IgG, IgM is largely involved in complement activation and is actually more efficient because of the pentameric arrangement of the antigen binding sites. The large size of the IgM pentamer prohibits it from diffusing into some tissues in the eye, such as the avascular central cornea.

IgE

Despite its extremely low serum concentration, IgE is a powerful activator in the allergic reaction. In both the early and late phases of the allergic reaction, IgE plays the crucial role of initiating mast cell degranulation in the presence of antigen. IgE molecules bound to the corresponding Fc regions on the mast cell surface are presented with antigen that initiates the biochemical cascade, resulting in the degranulation of the mast cell and the release of its chemical mediators.[5, 7] This immunoglobulin is perhaps the most important to the understanding of the allergic reaction because it is this molecule that is specific to allergens. After exposure, an individual becomes sensitized to an environmental antigen. When that occurs, specific IgE molecules are produced. Upon sensitization, inflammatory mediators are released that cause inflammation. This chain of reactions results in hyperresponsiveness. The severity of a response (specific IgE production) is determined by the duration and dose of exposure to the allergen. A longer exposure to a high dose results in a more severe allergic response. The detection of IgE is an important tool used to determine the specific allergen that an individual is allergic to. The test must be able to detect the specific IgE antibody as opposed to total IgE, which is a measurement of all IgE molecules, independent of their specificity, in the serum or tears.

IgD

IgD is another immunoglobulin that appears in low concentrations, representing only 0.2% of total serum immunoglobulin.[7] IgD is found on the surface of B cells and plays no role as a biological effector.[5, 7]

REFERENCES

1. McClellan LA, et al. Mucosal defense of the outer eye. Surv Ophthalmol. 42:233, 1997.
2. Pleyer U, Baatz H. Antibacterial protection of the ocular surface. Ophthalmalogica 211(Suppl 1):2, 1997.
3. Dekaris I, Zhu S, Dana MR. TNF-α regulates corneal Langerhans cell migration. J Immunol 162: 4235, 1999.
4. www.eb.com: MAST CELLS
5. Katzung BG. Basic and clinical pharmacology, 7th ed. Stamford, CT, Appleton and Lange, 1998.
6. Kuby J. Immunology, 3rd ed. New York, W. H. Freeman and Company, 1997.
7. Robinson NL. Principles and practices of ophthalmology, 2nd ed. Philadelphia, WB Saunders, 1994.
8. Friedlander MH. Allergy and immunology of the eye. Hagerstown, MD, Harper and Row, 1979.
9. Ballow M, et al. Pollen specific IgG antibodies in the tears of patients with allergic-like conjunctivitis. J Allergy Clin Immunol 66:112–118, 1980.

CHAPTER 4

T Lymphocytes

DENISE DE FREITAS ■ **ELCIO H. SATO** ■ **LUIZ RIZZO**

DEFINITION AND ORIGIN

The immune response is the result of interactions among different cell types, including lymphocytes, macrophages, and polymorphonuclear cells. T lymphocytes originate from pluripotent stem cells within the bone marrow (Fig. 4.1). T-cell precursors (pre-T cells) become committed to the T-lymphocytic pathway of differentiation before emergence from the bone marrow. These pre-T cells then leave the bone marrow and migrate via the circulation to the thymus. Pre-T cells enter the cortex of the thymus, where immature lymphocytes differentiate. The maturing lymphocytes migrate through the medulla of the thymus. During this migration, maturing T-cells undergo positive and negative selection. T cells unable to recognize foreign antigen bound to self-major histocompatibility complex (MHC), as well as cells that recognize self-antigens bound to self-MHC are eliminated. This process ensures selection of T lymphocytes that will only recognize foreign antigen in association with self-MHC molecules (MHC restriction).

ACTIVATION PATHWAYS

T cells only execute their functions when activated. Activation occurs through a two-signal process. The first signal is the recognition by the T-cell receptor (TCR) of an antigen bound to the appropriate MHC molecule on the surface of an antigen-presenting cell. The crosslinking of the TCR results in a series of signals transmitted via the cluster of differentiation (CD) 3 molecule. These signals cause phosphorylation of intracellular proteins,

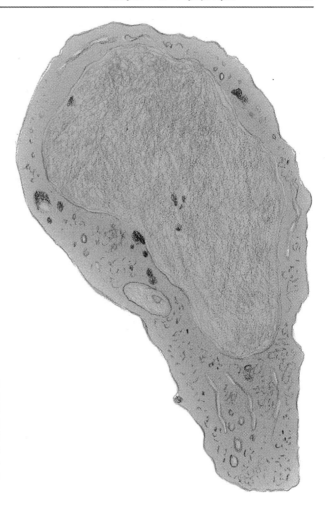

FIGURE 4.1 T lymphocytes (T cells) originate from the pluripotent stem cells in the bone marrow. Once produced, the T cells leave the bone marrow and migrate via the circulation to the thymus. Following the maturation process within the thymus, T cells express a unique membrane receptor that recognizes antigen only in association with cell-membrane proteins known as major histocompatibility complex (MHC) molecules.

phosphatidylinositol turnover, and calcium influx. A second signal is necessary to advance the T cell through the cell cycle. This second signal results from the crosslinking of other surface molecules, known as accessory molecules. Apparently, an interaction between CD28 and B7 provides the second signal for most T cells. Once a T cell is activated, it proliferates, expressing certain surface markers and secreting cytokines. The combination of cytokines that it secretes and the surface markers that it expresses define the T cell's function in an immune response.

CLASSIFICATION AND FUNCTIONS

T lymphocytes can be classified based on their surface markers and cytokine profile and function. Classic T-cell subsets are CD4+ and CD8+ cells. CD4+ cells recognize antigen in association with MHC class II molecules and are thought to play a regulatory role in the immune response, providing help for antibody production by B cells and coordinating events that lead to delayed-type hypersensitivity. CD8+ cells recognize antigen in association with MHC class I molecules and are thought to be responsible for cytotoxicity and immunological surveillance.

A subpopulation of T lymphocytes known as T-suppressor (T_S) cells has been hypothesized. The T_S cells are believed to be capable of mediating suppression of the humoral and the cell-mediated branches of the immune system. T_S cells have been shown to release suppressor factors that are antigen-specific, in contrast to cytokines, which are not antigen-specific. The suppressor factors may bind to peptides and MHC displayed on antigen-presenting cells, thereby blocking the interaction of antigen-presenting cells with other T cells. Some T_S cells have demonstrated idiotype-specificity, whereas others are MHC restricted, a finding that suggests that the T_S cells may be soluble released forms of the TCR.

T cells can also be classified as T_1 or T_2, depending on their cytokine profile. T_1 cells (irrespective of surface markers) secrete interleukin (IL)-2, interferon (IFN)-gamma, and lymphotoxin (tumor necrosis factor (TNF)-beta). T_2 cells secrete IL-4, IL-5, and IL-10, although secretion of IL-10 does not seem to be characteristic of the T_2 phenotype in humans. These two subsets appear to be mutually regulated; thus, IFN-gamma (secreted by T_1 cells) inhibits the differentiation and proliferation of T_2 cells. On the other hand, IL-4 and IL-10 (secreted by T_2 cells) prevent the differentiation and activation of T_1 cells. Additional cytokines such as IL-12 and IL-1 are secreted by other T-cell types and play a role in the differentiation process that leads a precursor cell to become either a T_1type cell or a T_2-type cell.

T cells can be categorized according to their developmental stage. Memory cells bear the CD29 marker or CD45RO, whereas naive cells are CD45RA positive. Another useful surface marker is the CD25, or IL-2 receptor, displayed on the surface of activated T cells.

T cells can be grouped according to the type of TCR chains that they carry. The TCRs belong to the immunoglobulin gene superfamily and have a similar structure to that of antibodies. The T cell is also assembled based on gene rearrangement. Alpha-beta T cells are the most common and follow the typical T-cell pathways described earlier. Gamma-delta T cells represent a minute subset found in the periphery, although they may be overrepresented in the skin and the mucosa-associated lymphoid tissue. These lymphocytes present differential MHC restriction and are generally double-negative cells (do not express either CD4 or CD8 molecules).

Functionally, T cells can be classified as either helper or cytotoxic T cells. Helper T cells are generally CD4+ cells and are involved in providing help for antibody syntheses. Crucial for this function is the interaction between CD40 and the CD40 ligand (GP39). Consequently, only T cells that can signal through the CD40 pathway can provide help for antibody syntheses. T-helper type 1 (T_H1) cells assist the syntheses of complement-fixing antibodies, whereas T_H2 cells assist the syntheses of opsonizing antibodies as well as immunoglobulin E (IgE). Thus, T_H2 cells are thought to be involved in allergic diseases and the immune response to helminths. CD4+ cells also induce delayed-type hypersensitivity response; those involved are frequently of the T_H1 type. Thus, these cells are thought to be involved in granuloma formation and the response against intracellular parasites. However, a more immediate type of cellular infiltrate can be induced by T_H2 cells, and granulomas seen in helminthic infections such as schistosomiasis are thought to be induced by T_H2-type cells. Several studies have indicated that the regulation of IgE is controlled essentially by the reciprocal activity of T_H1 and T_H2 cytokines, particularly IL-4 and INF-γ. It requires direct T-B interactions, combining both MHC-restricted and non-MHC−restricted events. However, the immune system has several redundant pathways, and no pathway is absolute. Furthermore, the immune responses are balanced, and although these subsets appear disconnected, they act in unison to maintain the body homeostasis.

The immune system can eliminate foreign or altered self-cells by mounting a cytotoxic reaction that results in lysis of target cells. One of the cytotoxic effector mechanisms involves immune activation of T-cytotoxic (T_C) cells that generate antigen-specific cytotoxic T lymphocytes (CTLs) with lytic capability. Typically, CTLs are CD8+ and are class I MHC restricted, although uncommon CD4+ class II−restricted T cells have functioned as CTLs.

ROLE IN ALLERGY

The various T-cell types play a number of roles in the allergic response, particularly type I and type IV hypersensitivity reactions. During type I hypersensitivity reactions, mast cells release inflammatory mediators in response to allergens. Mucosal mast cell proliferation is dependent on T-cell−derived lymphokines, including IL-3 and IL-4. Connective tissue mast cells are not dependent on T cells for proliferation. An antigen-specific T-cell factor can sensitize any mast cell to the specific antigen. Unlike IgE sensitization of mast cells, which can last for months, T-cell sensitization lasts only a few hours. T cells can also stimulate histamine release from basophils.

T cells can directly affect IgE levels. T_H cells (CD4+) produce IgE-potentiating factor (IgE-PF). T_S cells produce IgE-suppressor factor (IgE-SF). The relative amounts of IgE-PF and IgE-SF present are controlled by factors derived from other antigen-specific T cells. The increase in IgE levels demonstrated in individuals with ocular allergic disorders cannot be solely attributed to IgE-PF and IgE-SF. A slight increase in T_H-cell function does occur in ocular allergy, but no decrease in T_S-cell function has been demonstrated. The increase in IgE is out of proportion with the increase in T_H-cell function.

Some T cells express a low-affinity receptor for the Fc portion/IgE molecules. The function of this receptor is unknown; however, atopic individuals display an increased expression of this receptor.

T cells are essential to type IV hypersensitivity reactions. In contact-sensitivity reactions, antigen is presented to the T cell by antigen-presenting cells such as Langerhans' cells. Certain T cells, called T−delayed hypersensitivity (T_D) cells, become sensitized with the initial exposure to specific allergens. Subsequent exposure activates the T_D cells, via lymphokines such as macrophage-activating factor, to recruit macrophages. These macrophages are responsible for most of the symptoms seen in delayed hypersensitivity reactions. This series of events explains why these symptoms occur 24 or more hours after exposure.

T cells may develop a tolerance to particular antigenic determinants at fairly low antigen dose levels. Stimulation of B-cell tolerance typically requires 100 to 1,000 times as much antigen. T_H and T_C subsets may be deleted separately, resulting in tolerance with respect to only one of the T-cell functions. Immature T cells are subject to clonal abortion, whereas mature T cells may be tolerated either by functional deletion or the action of T_S cells. T-cell toleration also lasts much longer than that of B-cells, more than 150 days as opposed to 40 to 50 days, respectively.

BIBLIOGRAPHY

1. Gallin JI, Goldstein IM, Snyderman R, eds. Inflammation: basic principles and clinical correlates. 2nd ed. New York, Raven Press, 1992.
2. Morrison LA, Lukacher AE, Braciale VL. Differences in antigen presentation to MHC class I and class II–restricted influenza virus-specific cytolic T lymphocyte clones. J Exp Med 163:903, 1986.
3. Pearce E, Caspar P, Grzych JM. Downregulation of T_H1 cytokine production accompanies induction of T_H2 responses by parasitic helminth: *Schistosoma mansoni.* J Exp Med 173:159, 1991.
4. Roitt I, Brostoff J, Male D. Immunology. 3rd ed. St. Louis, CV Mosby, 1993.
5. Saito H, Pardoll DM, Fowlkes BJ, et al. A murine thymocyte clone expressing gamma delta T-cell receptor mediates natural killer-like cytolytic functions and T_H1-like lymphokine productions. Cell Immunol 131:284, 1990.
6. Springer TA. Adhesion receptors of the immune system. Nature 346:425, 1990.
7. Hall T, Brostoff J. Hypersensitivity: type I. In: Immunology. Roitt IM, Brostoff J, Male DK, eds. London, Gower Medical Publishing, 1989.
8. Yuasa T. Lymphocytes in allergic conjunctival disorders. In: Advances in immunology and immunopathology of the eye. O'Connor GR, Chandler JW, eds. New York, Masson, 1985.
9. Barnetson R, Gawkrodger D. Hypersensitivity: type IV. In: Immunology. Roitt IM, Brostoff J, Male DK, eds. London, Gower Medical Publishing, 1989.
10. Huang S. Molecular modulation of allergic responses. J Allergy Clin Immunol 102:887, 1998.
11. Larché M, Kay AB. T lymphocytes. *In:* Kaliner MA, ed. Current Review of Allergic Diseases. Philadelphia, Current Medicine, Inc., 1999.

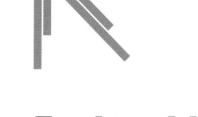

CHAPTER 5

Eosinophils

THOMAS JOHN

HISTORICAL ASPECTS

In 1846, Wharton-Jones first observed eosinophils in the peripheral blood.[1] Paul Ehrlich, inventor of the now standard techniques to stain human peripheral blood cells with aniline dyes, named this cell the eosinophil[2] because of the strong affinity of the granules for the acidic, rose-colored dye, eosin. It was not until the early part of the 20th century that an association was established between peripheral blood eosinophilia and allergic and parasitic disease. In the early 1900s, eosinophils were observed in the draining lymph nodes following experimental infection of parasites in animals.[3] Peribronchial eosinophilia also was observed in the draining lymph node following experimental infection of parasites in animals.[4] The role of eosinophils in ocular allergic and nonallergic diseases was not recognized until much later.

As research efforts have disclosed various characteristics of eosinophils, we have learned both positive and negative aspects of their function. On the positive side, eosinophils play a definitive role in defense mechanisms against infection; specifically, they can destroy many species of helminths and other parasites that invade tissues. On the negative side, eosinophils may play an undesirable role in inflammatory responses in the eye, the lung, the skin, and the heart when stimuli such as pollen granules are recognized as threatening.

EOSINOPHIL STRUCTURE AND FUNCTION

In humans, the eosinophil is slightly larger than the neutrophil, ranging from 12 to 17 mm in diameter.[5] The eosinophil found in the circulation is circular or ovoid, with a bi-lobed nucleus[6] and characteristic cytoplasmic granules (Fig. 5.1).

The eosinophil cell membrane is morphologically similar to that of neutrophils and lymphocytes. Under the scanning electron microscope, eosinophils appear spherical with surface microvilli; a few cells may have ridges, ruffles, or blebs.[7] The eosinophil membrane, which contains Charcot-Leyden crystal (CLC) protein (lysophospholipase) was described in the 1800s.[8–10] Although CLC protein, observed as hexagonal bi-pyramidal crystals, was thought to be specific for eosinophils, it has since been associated with basophils as well.

In humans, the eosinophil nucleus has a lobular shape and a bi-lobed nuclei, with an average of 2.06 nuclear lobes per cell (Fig. 5.2). In eosinophilia, one may see increased nuclear segmentation, with the nuclei having three or four lobes. This phenomenon is thought to be a reflection of increased age of the eosinophil.[6]

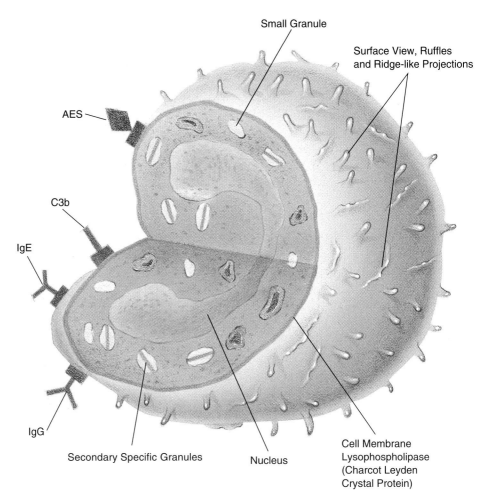

FIGURE 5.1 The eosinophil is circular or ovoid and 12 to 17 mm in diameter. The cell has a bilobed nucleus and cytoplasmic granules. The membrane contains surface micirovilli.

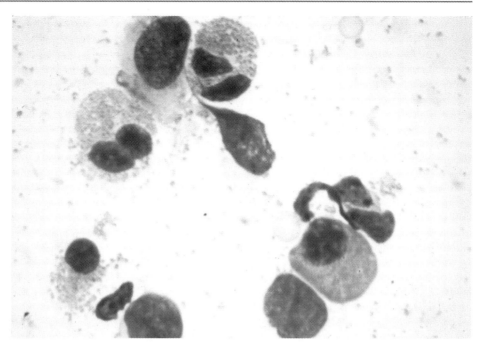

FIGURE 5.2 Typical eosinophilic granules are clearly visible. Each granule has a disc-shaped crystal that is electron dense and is surrounded by a matrix enveloped in a unit membrane.

The distinctive morphological features of the eosinophil are its granules. Eosinophil granules stain orange to deep red, depending on the species, with standard stains (Wright's, Leishman's, May-Grunwald, Giemsa's).[11] However, after degranulation, eosinophils may be undetected by standard histological staining methods. Eosinophil cytoplasmic granules consist of three types: primary, secondary (specific), and small dense.

The primary granules are round, uniformly electron dense, and seen mainly in eosinophil promyelocytes.[12, 13] The secondary granules display characteristic features under the electron microscope, namely, an electron-dense crystalloid core surrounded by an electron-radiolucent matrix.[14, 15] In humans, the granules, which are ovoid, have a longer diameter of 0.5 to 1.5 mm and a shorter diameter of 0.3 to 1.0 mm.[5] The granule core (electron dense) contains the major basic protein (MBP). The surrounding matrix (electron radiolucent) has two proteins, eosinophil cationic protein (ECP) and eosinophil-derived neurotoxin (EDN), and one enzyme, eosinophil peroxidase (EPO) (Table 5.1). Another protein, eosinophil protein X (EPX), may actually be the same as EDN. The small, dense granules have a density similar to that of the primary and secondary granules, and they contain acid phosphatase and arylsulfatase.[14, 15]

PROPERTIES OF SECONDARY EOSINOPHIL GRANULES

Major Basic Protein

Under higher magnification, the core reveals a crystalline lattice structure. The protein contents of these granules are described as "major" because

TABLE 5.1 Human Eosinophil Granule Proteins*

Name	Location	Molecular Weight ($\times 10^{-3}$)	Actions
MBP	Core	14	Toxic to parasites, epithelial cells; neutralizes heparin; releases histamine from basophils and rat mast cell
ECP	Matrix	21	Shortens coagulation time and alters fibrinolysis; toxic to parasites; potent neurotoxin; releases histamine from rat mast cells
EDN (EPX)	Matrix	18–19	Toxic to parasites, potent neurotoxin; has RNase activity
EPO	Matrix	71–77	Kills microorganisms in the presence of H_2O_2 + halide; releases histamine from rat mast cells; inactivates leukotrienes

* Eosinophil cytoplasmic granules consist of several different proteins that have a wide range of activities. The granule core (electron dense) contains the major basic protein (MBP). The surrounding matrix (electron-radiolucent) has two proteins, eosinophil cationic protein (ECP) and eosinophil-derived neurotoxin (EDN), and one enzyme, eosinophil peroxidase (EPO). Another protein, eosinophil protein X (EPX), may actually be the same as EDN.

they comprise 55% of guinea pig eosinophil granule protein; they are described as "basic" because their isolelectric point is too high to measure. Unlike other proteins in the granule, MBP lacks any know enzymatic property.[13]

The activity of MBP differs depending on its concentration. At high concentrations, it is cytotoxic in vitro to a number of mammalian cell types.[16, 17] However, in lower (nontoxic) concentrations, MBP stimulates the release of histamine from rat mast cells and human basophils.[18] At this reduced concentration, MBP can also activate neutrophils.[19] Eosinophil MBP has been detected in a number of ocular conditions including vernal keratoconjunctivitis (VKC), contact lens–associated giant papillary conjunctivitis (GPC),[20] Wegener's granulomatosis,[21] and active ocular cicatricial pemphigoid.[22] Elevated levels have been detected in tears of patients with VKC.[23]

Eosinophil MBP is toxic to parasites, including *Schistosoma mansoni*,[24, 25] *Brugia pahangi*, *Brugia malayi*,[26] *Trichinella spiralis*,[27, 28] *Ascaris suum*, and *Toxocara canis*.[29, 30] Eosinophils adhere to *A. suum* and *T. canis* larvae. Eosinophil granules are dispersed over the larval surfaces, followed by rupture of the larval sheath, which is engulfed by eosinophils.[30] The killing of *S. mansoni* is a two-step process involving an initial adherence to the organism's surface involving the Fc receptors followed by an irreversible binding to the parasite and subsequent degranulation.

Eosinophil Cationic Protein

Eosinophil cationic protein is a zinc-containing, single polypeptide chain within the granule matrix.[31] This protein has a high isoelectric point (pI > 11). ECP enhances blood coagulation by forming a complex with and inactivating heparin.[32] Like MBP, ECP plays a role in the defense against parasites.[26, 33] ECP can release histamine from rat mast cells, but unlike MBP, it cannot induce histamine release from basophils. ECP is also neurotoxic.

Eosinophil-Derived Neurotoxin

When injected into the rabbit or guinea pig brain or cerebrospinal fluid, EDN causes neurotoxicity, producing Gordon's phenomenon in these animals. EDN, like ECP, is toxic to parasites.[28, 34]

Eosinophil Peroxidase

EPO, which constitutes 25% of the specific granule protein,[35] has cytotoxic activity against a variety of targets, including parasites, tumor cells, and mast cells.[15] EPO is also toxic to a variety of other cells. It has been shown to affect the viability of corneal epithelial cells and may contribute to keratopathy associated with severe ocular allergy.[36] EPO was also shown to be toxic to urinary bladder epithelium via a mechanism that involves an increase in membrane permeability.[37] Although EPO alone has cytotoxic capabilities against parasites and mammalian cells, its activity is greatly enhanced in the presence of hydrogen peroxide and halide.[38, 39]

The eosinophil granule also contains a number of enzymes including peroxidase, phospholipase, lysophospholipase, acid phosphatase, beta-glucuronidase, acid beta-glycerophosphatase, cathepsin, ribonuclease, arylsulfatase, collagenase, histaminase, and peroxisomes.[40–42]

Eosinophil peroxidase is a useful activation marker in allergic diseases. Studies have shown a positive correlation between clinical symptoms and EPO levels in asthmatic patients.[43] The major products of protein oxidation by EPO, 3-bromotyrosine, and 3,5-dibromotyrosine have the potential for being markers for eosinophil-dependent tissue injury in vivo.[44] EPO expression has been shown to occur in an immature basophil cell line. The function of EPO in basophils is unknown.[45]

Eosinophils possess a number of surface receptors for immunoglobulin G (IgG), complement 11 to 15, and the Fc portion of IgE.[46, 47] Activation by specific antigen or anti-IgE antibodies results in the release of eosinophil MBP. However, IgG activation fails to do the same.[48] In addition, receptors for IgM[49] and cytokines, namely, interleukin (IL)-3, IL-5, and granulocyte-macrophage–colony-stimulating factor (GM-CSF), which can enhance eosinophil's helmintoxicity,[50] have also been found.

Antieosinophil serum (AES) can act against both mature and immature eosinophils,[51] blood and mature marrow eosinophils,[52] or marrow eosinophils without altering circulating eosinophils.[53] These antisera are a valuable research tool for the selective ablation of eosinophils and have provided evidence that the eosinophil may play a significant defense role against tissue-invasive parasites.[24, 25]

EOSINOPHILS IN TISSUE

Eosinophils are usually produced in the bone marrow, although occasional eosinophil mitoses may occur in extramedullary sites such as the thymus.[54] Once in the blood, eosinophils seem to be removed randomly, independent of their age, and have a half-life of 3 to 8 hours in humans.[55] They appear to have a diurnal variation, with the highest number of circulating eosinophils observed late at night during sleep; the number decreases during the morning and rises in midafternoon.[56] Following a brief period in the circulation, eosinophils migrate into tissues. Most eosinophils do not reenter the circulation, although some may recirculate and may be found in the thoracic duct lymph.[57] In humans, the ratio of tissue to blood eosinophils is about 200 to 300:1. Hence, circulating eosinophils may be considered as "passing through" the blood en route to tissue. In humans, eosinophils normally are present in the gut, especially in the colonic epithelium. Few are present in the normal human lung, and none is seen in normal human skin.[58] Eosinophils are absent from the normal human conjunctiva.[59]

EOSINOPHIL CHEMOTACTIC FACTOR

Eosinophil chemotactic factor (ECF), which is released from T cells, mast cells, and basophils, is a potent chemoattractant for eosinophil migration into the conjunctiva.[60] In vitro, several eosinophil chemotactic factors have been described, including histamine, leukotriene B_4, ECF of anaphylaxis, platelet-activating factor, T-cell derived eosinophil-stimulation promoter, some proteolytic fragments of the complement system, substances extracted from parasites, and factors present in tissues associated with eosinophilia.[58]

The old belief that eosinophils are simple effector cells has changed because of the discovery that eosinophils can produce cytokines.[60-65] The cytokines are classically products of activated lymphocytes and monocytes and possess a number of biological activities. Investigators have shown that eosinophils are an important source of IL-8 in serious allergic ocular disease and that IL-8 production by eosinophils was greater in atopic keratoconjunctivitis (AKC) than in VKC.[65]

ROLE OF EOSINOPHILS IN OCULAR ALLERGIC DISEASES

Hay Fever Conjunctivitis

Eosinophil infiltration is the hallmark of allergic ocular disease.[66] Hay fever conjunctivitis is the most common ocular allergic condition, and depending on the involved allergen, the symptoms may be seasonal or perennial. The presence of eosinophils in the conjunctiva confirms the clinical diagnosis of allergic conjunctivitis, but their apparent absence cannot rule out the diagnosis because they may be residing in deeper tissues.[67, 68] Eosinophil granule proteins that are released may have cytotoxic effects on the conjunctival cells and may cause further release of histamine from mast cells.[69] Like other organs, the eye also demonstrates a bi-phasic immediate hypersensitivity reaction (early-phase and late-phase reactions).[70-72]

Vernal Keratoconjunctivitis

The role of eosinophils in VKC has been well established in a guinea pig model of VKC.[73] Human studies have shown the presence of eosinophils located more superficially in the conjunctiva in VKC, and hence they are often recovered on conjunctival scrapings. Mast cells (80% degranulated), lymphocytes, macrophages, basophils, and occasionally, polymorphonuclear cells are also seen.[75] The substantia propria of patients with VKC has significantly fewer lymphocytes but more eosinophils, basophils, and mast cells.[75] Eosinophil MBP has been recovered from VKC shield ulcers.[23] This toxic material is thought to play a role in the development of VKC keratitis and shield ulcers.[23] Additionally, eosinophils and their granules have been demonstrated in the mucoid plaque overlying the VKC shield ulcer.[76] Eosinophils are an important source of IL-8 in serous allergic ocular disease, and the IL-8 production is greater in AKC than in VKC.[65]

Atopic Keratoconjunctivitis

The conjunctiva in patients with AKC has degranulating mast cells, eosinophils, and tissue deposition of MBP.[77] The significance of finding a greater amount of IL-8 in AKC compared with VKC is yet to be fully understood. Conjunctival eosinophil IL-8 expression correlated with the degree of neutrophil, but not eosinophil, infiltration.[65] Such differences may be exploited in the future to allow the development of more specific therapy for chronic allergic disease.

Giant Papillary Conjunctivitis

Histopathologically, similarities exist between GPC and VKC: both conditions are associated with tissue eosinophils, although these cells are more numerous in VKC compared with GPC.[75, 78] Conjunctival eosinophil MBP has been detected in patients with GPC.[78] The cytotoxic effects of these cationic proteins are thought to play a significant role in the conjunctival inflammatory reaction and the subsequent deposition of collagen in GPC and VKC.[74]

SUMMARY

The eosinophil is a fascinating cell with multiple functions in the eye and elsewhere in the body. Eosinophils, by virtue of their proinflammatory activity in combination with the release of various toxic products, play a definitive role in the tissue damage seen in various ocular allergic conditions and orbital diseases. In addition to the well-known role of eosinophils in anterior segment disease, apparently they also play a role in certain posterior segment ocular diseases. Continued research will unveil the importance of cytokine release by eosinophils and other as yet unknown properties of this functionally complex cell.

REFERENCES

1. Jones TW. The blood corpuscle considered in its different phases of development in the animal series. Memoir I. Vertebrate. Philos Trans R Soc Lond 136:63, 1846.
2. Hirsch JG, Hirsch BI. Paul Ehrlich and the discovery of the eosinophil. In: The eosinophil in health and disease. Mahmoud AAF, Austen KF, eds. New York, Grune & Stratton, 1980, p 2.
3. Opie EL. An experimental study of the relation of cells with eosinophil granulation to infection with an animal parasite, *Trichina spiralis*. Am J Med Sci 127:477, 1904.
4. Schlecht H, Schwenker G. Ueber die beziehungen der eosinophilie zur anaphylaxie. Dtsch Arch Klin Med 108:405, 1912.
5. Zucker-Franklin D. Electron microscopic studies of human granulocytes: structural variations related to function. Semin Hematol 5:109, 1968.

6. Sparrevohn S, Wulff HR. The nuclear segmentation of eosinophils under normal and pathological conditions. Acta Hematol 37:120, 1967.

7. Polliack A, Douglas SD. Surface features of human eosinophils: a scanning and transmission electron microscopic study of a case of eosinophilia. Br J Haematol 30:303, 1975.

8. Charcot JM, Robin C. Observation de leucocythemie. Mem Soc Biol 5:44, 1853.

9. Leyden E. Zur Kenntniss des Bronchial-Asthma. Virchows Arch (Pathol Anat) 54:324, 1872.

10. Schwarz E. Die Lehre von der allgemeinen und ortlichen Eosinophilie. Ergebn Allg Pathol Anat 17:137, 1914.

11. Sur S, Adolphson CR, Gleich, GJ. Eosinophils: biochemical and cellular aspects. In: Allergy: principles and practice. 4th ed. Vol. 1. Middleton E, ed. St. Louis, CV Mosby, 1993, p 169.

12. Zucker-Franklin D. Eosinophil structure and maturation. In: The eosinophil in health and disease. Mahmoud AAF, Austen KF, eds. New York, Grune & Stratton, 1980, p 43.

13. Gleich GJ, Adolphson CR. The eosinophil leukocyte: structure and function. Adv Immunol 39: 177, 1986.

14. Dvorak AM, Ackerman SJ, Weller PF. Subcellular morphology and biochemistry of eosinophils. In: Ocular immunology. 2nd ed. Smolin GS, O'Connor GR, eds. Boston, Little, Brown, 1986, p 237.

15. Beeson PB, Bass DA. Structure. In: The eosinophil. Smith LH, ed. Philadelphia, WB Saunders, 1977, p 17.

16. Gleich GJ, Frigas E, Loegering DA, et al. Cytotoxic properties of the eosinophil granule major basic protein. J Immunol 123:2925, 1979.

17. Frigas E, Gleich GJ. The eosinophil and the pathophysiology of asthma. J Allergy Clin Immunol 77:527, 1986.

18. Thomas LL, Zheutlin LM, Gleich GJ. Pharmacological control of human basophil histamine releaes stimulated by eosinophil granule major basic protein. Immunology 66:611, 1989.

19. Moy JN, Gleich GJ, Thomas LL. Noncytotoxic activation of neutrophils by eosinophil granule major basic protein: effect on superoxide anion generation and lysosomal enzyme release. J Immunol 145:2626, 1990.

20. Trocme SD, Kephart GM, Allansmith MR, et al. Conjunctival deposition of eosinophil major basic protein in vernal keratoconjunctivitis and contact lens–associated giant papillary conjunctivitis. Am J Ophthalmol 108:57, 1989.

21. Trocme SD, Bartley GB, Campbell J, et al. Eosinophil and neutrophil degranulation in ophthalmic lesions of Wegener's granulomatosis. Arch Ophthalmol 109:1585, 1989.

22. Heiligenhaus A, Schaller J, Maub S, et al. Eosinophil granule proteins expressed in active ocular cicatricial pemphigoid. Invest Ophthalmol Vis Sci 37 Suppl:1023, 1996.

23. Udell IJ, Gleich GJ, Allsnsmith MR, et al. Eosinophil granule major basic protein and Charcot-Leyden crystal protein in human tears. Am J Ophthalmol 92:824, 1981.

24. Butterworth AE, Sturrock RF, Houba V, et al. Eosinophils as mediators of antibody-dependent damage to schistosomula. Nature 256:727, 1975.

25. Butterworth AE, Wassom DL, Gleich GJ, et al. Damage to schistosomula of *Schistosoma mansoni* induced directly by eosinophil major basic protein. J Immunol 122:221, 1979.

26. Hamann KJ, Gleich GJ, Checkel JL, et al. In vitro killing of microfilariae of *Brugia pahangi* and *Brugia malayi* by eosinophil granule proteins. J Immunol 144:3166, 1990.

27. Wassom DL, Gleich GJ. Damage to *Trichinella spiralis* newborn larvae by eosinophil major basic protein. Am J Trop Med Hyg 28:860, 1979.

28. Hamman KJ, Barker RL, Loegering DA, et al. Comparative toxicity of purified human eosinophil granule proteins for newborn larvae of *Trichinella spiralis*. J Parasitol 73:523, 1987.

29. John T, Donnelly JJ, Rockey JH. Experimental ocular *Toxocara canis* and *Ascaris suum* infection: in vivo and in vitro study. Trans Penn Acad Ophthalmol Otolaryngol 36:131, 1983.

30. Rockey JH, John T, Donnelly JJ, et al. In vitro interaction of eosinophils from ascarid infected eyes with *A. suum* and *T. canis* larvae. Invest Ophthalmol Vis Sci 24:1346, 1983.

31. Olsson I, Venge P, Spitznager JK, et al. Arginine-rich cationic proteins of human eosinophil granules: comparison of the constituents of the eosinophilic and neutrophilic leukocytes. Lab Invest 36:493, 1977.

32. Fredens K, Dahl R, Venge P. In vitro studies of the interaction between heparin and eosinophil cationic protein. Allergy 46:27, 1991.

33. Yazdanbakhsh M, Tai PC, Spry CJF, et al. Synergism between eosinophil cationic protein and oxygen metabolites in killing of schistosomula of *Schistosoma mansoni*. J Immunol 138:3443, 1987.

34. Fredens K, Dahl R, Venge P. The Gordon phenomenon induced by the eosinophil cationic protein and eosinophil protein X. J Allergy Clin Immunol 70:361, 1982.

35. Carlson MG, Peterson CGB, Venge P. Human eosinophil peroxidase: purification and characterization. J Immunol 134:1875, 1985.

36. Trocme SD, Hallberg CK, Gills KS, et al. Effects of eosinophil granule proteins on human corneal epithelial cell viability and morphology. Invest Ophthalmol Vis Sci 38:593, 1997.

37. Kleine TJ, Gleich GJ, Lewis SA. Eosinophil peroxidase increases membrane permeability to mammalian urinary bladder epithelium. Am J Physiol 267:C638, 1999.

38. Slungaard A, Mahoney JJR. Thiocynate is the major substrate for eosinophil peroxidase in physiologic fluids: implications for cytotoxicity. J Biol Chem 266:4903, 1991.

39. Klebanoff SJ, Jong EC, Henderson WR. The eosinophil peroxidase: purification and biological properties. In: The eosinophil in health and disease. Mahmoud AAF, Austen KF, eds. New York, Grune & Stratton, 1980, p 99.

40. Archer GT, Hirsch JG. Isolation of granules from eosinophil leukocytes and study of their enzyme content. J Exp Med 118:277, 1963.

41. Hirsch JG. Neutrophil and eosinophil leukocytes. In: The inflammatory process. Zweifach BS, Grant L, McCluskey RT, eds. New York, Academic Press, 1965, p 245.

42. West BC, Gelb NA, Rosenthal AS. Isolation and partial characterization of human eosinophil granules. Am J Pathol 81: 575, 1975.

43. Parra A, Sanz ML, Vila L. Eosinophil soluble protein levels, eosinophil peroxidase and eosinophil cationic protein in asthmatic patients. J Investig Allergol Clin Immunol 9:27, 1999.

44. Wu W, Chen Y, d'Avignon A, et al. 3-Bromotyrosine and 3,5-dibromotyrosine are major products of protein oxidation by eosinophil peroxidase: potential markers for eosinophil-dependent tissue injury in vivo. Biochemistry 38:3538, 1999.

45. Masuko M, Koike T, Toba K, et al. Expression of eosinophil peroxidase in the immature basophil cell line KU812–F. Leuk Res 23:99, 1999.

46. Capron M, Capron A, Dessaint J-P, et al. Fc receptors for IgE on human and rat eosinophils. J Immunol 126:2087, 1981.

47. Capron M, Spiegelberg HL, Prin L, et al. Role of IgE receptors in effector function of human eosinophils. J Immunol 132:462, 1984.

48. Capron M. Eosinophils: receptors and mediators in hypersensitivity. Clin Exp Allergy 19 Suppl:3, 1989.

49. DeSimone C, Donelli G, Meli D, et al. Human peripheral eosinophils with receptors for IgM: demonstration and ultrastructural morphology. Immunobiology 162:116, 1982.

50. Weller PF. Cytokine regulation of eosinophil function. Clin Immunol Immunopathol 62:S55, 1992.

51. Gleich GJ, Loegering DA, Olson GM. Reactivity of rabbit antiserum to guinea pig eosinophils. J Immunol 115:950, 1975.

52. Mahmoud AAF, Warren KS, Boros DL. Brief definite reports: production of a rabbit antimouse eosinophil serum with no cross-reactivity to neutrophils. J Exp Med 137:1526, 1973.

53. Mahmoud AAF, Warren KS. Anti-precursor eosinophil serum: comparison with anti-mature eosinophil serum. Clin Res 25:478A, 1977.

54. Bhathal PS, Campbell PE. Eosinophil leukocytes in the child's thymus. Aust Ann Med 14:210, 1965.

55. Parwaresch MR, Walle AJ, Arndt D. The peripheral kinetics of human radiolabelled eosinophils. Virchows Arch (Cell Pathol) 21:57, 1976.

56. Beeson PB, Bass DA. Numbers in blood and marrow. In: The eosinophil. Smith LH, ed. Philadelphia, WB Saunders, 1977, p 10.

57. Zucker-Franklin D. The ultrastructure of cells in human thoracic duct lymph. J Ultrastruct Res 9: 325, 1963.

58. Gleich GJ. Current understanding of eosinophil function. Hosp Pract 23:137, 1988.

59. Allansmith MR, Greiner JV, Baird RS. Number of inflammatory cells in the normal conjunctiva. Am J Ophthalmol 86:250, 1978.

60. Reiss J, Abelson MB, George MA, et al. Allergic conjunctivitis. In: Ocular infection and immunity. Pepose JS, Holland GN, Wilhelmus KR, eds. St. Louis, CV Mosby, 1996, p 345.

61. Moqbel R, Levi-Schaffer F, Kay AB. Cytokine generation by eosinophils. J Allergy Clin Immunol 94:1183, 1994.

62. Venge P, Hakanson L. Current understanding of the role of the eosinophil granulocyte in asthma. Clin Exp Allergy 21 Suppl 3:31, 1991.

63. Kay AB, Young S, Durham SR. Phenotype of cells positive for interleukin-4 and interleukin-5 MRNA in allergic tissue reactions. Int Arch Allergy Immunol 107:208, 1995.

64. Costa JJ, Matossian K, Resnick MB, et al. Human eosinophils can express the cytokines tumor necrosis factor-alpha and macrophage inflammatory protein-1 alpha. J Clin Invest 91:2673, 1993.

65. Hingorani M, Calder V, Buckley RJ, et al. Eosinophil production of interleukin 8 in chronic allergic eye disease. Invest Ophthalmol Vis Sci 37: S1021, 1996.

66. Abelson MB, Schaefer K. Conjunctivitis of allergic origin: immunologic mechanisms and current approaches to therapy. Surv Ophthalmol 38 Suppl:115, 1993.

67. Abelson MB, Madiwale N, Weston JH. Conjunctival eosinophils in allergic ocular disease. Arch Ophthalmol 101:555, 1983.

68. Friedlaender MH, Okumoto M, Kelly J. Diagnosis of allergic conjunctivitis. Arch Ophthalmol 102:11989, 1984.

69. O'Donnell MC, Ackerman SJ, Gleich GJ, et al. Activation of basophil and mast cell histamine release by eosinophil granule major basic protein. J Exp Med 157:1981, 1983.

70. Bonini S, Bonini S, Berruto A, et al. Conjunctival provocation test as a model for the study of allergy and inflmmation in humans. Int Arch Allergy Appl Immunol 88:144, 1989.

71. Bonini S, Bonini S, Bucci MG, et al. Allergen dose response and late symptoms in a human model of ocular allergy. J Allergy Clin Immunol 86:869, 1990.

72. Saiga T, Briggs RM, Allansmith MR. Clinical and cytologic aspects of ocular late-phase reaction in the guinea pig. Ophthalmic Res 24:45, 1992.

73. Khatami M, Donnelly JJ, John T, et al. Vernal conjunctivitis: model studies in guinea pigs immunized topically with fluoresceinyl ovalbumin. Arch Ophthalmol 102:1683, 1984.

74. Abelson MB, Udell IJ, Allansmith MR, et al. Allergic and toxic reactions. In: Principles and practice of ophthalmology. Vol. 1. Albert DM, Jakobiec FA, eds. Philadelphia, WB Saunders, 1994, p 77.

75. Allansmith MR, Baird RS, Greiner JV. Vernal conjunctivitis and contact lens-associated giant papillary conjunctivitis compared and contrasted. Am J Ophthalmol 87:544, 1979.

76. Golubovic S, Parunovic A. Vernal conjunctivitis: a cause of corneal mucoid plaque. Fortschr Ophthalmol 83:272, 1986.

77. Porter DP, Trocme SD, Foster CS, et al. Conjunctival deposition of eosinophil major basic protein, neutrophil elastase, and mast cell tryptase in atopic keratoconjunctivitis. Invest Ophthalmol Vis Sci 34 Suppl:855, 1993.

78. Henriquez AS, Kenyon KR, Allansmith MR. Mast cell ultrastructure: comparison in contact lens-associated giant papillary conjunctivitis and vernal conjunctivitis. Arch Ophthalmol 99:1266, 1981.

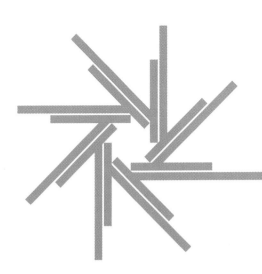

CHAPTER 6

Polymorphonuclear Leukocytes

MARK B. ABELSON ■ **KEVIN P. RICHARD**

Polymorphonuclear leukocytes (PMNs), or neutrophils, are the first cells of the host defense called in to contain, neutralize, and combat various endogenous or exogenous pathogens. PMNs mature in the bone marrow over a 2-week period and are released into the circulation, where they constitute approximately 60 to 70% of the circulating leukocytes. Approximately 12 to 15 μm in diameter, PMNs contain a multilobed nucleus, consisting of two to five lobes joined by thin strands of chromatin (Fig. 6.1). This arrangement is highly dynamic, regularly changing shape, position, and number.[1]

The chromatin of the neutrophil exhibits a characteristic pattern. Dense regions of heterochromatin are located primarily at the periphery of the nuclear envelope. Alternatively, the regions of euchromatin are located mainly in the center of the nucleus, with smaller regions in contact with the nuclear envelope. Alternatively, the regions of euchromatin are located mainly in the center of the nucleus, with smaller regions in contact with the nuclear envelope.[2]

The cytoplasm of the neutrophil contains two types of granules: specific granules and azurophilic granules, which differ in size and staining property. Specific granules are differentiated by the characteristic salmon-pink color they exhibit when stained with Romanovsky-type dyes. These granules are smaller and more numerous than azurophilic granules. Specific granules are surrounded by a typical membrane and contain alkaline phosphatase, collagenase, lactoferrin, some poorly characterized basic proteins (phagocytins), and two-thirds of the lysozyme found in neutrophils. Azurophilic granules, appearing deep reddish-purple when stained with the azure dyes, are

43

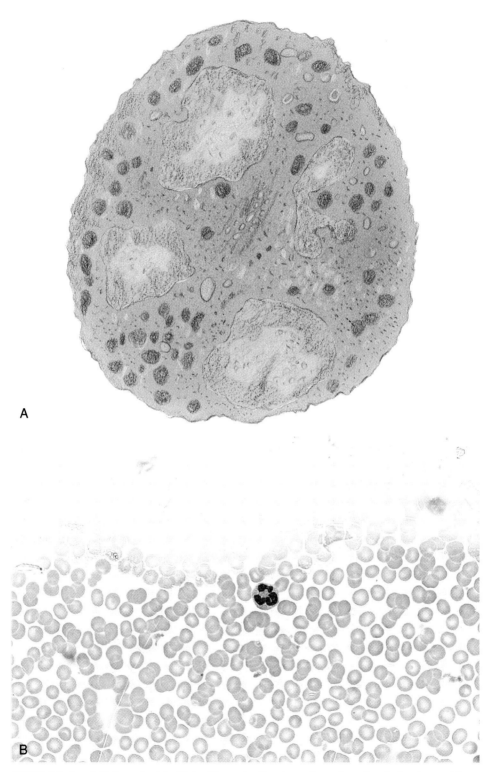

A

B

FIGURE 6.1 *A* and *B*, Approximately 12 to 15 μm in diameter, polymorphonuclear leukocytes contain a multilobed nucleus, consisting of two to five lobes that are joined by thin strands of chromatin. This arrangement is highly dynamic, regularly changing shape, position, and number.

TABLE 6.1 Granule Composition of the Neutrophil*

Specific Granules	Azurophilic Granules
Specific granules	Azurophilic granules
Alkaline phosphatase	Acid phosphatase
B_{12}-Binding protein	alpha-Mannosidase
Collagenase	Arylsulfatase
Cytochrome b558	Azurocidin
Formyl peptide receptor	beta-Galactosidase
Histaminase	beta-Glucuronidase
Lactoferrin	BPI
Lysozyme	Cathepsin
Mac-1/C3bi receptor	Defensins
	5'-Nucleotidase
	Elastase
	Collagenase
	Myeloperoxidase
	Lysozyme

* The cytoplasm of the neutrophil contains two types of granules: specific granules and azurophilic granules, that differ in size and staining property.

primarily lysosomes and contain a variety of enzymes (Table 6.1). Specific granules are released to the extracellular environment, where they induce inflammation. The azurophilic granules are released into the phagolysosomal vacuole, where they are involved in the killing and degradation of microorganisms and antigen-antibody complexes.

ROLE OF NEUTROPHILS

The various granular constituents of the neutrophil can either cause primary tissue injury or may perpetuate the injurious process. Proteolytic enzymes cause structural injury to vascular membranes. Collagenase is a neutral hydrolase that cleaves the protein polysaccharide of cartilage. Elastase is also capable of inducing primary structural changes in the elastin of affected tissue. PMNs release a procoagulant with thromboplastic activity, which leads to fibrin formation, collagen synthesis, and scarring. The cationic proteins, the leukotrienes, and the kinin-forming enzymes cause an evanescent increase in vascular permeability, whereas complement activation augments the accumulation of neutrophils.[3]

Neutrophils play a critical role in the scavenging of both inflammatory stimuli and damaged local connective tissue. On release from the bone marrow to the circulation, the cells are in an inactivated state and have a half-life of approximately 6 hours. Activation of the complement system by immune complexes or the stimulation of certain cell populations by specific antigens results in the release and production of neutrophil chemotactic factors. These chemoattractants bind to high-affinity receptors on the surface of the cell, thus resulting in activation (chemokinesis) with orientation (chemotaxis) toward a higher concentration of the stimulus.[4]

Studies on the role of closed-eye tears in ocular surface defense have provided evidence that IgA, secreted in greater quantities during the night, is a potent chemoattractant for neutrophils, calling them to the tears in large quantities during eye closure.[5, 6] This evidence suggests a physiological, protective role of neutrophils during sleep that disappears during the day in open-eye tears. Closed-eye tears have also been shown to contain much higher levels than open-eye tears of proinflammatory cytokines and lipid inflammatory mediators that serve to recruit these neutrophils and regulate the function of PMNs and IgA during sleep.[7] IL-6, IL-8, granulocyte macrophage–colony stimulating factor (GM–CSF), leukotriene B4 (LTB4), and platelet activating factor were all shown to be present in high levels in closed-eye tears compared with open-eye tears. Closed-eye tears were also shown to recruit neutrophils, maximally after 8 hours of sleep, suggesting that both IL-8 and LTB4 were active.[7] Furthermore, flow cytometric analysis revealed that incubation of neutrophils with closed-eye tears up-regulated the surface expression of IgA receptor, indicating that GM–CSF in closed tears was functionally active.[7] A nightly up-regulation of cytokines and LTB4, which have an established role in the initiation and amplification of the inflammatory response, as a normal occurrence during sleep has fascinating implications as to the role of inflammatory cells in homeostasis of the healthy eye. Another study, which has shown that MPO is a potent inhibitor of tryptase, lends even further support to the hypothesis that neutrophil proteins, such as MPO and lactoferrin, may play a regulatory role as endogenous suppressors of tryptase enzyme activity.[8]

NEUTROPHIL ACTIVATION AND DEGRANULATION

The activated neutrophil loses its round configuration in response to complex interactions of the cytoskeletal elements. Microtubules confer both stability and directionality to the cell, whereas the actin-myosin system provides the contractile forces and contributes to directionality. A defined lattice structure of actin filaments is seen at the leading edge of the cell, whereas a condensed rim of irregularly organized filaments is seen along the edges of the cell.[4]

In response to chemoattractant stimulation, sodium- and calcium-exchange channels are activated, leading to a transient decrease in cytosolic pH. The neutrophil membrane depolarizes; however, potassium efflux then leads membrane hyperpolarization. Intracellular calcium levels then increase. Serine esterases and proteases within the neutrophil are also activated by chemoattractants.

Neutrophils respond to chemotactic factors by adhering to endothelial cells (margination) on the inner wall of blood vessels (most commonly, postcapillary venules). Margination is mediated by various adhesion proteins that are expressed on both the neutrophil and endothelial cell membranes. Once the neutrophil is attached to the vessel wall, it insinuates itself between endothelial cells and migrates out of the venule and into the surrounding tissue (diapedesis).

Chemotactic factors in the tissues stimulate the neutrophils to move to the site of injury or infection. Once at the site, the neutrophils release more granule contents, cytotoxic enzymes, and toxic oxygen products (oxygen free radicals). This release leads to destruction of tissue and nonself matter. The continued release of chemoattractants and complement activators form the neutrophil serves to amplify the inflammatory reaction.

NEUTROPHILIC MEDIATORS

Mast cells, known to be the effector cells in immediate hypersensitivity reactions, also contain various mediators that regulate the tissue microenvironment and influence the development of an inflammatory response. Both preformed and newly synthesized mediators are involved in neutrophil activation.[9] Histamine has been shown to facilitate PMN adhesion to endothelial cells. Cytokines, such as interleukin-1 and tumor necrosis factor-alpha, can induce the expression of adhesion molecules for leukocytes on endothelial cells.[10] Platelet-activating factor can activate neutrophils.[11] Leukotriene B_4, by far the most potent chemotactic factor for human PMNs, has chemokinetic, degranulating, and aggregating activities on neutrophils as well.[12] In addition to leukotriene B_4, 5-HETE can recruit and regulate the PNM component of hypersensitivity responses.

ROLE OF NEUTROPHILS IN ALLERGIC REACTIONS

Neutrophils have a poorly defined role in allergic disorders of the eye. Studies have focused primarily on the role of the neutrophil in the early-phase and late-phase response. Several studies in both animals and humans have demonstrated a significant increase in neutrophils in both the acute phase and the late phase of allergic conjunctivitis induced by topical ocular challenge.[13–14] Although significant cellular changes have been demonstrated in both phases, correlation between the histopathological and clinical events is evident only at the acute stage. The neutrophil probably contributes to the pathophysiology of the late-phase response by releasing proinflammatory mediators such as leukotriene B_4, platelet-activating factor, prostaglandins, toxic oxygen radicals, enzymes, and neutrophil-derived histamine-releasing activity.[15] Additionally, investigators have hypothesized that this late-phase phenomenon depends on IgE and mast cell activation, thus implicating the mast cell as one of the key activators of the neutrophil in allergic disorders.[13]

Tissues from patients with giant papillary conjunctivitis have demonstrated a significant increase in the number of neutrophils in the substantia propria and epithelium.[18] This increase is thought to be the result of chronic lens trauma to the superior lid plate. Studies by Elgebaly et al.[19] and by Greiner et al.[20] support this theory. Elgebaly et al. demonstrated significantly increased levels of neutrophil chemotactic factors in the tears of patients with giant papillary conjunctivitis when compared with asymptomatic lens wearers. Interestingly, asymptomatic lens wearers also presented with slightly elevated levels of neutrophil chemotactic factors, a finding suggesting that subclinical abnormalities may be present.

The findings of Greiner et al. demonstrated that trauma results in a significant influx of neutrophils into the substantia propria and epithelium of the affected site. Further, they provide evidence that digital manipulation may influence the course of ocular allergic disease, resulting in both the clinical manifestations and the histopathological alteration noted on examination. The increase in the neutrophil population of the conjunctival tissue noted in these trials supports the theory that trauma plays a critical role in altering the cellular profile and disrupting the normally smooth epithelium, characteristics noted in various allergic disorders.

Patients with vernal keratoconjunctivitis have demonstrated a slight increase in neutrophil infiltration as compared with healthy controls. Neutrophils can be found in the substantia propria, the conjunctival epithelium, and the yellow, stringy mucus characteristic of this disease.[13–17] Pronounced degranulation of neutrophils has been reported in patients with atopic keratoconjunctivitis, undoubtedly contributing significantly to the clinical picture of the disease (e.g., vasodilation, corneal complications).[17–21]

All these ocular disorders demonstrate some degree of mast cell degranulation. The mast cell likely plays a significant role in neutrophil recruitment in all these disorders. Neutrophil recruitment in giant papillary conjunctivitis, although possibly secondarily influenced by mast cell degranulation, is more likely activated by the primary cause, trauma. Because neutrophils possess highly destructive properties (i.e., granular contents) and appear to play an important role in allergic disorders, further work evaluating their role is warranted.

One clinical study[22] determined the local and systemic levels of leukocyte markers in sera and tears of patients with various ocular inflammatory/allergic diseases: vernal keratoconjunctivitis (VKC), atopic keratoconjunctivitis (AKC), seasonal allergic conjunctivitis (SAC), giant papillary conjunctivitis (GPC), rosacea blepharoconjunctivitis (BKC), and bacterial conjunctivitis (BC), and normals. Neutrophil myeloperoxidase (MPO), a marker for neutrophil activation, was not found increased in serum of any allergic patient but was significantly increased in tears of VKC, AKC, and GPC, but not SAC, patients. MPO was one of the few markers that was significantly correlated with the allergic clinical score in VKC patients. Furthermore, MPO levels in tears, but not sera were significantly increased in the nonallergic diseases BC and BKC. This finding was correlated with signs and symptoms of the latter and mirrored the tear cytology results in BC and BKC, which showed a massive presence of neutrophils compared with controls.

Although the finding of local neutrophil activation was expected with BC, the active allergic eye diseases demonstrated notable neutrophil activity. The finding that this neutrophil activation was correlated with signs and symptoms of VKC and rosacea BKC suggests that the release of neutrophil, as well as eosinophil, stored enzymes and cytokines may have a role in the corneal involvement of ocular roseacea and VKC.

REFERENCES

1. Junqueira LC, Carneiro J, Long JA. Blood cells. In: Basic histology. Junqueira LC, Carneiro J, Long JA, eds. Norwalk, CT, Appleton-Century-Crofts, 1986.
2. Ross MH, Romrell LJ. Blood. In: Histology: a text and atlas. Kist K, Vaughn VM, Potler S, eds. Baltimore, Williams & Wilkins, 1989.
3. Cochrane CG, Dixon FJ. Antigen-antibody complex induced disease. In: Textbook of immunopathology. Muscher PA, Muller-Eberhard HJ, eds. New York, Grune & Stratton, 1976.
4. Gallin JI. Inflammation. In: Fundamental immunology. Paul WE, ed. New York, Raven Press, 1993.
5. Lan JX, Wilcox MD, Jackson GD, Thakur A. Effect of tear secretory IgA on chemotaxis of polymorphonuclear leukocytes. Aust N Z J Ophthalmol 26 (S1):S36–9, 1998.
6. Sakata M, Sack RA, Sathe S, et al. Polymorpho-

nuclear leukocyte cells and elastase in tears. Curr Eye Res 16:809, 1997.
7. Thakur A, Wilcox MD, Stapleton F. The proinflammatory cytokines and arachidonic acid metabolites in human overnight tears: homeostatic mechanisms. J Clin Immunol 18:61, 1998.
8. Cregar L, Elrod KC, Putnam D, Moore WR. Neutrophil myeloperoxidase is a potent and selective inhibitor of mast cell tryptase. Arch Biochem Biophys 366:125–130, 1999.
9. Zhang Y, Ramos BF, Jakschik BA. Mast cells enhance the antibody-mediated injury of skin basement membrane in mice. J Immunol 149:2482, 1992.
10. Zhang Y, Ramos BF, Jakschik BA. Neutrophil recruitment by tumor necrosis factor from mast cells in immune complex peritonitis. Science 258:1957, 1992.
11. Braquet P, Touqui L, Shen TY, et al. Perspec-

tives in platelet-activating factor research. Pharmacol Rev 39:97, 1987.

12. Ramos BF, Qureshi R, Olsen KM, et al. The importance of mast cells for the neutrophil influx in immune complex-induced peritonitis in mice. J Immunol 145:1868, 1990.

13. Bonini S, Bonini S, Vecchione A, et al. Imflammatory changes in conjunctival scrapings after allergen provocation in humans. J Allergy Clin Immunol 82:462, 1988.

14. Trocme SD, Bonini S, Barney NP, et al. Late-phase reaction in topically induced ocular anaphylaxis in the rat. Curr Eye Res 7:437, 1988.

15. Calonge M, Briggs RM, Levene RB, et al. Early and late phases of ocular anaphylaxis in actively immunized guinea pigs. Acta Ophthalmol 68:470, 1990.

16. Leonardi A, Bloch KJ, Briggs R, et al. Histology of ocular late-phase reaction in guinea pigs passively sensitized with IgG1 antibodies. Ophthalmic Res 22:209, 1990.

17. Saiga T, Briggs RM, Allansmith MR. Clinical and cytological aspects of ocular late-phase reaction in the guinea pig. Ophthalmic Res 24:45, 1992.

18. Allansmith MR, Baird RS, Greiner JV. Vernal conjunctivitis and contact lens–associated giant papillary conjunctivitis compared and contrasted. Am J Ophthalmol 87:544, 1979.

19. Elgebaly SA, Donshik PC, Rahhal F, et al. Neutrophil chemotactic factors in the tears of giant papillary conjunctivitis patients. Invest Ophthalmol Vis Sci 32:208, 1991.

20. Greiner JV, Peace DG, Baird RS, et al. Effects of eye rubbing on the conjunctiva as a model of ocular inflammation. Am J Ophthalmol 100:45, 1985.

21. Trocme AD, Raizman AM, Bartley GB. Medical therapy for ocular allergy. Mayo Clin Proc 67: 557, 1992.

22. Leonardi A, Borghesan F, Faggian D, et al: Leukocyte activation markers in allergic eye diseases. Am J Ophthalmol (In press.)

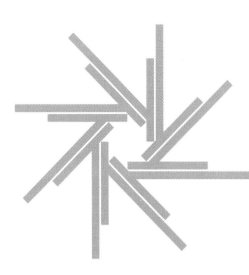

CHAPTER 7

Basophils

MARK B. ABELSON ■ **JIN PYUN**

Basophils are the least common granulocyte, accounting for only 0.5 to 1.0% of circulating leukocytes and 0.35% of nucleated cells in the bone marrow.[1] Basophils terminally differentiate in the bone marrow and circulate in mature form in the blood. Basophils are distinguished by their large, blue-staining, cytoplasmic granules. Similar to mast cells, basophils possess cell-surface receptors for the Fc portion of immunoglobulin E (IgE) antibodies. This granulocyte is activated when a membrane-bound IgE antibody crosslinks with a specific antigen.

BASOPHIL DEVELOPMENT

In bone marrow, basophil precursors undergo a progressive reduction in size. Nuclear chromatin condenses, Golgi and rough endoplasmic reticulum reduce in size, and mitosis occurs until a typical mature basophil results. Granulogenesis commences as small vacuoles of moderate density pinch off from the Golgi stacks. These immature granules migrate peripherally, enlarge, and display clusters of vesicles associated with the surfaces of their inner and outer membranes. The contents of the granules undergo condensation to produce more electron-dense matrices.

Mature basophils are approximately 12 to 15 μm in diameter.[2, 3] The nucleus is multilobed, and the chromatin is heavily condensed; the heterochromatin is located primarily in the periphery, whereas the euchromatin is centrally located. Granules of human basophils are surrounded by a membrane and contain a substructure composed of dense particles embedded in a less dense matrix. In addition to granules, the cytoplasm of mature basophils contains glycogen and a number of vesicles. Other organelles are inconspicuous (Fig. 7.1).

IMMUNOGLOBULIN E RECEPTORS

The presence of IgE receptors was indicated by the binding of radioactively labeled IgE myeloma protein or anti-IgE to the surface of blood basophils.[4] Initially, the IgE molecules appeared to be distributed diffusely throughout the membrane. Subsequent treatment with anti-IgE aggregated the IgE into patches, a finding suggesting that the IgE receptor can diffuse freely in the plane of the plasma membrane. Studies have revealed that human basophils contain between 40,000 and 90,000 IgE receptors per cell.[5] Fc fragments of IgE molecules bind to human basophils, whereas Fab fragments do not. The receptor, designated the FcϵRI receptor, exhibits a high affinity for the CH2/CH2 domain of the Fc fragment, with an association constant between 1.0 and 2.0×10^9 M^{-1}.

Isolation of the receptor revealed an 85,000-kd glycoprotein.[4] The hydrophobic properties of the receptor suggest that the molecule is embedded in the plasma membrane. The receptor contains four polypeptide chains: an alpha and a beta chain and two identical disulfide-linked gamma chains. The alpha chain is composed of two 90 amino acid domains that extend extracellularly to interact with the CH2/CH2 domain of the IgE molecule. The beta chain crosses the plasma membrane four times and is believed to link the alpha chain to the gamma homodimers, which extend into the cytoplasm. The binding of an IgE molecule alone to its receptor apparently does not have any effect on the target cell.

BASOPHIL DEGRANULATION

IgE-mediated degranulation begins when an allergen crosslinks receptor-bound IgE on the surface of the basophil. Methylation of various membrane phospholipids can be observed within 15 seconds after receptor crosslinkage. During this process, phosphatidylserine (PS) is converted into phosphatidylethanolamine, which, in turn, is converted to phosphatidylcholine. The methylation of phospholipids and the subsequent conversion of phosphatidylethanolamine to phosphatidylcholine facilitates the opening of calcium (Ca^{2+}) channels. Peak Ca^{2+} influx is observed within 2 minutes after receptor crosslinkage. The influx of Ca^{2+} produces a number of effects such as the activation of phospholipase A_2, promotion of microtubule assembly, and microfilament contraction. Intracellular cyclic adenosine monophosphate levels also increase 15 seconds after IgE receptor crosslinkage, resulting in the phosphorylation of granule-membrane proteins. Intracellular cyclic adenosine monophosphate levels peak after 2 to 3 minutes, then drop below baseline levels.[6]

IgE-mediated degranulation of human basophils proceeds by the extrusion of individual granules from widely scattered points on the plasma membrane.[3, 7] Basophils generally discharge their granules singly, not in multigranule clusters. Correspondingly, intracytoplasmic degranulation sacs

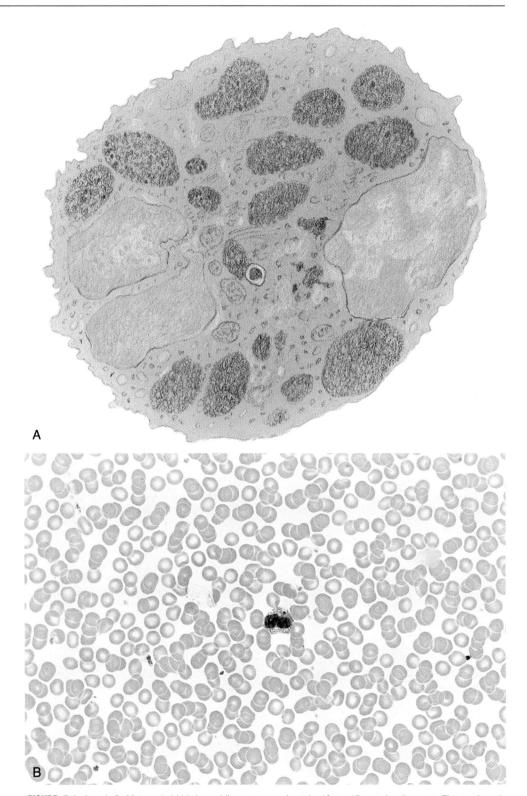

A

B

FIGURE 7.1 *A* and *B*, Mature (rabbit) basophils are approximately 12 to 15 μm in diameter. The nucleus is multilobed, and the chromatin is heavily condensed. Granules of human basophils are surrounded by a membrane and contain a substructure composed of dense particles embedded in a less dense matrix.

containing the contents of multiple fused basophilic granules, which release at a single site on the plasma membrane, are rare.

BASOPHIL SECRETAGOGUES

Certain secretagogues can induce basophil degranulation without stimulating the IgE receptor. Formylated bacterial peptides and complement fragments of C5a and C3a activate basophils through IgE-independent mechanisms.[8-10] Interleukin (IL)-1, IL-3, IL-5, stem-cell factor (SCF), and granulocyte-macrophage–colony-stimulating factor (GM-CSF) potentiate IgE-dependent mediator release from basophils.[11-13] IL-3 is a potent modifier of basophilic granule release that, at picomolar concentrations, increases mediator release in response to appropriate stimuli.

Relatively cell-specific peptides referred to as chemokines have been found to attract leukocytes. Chemokines are 6- to 10-kd proteins that are similar in amino acid sequence (20–55%).[14] These proteins are basic and bind strongly to heparin. Chemokines consist of histamine-releasing factors produced by monocytes, B cells, platelets, and endothelial cells. Chemokines have also been identified to induce mediator release from basophils. Of these proteins, monocyte chemotactic and activating factor and monocyte chemotactic protein-3 are the most potent activators of basophils.[15]

BASOPHILIC MEDIATORS

Basophils release a number of mediators on degranulation. Although some mediators are preformed, others are synthesized de novo on stimulation. Histamine, which is preformed, is the most widely studied mediator released by basophils. Evidence of histamine synthesis was obtained when basophils were cultured with ^{3}H-histidine, and newly synthesized histamine was measured.[16] In a spontaneous histamine release model, in which basophils from normal subjects were incubated at 37°C for 60 minutes, the mean histamine content per basophil was determined to be 1.48 ± 0.13 pg.[17]

Proteoglycans are a major constituent of basophil granules.[18] Most (approximately 85%) of these macromolecules are a mixture of chondroitin sulfate and dermatan sulfate. Release of proteoglycans, like that of histamine, has been shown to be Ca^{2+} dependent. However, allergen-induced release from atopic individuals exhibits a different time course and dose response from those of histamine.[17] Possible roles of proteoglycans include stabilization of the granule matrix and provision of a polyfunctional ligand for histamine.

Human basophils also contain major basic protein (MBP) and Charcot-Leyden crystal (CLC) protein. MBP stimulates the release of histamine.[19] In experiments using immunofluorescence, MBP in basophils appeared to be localized in the histamine-heparin containing granules. In normal subjects, the MBP content of basophils averaged 140 ng/10^6 cells in eosinophils. MBPs from basophils and eosinophils are immunochemically indistinguishable.[20] CLC protein possesses lysophospholipase activity.[21] These proteins were found to be uniquely associated with the main, particle-filled granules in human basophils. On occasion, CLC proteins were localized within small, smooth perigranular vesicles.[22]

Studies have demonstrated that mature human basophils may be a source of IL-4. IL-4 is partially responsible for stimulating B cells to synthesize IgE and is influential in the development of TH2-like lymphocytes.[23-25]

IL-4 is also a regulator of the selective endothelial transmigration of eosinophils. Basophils constitutively express mRNA for IL-4, perhaps accounting for its rapid translation.[26] IL-4 is believed to be generated de novo because its secretion is completely inhibited by cycloheximide. The mechanisms controlling IL-4 secretion and histamine release apparently diverge at some point in the signal transduction network, because the anti-IgE dose-response curves for the two mediators are clearly dissociated.[27] Furthermore, increases in Ca^{2+} from 1.4 to 5.0 mmol tripled the amount of IL-4 secretion without causing significant changes in histamine release.[28] Both N-formyl-methionyl-leucyl-phenylalanine and C5a, potent IgE-independent stimuli of basophil histamine release, induce little or no IL-4 secretion.[28]

ROLE OF BASOPHILS IN ALLERGIC REACTIONS

The basophil's active role in the late-phase allergic reaction has been inferred through differences in its mediator composition from that of mast cells. Both cell types contain histamine and can generate leukotriene C_4 and kinins. In the past, basophils were thought to differ from mast cells in their capacity to generate prostaglandin D_2 and tryptase.[29] Metachromatic cells in the circulation of patients with asthma, allergy, or allergic drug reaction, however, were compared with those found in normal individuals. The surface expression of the mast cell marker, c-kit, and of the basophil marker, Bsp-1, and the granule expression of mast cell proteases tryptase, chymase, and carboxypeptidase were determined. Consistent with other findings, the basophils present in normal subjects constituted less than 1% of the cells of peripheral blood. Very little, if any, mast cell proteases and c-kit were identified in them. In contrast, basophils in the peripheral circulation of allergic patients were increased in number, expressed Bsp-1 as in normals, but also expressed c-kit, tryptase, chymase, and carboxypeptidase.[30] The finding of peripheral metachromatic cells with properties of both mast cells and basophils suggests that they are derived from a common progenitor. Because mast cell proteases are now known to regulate numerous immunological and physiological mechanisms,[31] their expression only in the peripheral basophils and mast cells of allergic individuals may have important implications. The presence of histamine and leukotriene C_4 in the absence of measurable PGD_2, PGF_2, and tryptase suggests that the basophil may be the source of the histamine found in late-phase fluids. For example, in allergic rhinitis, one sees a bi-phasic increase in histamine levels. The first peak (approximately 30 ng/mL), which occurs 10 minutes after challenge, is accompanied by a corresponding rise in levels of PGD_2 (7,000 pg/mL), PGF_2 (2,500 pg/mL), and tryptase (250 ng/mL). The second peak in histamine levels (60 ng/mL) occurs 10 hours after challenge; however, PGD_2, PGF_2, and tryptase levels are minimal.[32, 33] IL-4 produced by basophils may contribute to the late-phase response by inducing endothelial expression of the adhesion molecule VCAM-1, thereby recruiting eosinophils into the target tissues.[34]

ROLE OF BASOPHILS IN OCULAR ALLERGY

Investigation into the role of basophils in ocular allergy has been limited. Basophils are prominent in ocular delayed hypersensitivity reactions.[35] Guinea pigs sensitized systemically with protein antigens in incomplete

Freund's adjuvant, then challenged intrastromally, elicited a cellular response predominated by basophils.

Basophil activity in vernal conjunctivitis has also been identified.[36] In one study, basophilic infiltration of the stroma as well as the corneal epithelium was observed in every specimen obtained from patients with vernal conjunctivitis. In their study, Collin and Allansmith[36] observed similar pathological features in vernal conjunctivitis, especially the presence of basophils, and cutaneous basophil hypersensitivity.[3] These investigators hypothesized that vernal conjunctivitis must be, at least in part, a manifestation of delayed-type basophil hypersensitivity.

REFERENCES

1. Juhlin L. Basophil leukocyte differential in blood and bone marrow. Acta Haematol 29:89, 1963.
2. Junqueira LC, Carneiro J, Long JA. Basic histology. 5th ed. Los Altos, CA, Lange Medical Publications, 1971.
3. Dvorak AM. Morphologic and immunologic characterization of human basophils. J Immunol Immunopharm 8:50, 1988.
4. Kuby J, ed. Immunology. New York, WH Freeman, 1992.
5. Malveaux FJ, Conroy MC, Adkinson NF Jr, et al. IgE receptors for basophils: relationship to serum IgE concentration. J Clin Invest 62:176, 1978.
6. Ishizaka T, White JR, Saito H. Activation of basophils and mast cells for mediator release. Int Arch Allergy Appl Immunol 82:327, 1987.
7. Dvorak AM, Galli SJ, Schulman ES, et al. Basophil and mast cell degranulation: ultrastructural analysis of mechanisms of mediator release. Fed Proc 42:2510, 1983.
8. Glovsky MM, Hugli TE, Ishizaka T, et al. Anaphylatoxin-induced histamine release with human leukocytes: studies of C3a leukocyte binding and histamine release. J Clin Invest 64:804, 1979.
9. Siraganian RP, Hook WA. Complement induced histamine release from human basophils. II. Mechanism of histamine release reaction. J Immunol 116:639, 1976.
10. Siraganian RP, Hook WA. Mechanism of histamine release by formyl methionine containing peptides. J Immunol 119:2078, 1977.
11. Alam R, Welter JB, Forsythe PA, et al. Comparative effects of recombinant IL-1, 2, 3, 4, and 6, IFN-gamma, granulocyte-macrophage colony stimulating factor, tumor necrosis factor alpha, and histamine releasing factor on the secretion of histamine from basophils. J Immunol 142:3431, 1989.
12. Bischoff SC, Brunner T, DeWeck AL, et al. Interleukin 5 modifies histamine release and leukotriene generation by human basophils in response to diverse agonists. J Exp Med 172:1577, 1990.
13. Columbo M, Horowitz EM, Botana LM, et al. The human recombinant c-kit receptor ligand, rh SCF, induces mediator release from human cutaneous mast cells and enhances IgE-dependent mediator release from both skin mast cells and peripheral blood basophils. J Immunol 149:599, 1992.
14. Oppenheim JJ, Zachariae CO, Mukaida N, et al. Properties of the novel pro-imflammatory supergene "intercrine cytokine family." Annu Rev Immunol 9:617, 1991.
15. Dahinden CA, Geiser T, Brunner T, et al. Monocyte chemotactic protein 3 is a most effective basophil and eosinophil activating chemokine. J Exp Med 179:751, 1994.
16. Galli SJ, Galli AS, Dvorak AM, et al. Metabolic studies of guinea pig basophilic leukocytes in short term culture. I. Measurement of histamine synthesizing capacity by using an isotopic thin layer chromatographic assay. J Immunol 117:1065, 1976.
17. Akagi K, Townley RG. Spontaneous histamine release and histamine content in normal subjects and subjects with asthma. J Allergy Clin Immunol 83:742, 1989.
18. Orenstein NS, Galli SJ, Dvorak AM, et al. Sulfated glycosaminoglycans of guinea pig basophilic leukocytes. J Immunol 121:586, 1978.
19. Zheutlin LM, Ackerman SJ, Gleich GJ, et al. Stimulation of basophil and rat mast cell histamine release by eosinophil granule derived cationic proteins. J Immunol 133:2180, 1984.
20. Ackerman SJ, Kephart GM, Habermann TM, et al. Localization of eosinophil granule major basic protein in human basophils. J Exp Med 158:946, 1983.
21. Weller PF, Bach D, Austen KF. Human eosinophil lysophospholipase: the sole protien component of Charcot-Leyden crystals. J Immunol 128:1346, 1982.
22. Dvorak AM, Ackerman SJ. Ultrastructural localization of the Charcot-Leyden crystal protein (lysophospholipase) to granules and intragranular crystals in mature human basophils. Lab Invest 60:557, 1989.
23. Vercelli D, Geha RS. Regulation of IgE synthesis in humans: a tale of two signals. J Allergy Clin Immunol 88:285, 1991.
24. Moser R, Fehr J. IL-4 controls the selective endothelium driven transmigration of eosinophils from allergic individuals. J Immunol 149:1423, 1992.
25. Swain SL, Weinberg AD, English M, et al. IL-4 directs the development of T_H2-like helper effectors. J Immunol 145:3796, 1990.
26. MacGlashan DW Jr, White JM, Huang SK, et al. Secretion of IL-4 from human basophils: the relationship between IL-4 mRNA and protein in

resting and stimulated basophils. J Immunol 152:3006, 1993.

27. Shroeder JT, MacGlashan DW Jr, Kagey-Sobotka A, et al. IgE dependent IL-4 secretion by human basophils: the relationship between cytokine production and histamine release in mixed leukocyte cultures. J Immunol 153:1808, 1994.

28. MacGlashan DW Jr, Warner JA. Stimulus-dependent leukotriene release from human basophils: a comparative study of C5a and Fmet-leuphe. J Leukoc Biol 49:29, 1991.

29. MacGlashan DW Jr, Schleimer RP, Peters SP, et al. Comparative studies of mast cells and basophils. Fed Proc 42:2504, 1983.

30. Li L, Li Y, Reddel SW, et al. Identification of basophilic cells that express mast cell granule proteases in the peripheral blood of asthma, allergy and drug-reactive patients. J Immunol 161: 5079–5086, 1998.

31. Compton SJ, Cairns JA, Holgate ST, Walls AF. The role of mast cell tryptase in regulating endothelial cell proliferation, cytokine release, and adhesion molecule expression: tryptase induces expression of mRNA for IL-1 beta and IL-8 and stimulates the selective release of IL-8 from human umbilical vein endothelial cells. J Immunol 16:1939–1946, 1998.

32. Naclerio RM, Meier HL, Kagey-Sabotka A, et al. Mediator release after nasal airway challenge with allergen. Am Rev Respir Dis 128:597, 1983.

33. Proud D, Bailey GS, Naclerio RM, et al. Tryptase and histamine as markers to evaluate mast cell activation during the responses to nasal challenge with allergen, cold, dry air, and hyperosmolar solutions. J Allergy Clin Immunol 89:1098, 1992.

34. Bochner B, Luscinskas FW, Gimbrane MA Jr, et al. Adhesion of human basophils, eosinophils, and neutrophils to IL-1 activated human vascular endothelial cells: contributions of endothelial cell adhesion molecules. J Exp Med 173:1553, 1991.

35. Friedlaender MH, Dvorak HF. Morphology of delayed-type reactions in the guinea pig cornea. J Immunol 118:1558, 1977.

36. Collin HB, Allansmith AR. Basophils in vernal conjunctivitis in humans: an electron microscopic study. Invest Ophthalmol Vis Sci 16:858, 1977.

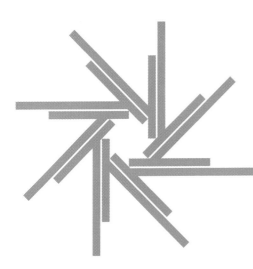

CHAPTER 8

Histamine

MARK B. ABELSON ■ **JIN PYUN**

Histamine (beta-imidazolylethylamine) was first synthesized in 1907. In 1911, Dale and Laidlaw observed bronchospastic and vasodilator activities in animals intravenously injected with histamine.[1] Eight years later, these same investigators noted that histamine applied locally to ocular tissues produced redness, swelling, and edema. Large doses of intravenous histamine also produced symptoms identical to those observed in systemic anaphylaxis.[2] Dale and Laidlaw later deduced that histamine was a humoral mediator involved in acute allergic reactions.[3] In 1953, histamine was identified in mast cells obtained from human skin.[4] This discovery led to a better understanding of histamine synthesis, secretion, metabolism, and activity.

HISTAMINE SYNTHESIS

Histamine (MW = 111) is an intercellular mediator exerting potent effects on several target tissues. The diamine is synthesized during a single-step decarboxylation of histidine by the pyridoxal phosphate-dependent enzyme, L-histidine decarboxylase.[5] Histamine is also synthesized from histidine by aromatic L-amino acid decarboxylase.[6] The bulk of histamine in tissues is stored in the secretory granules of mast cells, whereas circulating histamine is contained in basophils. Histamine in both cell types is preformed and is bound to the anionic side chains of proteoglycans composing the granule matrix.

HISTAMINE RELEASE

Antigen crosslinking of immunoglobulin E (IgE) receptors is the classic mast cell[7] and basophil[8] stimulus in allergic diseases. However, other physiological mediators can also induce histamine release. Some neuropeptides are mast cell secretatogues. The most widely studied neuropeptide, substance P, at micromolar concentrations, can induce histamine release. Conversely, histamine can cause the release of substance P from sensory nerve fibers, with both histamine and substance P contributing to histamine-induced vasodilation.[9] Opioids can cause degranulation through a naloxone-sensitive receptor; endogenous opioids, or endorphins, may stimulate a similar reaction.

Most inflammatory cells, including lymphocytes, neutrophils, platelets, macrophages, and eosinophils, produce or contain histamine-releasing factors, which can induce basophil or mast cell degranulation. Several cytokines, interleukin (IL)-1, IL-3, IL-8, and granulocyte-macrophage–colony-stimulating factor also cause basophil degranulation. Cross-desensitization, IgE stripping, and reconstituting experiments indicate that some, but not all, of these histamine-releasing factors act through IgE.[10]

HISTAMINE RECEPTORS

Histamine action is believed to be mediated by its binding to specific cell-surface receptors. Extensive pharmacological analysis using highly specific competitive antagonists and agonists has identified at least three different subtypes of histamine receptors: H_1, H_2, and H_3 receptors. Both H_1 and H_2 receptors have been identified in the eye.[11]

H_1 Receptor

The H_1 receptor was identified using the radiolabeled H_1 antagonist, [³H]-pyrilamine.[12] The presence of the H_1 receptor was indicated by the correlation between the level of pyrilamine binding and the degree of contractile response in guinea pig ileum. In addition, subclasses of the H_1 receptor have been identified using different radiolabeled ligands.[13] The molecular weight of the H_1 receptor on *differentiated cells* is approximately 68,000 kd, which, after being treated with *N*-glycanase, decreases to 40,000 kd, a weight similar to that of the H_1 receptor on *undifferentiated cells*.[14] *N*-glycosylation may therefore contribute to H_1 receptor heterogeneity. The number of disulfide bridges may also affect the molecular weight of the receptors.[15]

The H_1 receptor is coupled to phosphatidylinositol hydrolysis pathways. Receptor stimulation induces hydrolysis of phosphatidylinositol, leading to the activation of protein kinase C (PKC).[16] Multiple subtypes of PKC have been identified, and its action may vary because of differential allocation among different cells.[17]

Histamine H_1 receptors have been identified on human conjunctival epithelial cells in primary culture[17] and corneal epithelial cells in both primary[18] and immortalized cell lines.[19] Studies have shown that mRNA expression of the H_1 receptor is significantly increased in the mucosae of allergic patients versus normal subjects. This finding suggests that not only do allergic patients have increased levels of histamine at the target sites, but that the receptors are up-regulated and of increased density.[20] Whether this is a primary pathogenic phenomenon or a secondary event in response to high levels of histamine is unknown.

H$_2$ Receptor

The existence of an H$_2$ receptor was identified in 1972 by Black et al.,[22] who used a series of antagonists specific for H$_2$ receptors, but not for H$_1$ receptors. Black et al. also demonstrated that 2-methylhistamine acted on tissues considered to possess H$_1$ receptors, but it was relatively ineffective in tissues considered to possess H$_2$ receptors. Conversely, 4-methylhistamine had little effect on tissues with H$_1$ receptors, but it stimulated tissues with H$_2$ receptors. Black et al. also suggested that the effects of histamine on the cardiovascular system appear to be mediated by H$_1$ and H$_2$ receptors because both H$_1$ and H$_2$ antagonists were required to inhibit the depressor effect of histamine. Local edema produced by the injection of histamine is suppressed by burimamide (a H$_2$ antagonist) in combination with pyrilamine (a H$_2$ antagonist), but not by pyrilamine alone.

The H$_2$ receptor is coupled to adenylate cyclase; histamine stimulates increases in intracellular cyclic adenosine monophosphate (cAMP).[16] In neutrophils, H$_2$-specific stimulation consistently enhances the chemokinetic response, whereas the chemotactic response is inhibited in a H$_2$ receptor-dependent manner.[23] Although the inhibition of chemotaxis is due to the elevation of cAMP, the mechanism for the H$_2$ receptor-mediated stimulation of chemokinesis cannot be explained by the activation of secondary cAMP pathways. These data suggest that the H$_2$ receptor may stimulate multiple independent effects in early neutrophil activation. The H$_2$ receptor has been reported to increase calcium (Ca^{2+}) concentrations in parietal cells.[24] Therefore, the H$_2$ receptor may be capable of activating phosphatidylinositol hydrolysis pathways, much like the H$_1$ receptor (Fig. 8.1).

H$_3$ Receptor

The first strong evidence of a third type of histamine (H$_3$) receptor was provided in 1983.[25] Through the use of a range of agonists and antagonists, investigators demonstrated that the inhibition of histamine release involved neither H$_1$ nor H$_2$ receptors, but rather a third receptor. The discovery of highly selective ligands provided another breakthrough in the understanding of the H$_3$ receptor.[26] Alpha-methylhistamine exhibited high potency as a H$_3$ receptor agonist (15 times more potent than histamine) and only weak agonist activity for H$_1$ and H$_2$ receptors. Furthermore, thioperamide was found to be a potent and selective H$_3$ antagonist.

H$_3$ receptors are responsible for the negative feedback regulation of anaphylactic histamine release.[27] In one study, exogenously added histamine inhibited the anaphylactic histamine release, in a concentration-dependent fashion, from purified mast cells. Similarly, investigators revealed that H$_3$ antagonists, but not H$_1$ and H$_2$ antagonists, enhanced the anaphylactic histamine release. H$_3$ receptors are located directly on histaminergic terminals of nerves.[28] Autoinhibition can be apparently modulated in a complex manner by changes in extracellular Ca^{2+}, suggesting that H$_3$ receptors regulate histamine release via control of Ca^{2+} entry. These receptors have not been identified in ocular tissues, and selective therapeutic agents have yet to be determined.

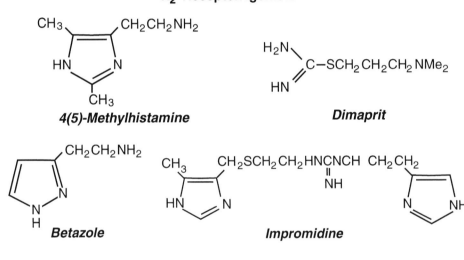

FIGURE 8.1 The use of receptor-specific histamine agonists led to the discovery of different histamine receptors.

HISTAMINE EFFECTS

Histamine has many functions including the down-modulation of mitogen- and antigen-induced lymphocyte proliferation, chemiluminescence, T-cell colony formation and cytotoxicity, inhibition of immunoglobulin production, and enhancement of natural killer cell activity. Histamine can associate with either the H_1 or H_2 receptor alone or in combination to produce a myriad of responses. When histamine associates with H_2 receptors, it decreases production of the complement component C2 in human monocytes[29] and reduces C2, C5, and factor B production in mouse peritoneal macrophages.[30] Interaction with H_2 receptors also down-regulates the biosynthesis of C3. C3 production is increased, however, when histamine stimulates H_1 receptors. Similar opposing regulation has been observed for phorbol ester–induced C2 production of the human monocytic-histocytic cell line.[31]

Histamine modifies cytokine-induced complement and fibrinogen synthesis, enhancing IL-6–stimulated C3 and fibrinogen expression. Constitutive biosynthesis of factor B is down-modulated by histamine via the H_2 receptor, whereas histamine acts through the H_1 receptor in IL-1–activated cells to stimulate factor B synthesis. In neutrophils, histamine interaction with either H_1 or H_2 receptors suppresses the function of Fc and complement receptors.[32] Both types of histamine receptors also stimulate eosinophil chemotaxis.[33]

Histamine influences the cytokine network, acting both as a modulator of cytokine-receptor interactions and as a target of cytokine action. When bound to the H_2 receptor, histamine retards endotoxin-induced Il-1[34] and tumor necrosis factor-alpha production in human monocytes.[35] Histamine directly inhibits the production of IL-2 and has an inhibitory effect on interferon-gamma, although this effect may be due to the IL-2 suppression.[36] The diamine also enhances the production of corticotropin, beta-endorphin, alpha-melanocyte–stimulating hormone, and prolactin, and it suppresses thyroid-stimulating hormone, all of which modulate the cytokine network.[37]

The synthesis and release of histamine is, in turn, influenced by cytokines. IL-3 induces histamine production, which can be enhanced further by IL-8.[38] IL-5 can also prime human basophils for histamine release induced by C5a, anti-IgE, and the chemotactic peptide *N*-formyl-methionyl-leucyl-phenylalanine.[39] IL-1 enhances histamine production, which, in turn, may inhibit the production of IL-1 and tumor necrosis factor-alpha through negative feedback.

Histamine causes significant vascular effects, such as transient flushing of the face and neck, reduced blood pressure, and edema. Pooling of blood and hypotension result from dilation of the small precapillary blood vessels and the constriction of larger venules.[40] Histamine induces edema by constricting the endothelial cells of the small venules, exposing the basement membrane, thus allowing plasma to pass into the extracellular space.

Itching, hyperemia, tearing, and chemosis are classic ocular manifestations resulting from histamine release. Ocular signs constitute conjunctival and lid edema, dilation of conjunctival blood vessels, and a papillary reaction.[41] Vasodilation results from the stimulation of H_2 receptors in blood vessels,[42] whereas H_1 stimulation leads to vasoconstriction. Stimulation of the H_1 receptor also induces ocular itching.[43] Topical and intrastromal administration of histamine has induced increased intraocular pressure, pupillary constriction,[44] and hyperemia and chemosis in the conjunctiva and uvea. Histamine also participates in the synthesis and release of prostacyclin, a potentially important mediator in allergic conjunctivitis.[45] Retinal blood vessels are unaffected by histamine (Fig. 8.2).

In addition to inducing vascular permeability, histamine binds to H_1 receptors on nociceptive type-C nerves, which are extensively branched into the epithelial and submucosal regions. Depolarization of these neurons in the submucosa leads to the release of substance P, calcitonin gene-related peptide, neurokinin A, gastrin-releasing peptide, and possibly others by what is known as the axon response mechanism.[46] Although extensively

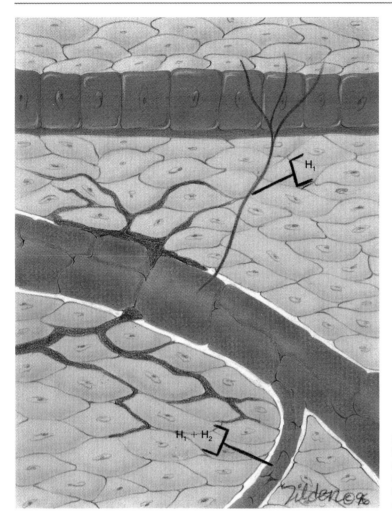

FIGURE 8.2 Vasodilation results from the stimulation of histamine (H_2) receptors in blood vessels, whereas H_1 stimulation leads to vasoconstriction. Stimulation of the H_1 receptor also induces ocular itching.

studied in laboratory animals (rodents, rabbits),[47] in human beings the axon response may actually have little effect on vascular permeability.[48] Other actions of the axon response, such as glandular secretion and endothelial adhesion marker expression, have been shown to occur in humans, since substance P and calcitonin gene-related peptide are released within 3 minutes after an allergen challenge to the nasal mucosa.[49] In a study in the guinea pig egg albumin model for allergic conjunctivitis, the conjunctival hyperpermeability induced by substance P seemed to occur through the neurokinin-1 receptor activation on blood vessels instead of through direct action on mast cells.[50] The direct effects of substance P have not yet been clearly distinguished from its indirect effects via histamine release in the human conjunctiva.

HISTAMINE METABOLISM¡

Histamine is metabolized by two enzymes. Diamine oxidase, also known as histaminase, oxidizes diamines with molecular oxygen, producing aminoaldehyde, ammonia, and hydrogen peroxide.[51] Histamine is initially bound by the enzyme, followed by aminoaldehyde release. Oxygen then binds to the complex and hydrogen peroxide and ammonia are released. The reaction is as follows:

$$H_2N - [CH_2]_n - NH_2 + O_2 + H_2O \; H_2N - [CH_2)_{n-1} - CHO + H_2O_2 + NH_3$$

Transglutaminase, a Ca^{2+}-dependent enzyme catalyzing the acyl transfer reaction, has been demonstrated to catalyze the formation of isopeptide crosslinks in the lens and may be involved in the development of senile cataracts.[52]

N-methyltransferase (HMT) accounts for approximately 70% of histamine degradation.[53] HMT metabolizes histamine by methylating the nitrogen in the imidazole ring in an S-adenosylmethionine–dependent reaction.[53] The cDNA clone of human HMT has been isolated from a cDNA library of human kidney, and the amino acid sequences have been determined. Human HMT consists of 292 amino acid residues (MW = 33,279) and shares 82% identity with rat HMT (Fig. 8.3).[12]

OCULAR HISTAMINE DISTRIBUTION

Histamine is widely distributed throughout the mammalian eye. In normal, nonhuman ocular tissues, histamine is present in highest concentrations in the lids, conjunctiva, subconjunctiva, episclera, and limbus. Uveal tissue has low but measurable concentrations of histamine, whereas histamine has not been detected in the lens, aqueous humor, retina, and other internal ocular structures.[54] In ocular structures (iris, ciliary body, choroid, retina, sclera, and optic nerve) enucleated from patients suffering from endophthalmitis, perforative wounds of cornea or sclera, or uncontrolled glaucoma, the highest levels of histamine were always detected in the uvea. The lowest values were always detected in the retina and sclera.[44] The relatively low levels of histamine in the sclera, optic nerve, and retina most likely result from the finding that these structures are not as affected by inflammation as the uveal tissue. Mast cells, which contain histamine, have been identified in the choroid and iris-ciliary body of many mammalian species.[55]

HISTAMINE AND OCULAR ALLERGIC DISEASES

Histamine has been used for ocular challenges in humans to create signs and symptoms of allergic diseases.[43] In one study, 10 μL of increasing concentrations of histamine ranging from 5 to 100 ng/mL was topically instilled into the eye, and the resulting clinical manifestations were monitored. Eyes challenged with 5 ng/mL of histamine displayed manifestations comparable to those challenged with control (10% of patients or subjects reported itching, 10% presented grossly detectable redness). The investigators noted an increase in the number of eyes with itching and conjunctival injection with each increase in antigen dosage. At 100 ng/mL, 80% of the subjects reported ocular itching, and 100% of the subjects presented with obvious redness. The conjunctival injection included ciliary flush, dilatation of the deep straight vessels of the episclera, and dilatation of the superficial vessels of the conjunctiva. This study also indicated individual differences in the level of histamine necessary to induce conjunctival vascular and itching responses.

Histamine plays a pivotal role in allergic ocular diseases. The four types

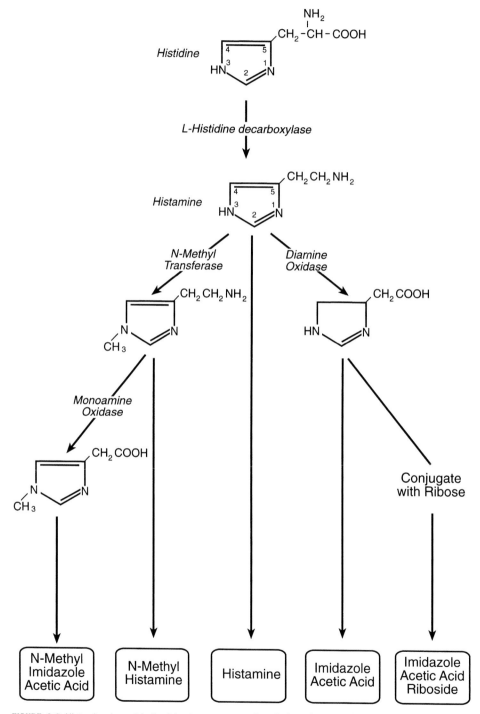

FIGURE 8.3 Histamine is metabolized by two enzymes, *N*-methyltransferase and diamine oxidase. *N*-methyltransferase accounts for approximately 46 to 55% of histamine metabolism, whereas diamine oxidase accounts for approximately 25 to 34%.

of allergic disorders of the eye are allergic rhinoconjunctivitis, atopic kerato-conjunctivitis, vernal keratoconjunctivitis (VKC), and giant papillary conjunctivitis (GPC).

ALLERGIC CONJUNCTIVITIS

Allergic rhinoconjunctivitis is a type I hypersensitivity response to airborne allergens. Degranulated mast cells have been identified in the conjunctiva of allergic rhinoconjunctivitis sufferers, indicating the release of histamine.[56] H_1 and H_2 associated signs are evident, such as conjunctival edema, vessel dilation, and minor lid swelling. Papillary reaction may occur, but without giant papillae formation.

A clinical study found histamine levels in conjunctival epithelial cell suspensions to be 0.8 ± 1.2 ng/mL in allergic conjunctivitis sufferers, versus 0.02 ± 0.02 ng/mL in controls.[57] Histamine is present in both the fluid portion and the cellular fragments of human tears.[58] Histamine levels in tears from subjects with drug-induced and nonatopic induced allergic conjunctivitis or with dust allergy were determined to be 0.8 to 3.7 ng/mL.[59] All studies, however, reported wide interindividual variation in histamine levels. Furthermore, the level of tear histamine increased in both the challenged and the unchallenged, contralateral eye, which may have been caused by a sympathetic reaction, mediated via a neural pathway.[60] Tear histamine values have been reported to peak 5 minutes after challenge.

In one study, elevated tear histamine levels were reported in allergic conjunctivitis patients after ocular allergen challenge during both the early and late phase reactions but only when histaminase enzymes were immediately inactivated in tear samples.[61] Certainly the need to immediately inactivate the rapid enzymatic destruction of histamine must account, at least in part, for the problems and inconsistencies in tear histamine determination over the years.

Atopic Keratoconjunctivitis

Atopy demonstrates the ability of an individual to produce an IgE-mediated hypersensitivity reaction against common environmental allergens. Atopic keratoconjunctivitis is a perennial disorder that usually develops in persons beyond their teenage years. Histamine-induced manifestations include moderate to severe itching, burning, hyperemia, and tearing with a watery or mucoid discharge.

Vernal Keratoconjunctivitis

VKC is a bilateral, chronic inflammatory disease initially presenting in young children. It may recur annually in spring and summer or, depending on the climate and allergic disposition of the patient, may persist throughout the year. Manifested as a limbal or tarsal allergic inflammation, VKC has always been considered as one entity with respect to its immunopathogenesis and histopathological features. Symptoms include intense itching, which increases toward the evening, tearing, photophobia, and increased corneal sensitivity. Histamine levels in conjunctival cell suspensions of VKC sufferers were determined to be 3.3 ng/mL,[60] whereas that in tears was measured to be 11.05 ng/mL.[62] The classic histological profile is an increased number of conjunctival mast cells, which is partly responsible for the elevated histamine levels found in VKC.

One study suggested another cause for elevated histamine levels in patients with VKC.[62] After determining that tear histamine level in patients with VKC to be 11.05 ng/mL, samples from the same collection were treated with 1 N perchloric acid to deactivate the histaminase in tears. Tears collected from normal volunteers were treated in the same manner. Histamine levels before and after treatment with the acid were then compared.

Histamine level in tears collected from VKC sufferers increased 2-fold, from 11.05 ng/mL to 22.25 ng/mL, whereas histamine level in tears in normal volunteers increased from 0.855 ng/mL to 10.64 ng/mL, a more than 10-fold increase. The results suggest that although histaminase in normal individuals is effective in degrading histamine, the enzyme in those with VKC does not demonstrate nearly the same level of activity. Whether this finding is due to a lower amount of histaminase in VKC sufferers overall or to a reduced capacity of the enzyme itself is unclear. Regardless, difficulties with this enzyme pathway appear to play an integral role in the disease process.

Fibroblasts isolated from VKC patients have been shown to have an enhanced reactivity to histamine, producing greater quantities of procollagen I than fibroblasts from normal individuals. This finding suggests that the structural remodeling that occurs in chronic allergic diseases, such as VKC, may be attributed to an exaggerated sensitivity of fibroblasts to this mediator.[63]

Giant Papillary Conjunctivitis

Giant papillary conjunctivitis (GPC) is a direct consequence of wearing contact lenses. The symptoms of GPC include itching, blurred vision, contact lens intolerance, and conjunctival injection. Increased inflammation leads to an abnormal coating of the contact lens, resulting in further trauma to the conjunctiva and continuous activation of the immune response. Signs of conjunctival inflammation consist of tarsal conjunctival hyperemia, and thickening and edema of the tarsus, in addition to a tarsal papillary reaction. Mast cells, eosinophils, and basophils are found in significant quantities in the conjunctival tissues.

Tear histamine levels of patients with GPC are equal to or lower than those found in normal subjects. Histamine levels of 3.3 to 19.4 ng/mL have been identified in soft contact lens–associated GPC, whereas levels of 1.2 to 6.3 ng/mL have been measured in hard contact lens–associated GPC.[59] Tear samples obtained from healthy volunteers contained 2.6 to 15.9 ng/mL of histamine.

REFERENCES

1. Dale HH, Laidlaw PP. The physiologic action of beta-imidazolethyamine. J Physiol (Lond) 41:318, 1910.
2. Dale HH, Laidlaw PP. Histamine shock. J Physiol (Lond) 52:355, 1919.
3. Best CH. The nature of vasodilator constituents of certain tissue extracts. J Physiol (Lond) 62: 397, 1927.
4. Riley JF, West GB. The presence of histamine in tissue mast cells. J Physiol (Lond) 120:528, 1953.
5. Douglas WW. Histamine and 5-hydroxytryptamine (serotonin) and their antagonists. In: The pharmacologic basis of therapeutics. 6th ed. Gilman AG, Goodman LS, Gilman A, eds. New York, Macmillan, 1980, p 609.

6. Green JP, Prell GD, Khandelwal JK, et al. Aspects of histamine metabolism. Agents Actions 22:1, 1987.

7. Ishizaka T. Role of GTP-binding protein in histamine release from mast cells. Clin Immunol Immunopath 50:20, 1989.

8. Merget RD, Maurer AB, Koch U, et al. Histamine release from basophils after in vivo application of recombinant human interleukin-3 in man. Int Arch Allergy Appl Immunol 92:366, 1990.

9. White MV. The role of histamine in allergic diseases. J Allergy Clin Immunol 86:599, 1990.

10. White MV, Kaliner MA. Histamine. In: The lung: scientific foundations. Barnes PJ, Cherniack NS, Weibel ER, eds. New York, Raven Press, 1997.

11. Hill SJ. Distribution, properties, and functional characteristics of three classes of histamine receptor. Pharmavol Rev 42:45, 1990.

12. Hill SJ, Young JM, Marrian DH. Specific binding of ^{3}H-mepyramine to histamine H_1 receptors in intestinal smooth muscle. Nature 270:261, 1977.

13. Mitsuhashi M, Payan DG. Molecular and cellular analysis of histamine H_1 receptors on cultured smooth muscle cells. J Cell Biochem 40:183, 1989.

14. Mitsuhashi M, Payan DG. Receptor-glycosylation regulates the affinity of histamine H_1 receptors during smooth muscle cell differentiation. 35:311, 1989.

15. Mitsuhashi M, Payan DG. Solubilization and purification of the pyrilamine binding protein from cultured smooth muscle cells. Proc Natl Acad Sci U S A 85:2743, 1989.

16. Boyer JL, Hepler JR, Harden TK. Hormone and growth factor receptor-mediated regulation of phospholipase C activity. Trends Pharm Sci 10:360, 1989.

17. Sharif NA, Xu SX, Magnini PE, Pang IH. Human conjunctival epithelial cells express histamine-$_1$ receptors coupled to phosphoinositide turnover and intracellular calcium mobilization: role in ocular allergic and inflammatory diseases. Exp Eye Res 63:169, 1996.

18. Sharif NA, Wiernas TK, Griffin BW, Davis TL. Pharmacology of [3H]-pyrilamine binding and of histamine-induced inositol phosphates generation, intracellular Ca^{2+}-mobilization and cytokine release from human corneal epithelial cells. Br J Pharmacol 125:1336, 1998.

19. Sharif NA, Wiernas TK, Howe WE, et al. Human corneal epithelial cell functional responses to inflammatory agents and their antagonists. Invest Ophthalmol Vis Sci 39:2562, 1998.

20. Iriyoshi N, Takeuchi K, Yuta A, et al. Increased expression of histamine H_1 receptor mRNA in allergic rhinitis. Clin Exp Allergy 26:379, 1996.

21. Abelson MB, Udell IJ. H_2 receptors in the human ocular surface. Arch Ophthalmol 99:302, 1981.

22. Black JW, Duncan WA, Durant CJ. Definition and antagonism of histamine H_2 receptors. Nature 236:385, 1972.

23. Anderson R, Glover A, Rabson AR. The in vitro effects of histamine and metiamide on neutrophil motility and their relationship to intracellular cyclic nucleotide levels. J Immunol 118:1690, 1977.

24. Chew CS. Cholecytokinin, carbachol, gastrin, histamine, and forskoline increase [Ca^{2+}] in gastric glands. Am J Physiol 250:G814, 1986.

25. Arrang JM, Garbarg M, Schwartz JC. Auto-inhibition of brain histamine release mediated by a novel class (H_3) of histamine receptor. Nature 302:832, 1983.

26. Arrang JM, Garbarg M, Lancelot JC. Highly potent and selective ligands for histamine H_3 receptors. Nature 327:117, 1987.

27. Kohno S, Nakao S, Ogawa K. Possible participation of histamine H_3 receptors in the regulation of anaphylactic histamine release from isolated rat peritoneal mast cells. Jpn J Pharmacol 66:173, 1994.

28. Arrang JM, Garbarg M, Schwartz JC. Autoregulation of histamine release in brain by presynaptic H_3 receptors. Neuroscience 15:553, 1985.

29. Lappin D, Whaley K. Effects of histamine on monocyte complement production. I. Inhibition of C2 production mediated by its action on H_2 receptors. Clin Exp Immunol 41:497, 1980.

30. Falus A, Meretey K. Effect of histamine on the gene expression and biosynthesis of complement components C2, factor B and C3 in mouse peritoneal macrophages. Immunology 60:547, 1987.

31. Falus A, Walcz E, Brozik M. Stimulation of histamine receptors of human monocytoid and hepatoma-derived cell lines and mouse hepatocytes modulates the production of the complement components C3, C4, factor B, and C2. Scand J Immunol 30:241, 1989.

32. Hsieh KH. The effects of histamine, antihistamines, isoproterenol and theophylline on the Fc and complement receptor functions of polymorphonuclear leukocytes in asthmatic children. Ann Allergy 47:38, 1981.

33. Clark RAR, Sandler JA, Gallin JI. Histamine modulation of eosinophil migration. J Immunol 118:137, 1977.

34. Dohlsten M, Kalland T, Sjugren HO. Histamine inhibits interleukin-1 production by lipopolysaccharide-stimulated human peripheral blood monocytes. Scand J Immunol 27:527, 1988.

35. Vannier E, Miller LC, Dinarello CA. Histamine suppresses gene expression and synthesis of tumor necrosis factor alpha via histamine H_2 receptors. J Exp Med 174:281, 1991.

36. Carlsson R, Dohlsten M, Sjorgen HO. Histamine modulates the production of interferon gamma and interleukin 2 by mitogen activated human mononuclear blood cells. Cell Immunol 96:104, 1985.

37. Knigge U, Warberg J. The role of histamine in the neuroendocrine regulation of pituitary hormone secretion. Acta Endocrinol 124:609, 1991.

38. Bischoff SC, Baggiolini M, DeWeck AL. Interleukin 8 inhibitor and inducer of histamine and leukotriene release in human basophils. Biochem Biophys Res Commun 179:628, 1991.

39. Bischoff SC, Brunner T, DeWeck AL. Interleukin 5 modifies histamine release and leukotriene generation by human basophils in response to diverse agonists. J Exp Med 172:1577, 1990.

40. Owen DAA, Poy E, Woodward DF. Evaluation of the role of histamine H_1 and H_2 receptors in cutaneous inflammation in the guinea pig produced by histamine and mast cell degranulation. Br J Pharmacol 69:615, 1980.

41. Allansmith MR, Ross RN. Ocular allergy and mast cell stabilizers. Surv Ophthalmol 30:229, 1986.

42. Chand N, Eyre P. Classification and biological distribution of histamine receptor subtypes. Agents Actions 5:277, 1975.

43. Abelson MB, Allansmith MR. Histamine and the eye. In: Immunology and immunopathology of the eye. Silverstein A, O'Connor G, eds. New York, Masson, 1979.

44. Nowak JZ, Nawrocki J. Histamine in the human eye. Ophthalmic Res 19:72, 1987.

45. Helleboid L, Khatami M, Wei ZG. Histamine and prostacyclin: primary and secondary release in allergic conjunctivitis. Invest Ophthalmol Vis Sci 32:2281, 1991.

46. Baraniuk JN. Pathogenesis of allergic rhinitis. J Allergy Clin Immunol 99:S763, 1997.

47. McDonald DM. Neurogenic inflammation in the respiratory tract: actions of sensory nerve mediators on blood vessels and epithelium of the airway mucosa. Am Rev Respir Dis 136:S65, 1987.

48. Svensson C, Anderson M, Greiff L, et al. Exudative hyperresponsiveness of the airway microcirculation in seasonal allergic rhinitis. Clin Exp Allergy 25:942, 1995.

49. Mossiman BL, White MV, Hohman RJ, et al. Substance P, calcitonin gene–related peptide, and vasoactive intestinal peptide increase in nasal secretions after allergen challenge in atopic patients. J Allergy Clin Immunol 92:95, 1993.

50. Yamaji M, Takada M, Fumiwara R, et al. Role of substance P in experimental allergic conjunctivitis in guinea pigs. Methods Find Exp Clin Pharmacol 19:637, 1997.

51. Bardsley WG, Crabbe MJ, Shindler JS. Kinetics of the diamine oxidase reaction. Biochem J 131:459, 1973.

52. Lorand L, Hsu LK, Siefring GE Jr, Rafferty NS. Lens transglutaminase and cataract formation. Proc Natl Acad Sci U S A 78:1356, 1981.

53. Yamauchi K, Sekizawa K, Suzuki H. Structure and function of human histamine N-methyltransferase: critical enzyme in histamine metabolism in airway. Am J Physiol 267:L342, 1994.

54. Stjernschantz J. Autocoids and neuropeptides. In: Pharmacology of the eye. Handbook of experimental pharmacology. Vol 69. Sears ML, ed. Berlin, Springer-Verlag, 1984, p 311.

55. Levene RZ. Mast cells and amines in normal ocular tissues. Invest Ophthalmol Vis Sci 1:532, 1962.

56. Allansmith MR, Ross RN. Ocular allergy and mast cell stabilizers. Surv Ophthalmol 30:229, 1986.

57. Fukagawa K, Saito H, Azuma N. Histamine and tryptase levels in allergic conjunctivitis and vernal keratoconjunctivitis. Cornea 13:345, 1994.

58. Abelson MB, Suter NA, Simon MA. Histamine in human tears. Am J Ophthalmol 83:417, 1977.

59. Abelson MB, Baird RS, Allansmith MR. Tear histamine levels in vernal conjunctivitis and other ocular inflammations. Ophthalmology 87:812, 1980.

60. Kari O, Salo OP, Hamepuro L. Tear histamine during allergic conjunctivitis challenge. Graefes Arch Clin Exp Ophthalmol 223:60, 1985.

61. Leonardi A, Smith LM, Fregona IA, et al. Tear histamine and histaminase during the early (EPR) and late (LPR) phases of the allergic reaction and the effects of lodoxamide. Eur J Ophthalmol 6:106, 1996.

62. Abelson MB, Leonardi AA, Smith LM. Histaminase activity in patients with vernal keratoconjunctivitis. Ophthalmology 102:1958, 1995.

63. Leonardi A, Radice M, Fregona IA. Histamine effects on conjunctival fibroblasts from patients with vernal conjunctivitis. Exp Eye Res (in press.)

CHAPTER 9

Immunoglobulins and Allergic Inflammation in the Eye

SUSAN SCHUKAR BERDY ■ **GREGG J. BERDY**

An effective immune response depends on recognition of foreign antigens and subsequent communication between immune cells. Recognition is accomplished by antibodies, T lymphocytes, and the major histocompatibility complex. Antibodies, the most important of these, also happen to be the most diverse. Antibodies are proteins synthesized by specialized B lymphocytes (plasma cells) that are capable of recognizing foreign substances, such as microbial pathogens, drugs, and toxins.

In 1890, Behring and Kitasato detected tetanus antitoxins. In the late 19th century, investigators demonstrated that protective immunity could be transferred with serum of recovering animals administered to noninfected recipients.[1] With electrophoresis, these proteins have been demonstrated to be contained in the third migrating globulin (gamma globulin) peak and hence are termed immunoglobulins.[2] In 1955, Niels Jerne proposed the selective theory of antibody formation, which laid the foundation for future studies and investigation. Later in that decade, Landsteiner performed his classic studies dealing with the specificity of antibodies to synthetic haptens. These studies demonstrated that antisera possessed the following four characteristics: universality, specificity, cross-reactivity, and diversity.[3] During the past three decades, the complex nature of antibodies has slowly been unraveled, revealing information about immunoglobulin structure,

69

physical and biological properties, mechanisms of gene diversity, and function.

IMMUNOGLOBULIN STRUCTURE

An antibody molecule is composed of four polypeptide chains. Each molecule contains a pair of identical heavy (H) chains and a pair of identical light (L) chains[4] (Fig. 9.1). All heavy and light chains share similar structural characteristics called the immunoglobulin domain, which is a core structure of approximately 110 amino acids that is directly involved with the folding of the protein molecule.[5] Light chains possess 2 immunoglobulin domains, whereas heavy chains may contain 4 or 5 domains.

Peptide sequencing of antibodies reveals that each immunoglobulin chain is composed of two regions called variable (V) and constant (C) regions. The amino (NH_2) terminus of both the heavy and light chains shows peptide sequence variation, whereas the carboxy (COO) terminus of both heavy and light chains is identical in peptide sequence. Within the variable regions, three areas of sequence hypervariability (idiotype) form the major contact areas for antigen. These hypervariable regions are called complementarity determining regions.[6] Therefore, the function of the amino

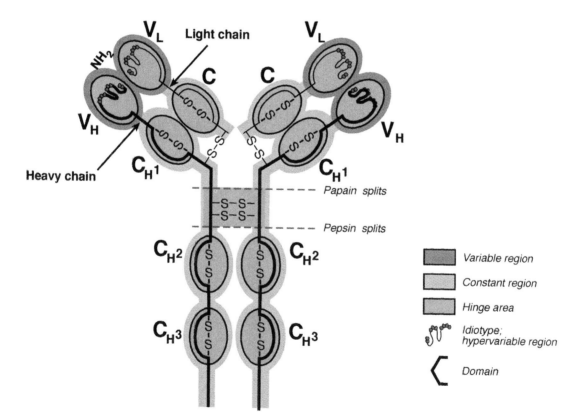

FIGURE 9.1 Immunoglobulin molecule. An antibody molecule is composed of four polypeptide chains. Each molecule contains a pair of identical heavy (H) chains and a pair of identical light (L) chains. (From Edelman GM. Dissociation of gamma globulin. J Chem Soc 81:3155, 1959.)

terminus or variable regions of both H and L chains is to bind antigen. The carboxy terminus of H chains forms the constant region and allows for effector functions, such as complement fixation and binding to Fc receptors. The constant region of the L chain primarily functions to join and bind the L chain to the constant region of the H chain. The constant region of the H chain determines the function of the immunoglobulin molecule.

Light and heavy chains are bound to one another by covalent and noncovalent interactions. The amino acid cysteine, which is present in both polypeptide chains, is responsible for disulfide bond formation. Similar disulfide binding occurs between the H chains in the hinge region.

Immunoglobulin molecules are proteins and hence can be cleaved by proteolytic enzymes. Papain cleaves within the hinge region to leave two identical antigen-binding (Fab) units and a third fragment (Fc) containing the carboxy terminus. Pepsin proteolysis occurs within the constant region of the H chains and yields only an amino terminal fragment composed of two Fab units. The carboxy terminus is enzymatically degraded.[7]

Antibodies can be either membrane bound on the surface of B cells or secreted into the systemic circulation by plasma cells. Membrane-bound antibodies possess H chains that contain a hydrophobic segment of amino acids that allow binding to and existing within the B-cell membrane. Secreted antibodies possess H chains lacking the hydrophobic regions. Some H chains possess a short tail segment on the carboxy terminus that permits the formation of immunoglobulin multimers[8] (Fig. 9.2). Antibodies may exist in dimeric and multimeric forms, with polymerization mediated by a series of proteins, called the J chain, the purpose of which is to maintain antibody structure.

PHYSICAL AND BIOLOGICAL PROPERTIES OF IMMUNOGLOBULINS

Both heavy and light chains of immunoglobulin molecules can be subdivided into classes or isotypes that share extensive homology in peptide sequencing. The two classes of light chains are kappa (κ) and lambda (λ). Five heavy-chain isotypes have been described and are designated alpha (α), delta (δ), epsilon (ϵ), gamma (γ), and mu (μ). Because the H chain of an antibody is responsible for effector function, immunoglobulins are named by their heavy-chain isotype: IgA (alpha chain), IgD (delta chain), IgE (epsilon chain), IgG (gamma chain), and IgM (mu chain) (Table 9.1).

The physical and biological properties of immunoglobulin are presented in Table 9.1. IgG is the most abundant antibody found in blood and may account for up to 85% of serum antibody. Four subclasses of IgG are known. Most are able to fix complement. The IgG molecule binds to Fc receptors on inflammatory cells, such as macrophages and neutrophils, thus allowing subsequent phagocytosis of the antigen. IgG molecules are able to cross the placenta and provide newborns with passive protection.[9]

IgA comprises approximately 10% of serum immunoglobulins and is found in secretions of mucosal surfaces. IgA exists in both monomeric and dimeric forms, which are coupled by the J chain and are stabilized by a protein component (secretory piece)[10] (Fig. 9.3). Secretory IgA is found in the mucosal surfaces of the gut, respiratory tract, mammary gland, and conjunctiva. The secretory piece appears to provide resistance to degradation by proteolytic enzymes present in the mucosal surface environment. IgA participates in the immune system by complexing with antigens in

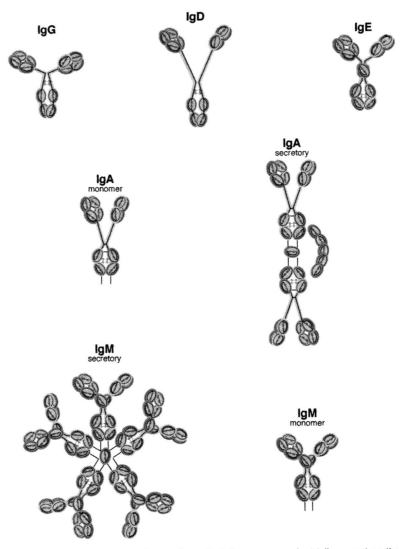

FIGURE 9.2 Immunoglobulin subtypes. Some H chains possess a short tail segment on the carboxy terminus that permits the formation of immunoglobulin multimers. (From Gally JA. The structure, genetics, and biological properties of immunoglobulins. In: Immunological diseases. Semter M, ed. Boston, Little, Brown, 1978.)

mucous secretions, thereby reducing absorption into local tissues. This immunoglobulin also provides immunological surveillance at the site of first contact with antigens. Mucosal IgA specifically acts to neutralize noxious agents at the initial site of antigen interaction.

IgM accounts for about 5% of serum immunoglobulin. The IgM antibody exists as a monomer, which is found affixed to the surface membrane of B-cell lymphocytes. In addition, IgM exists as a pentamer, which serves as the primary immunoglobulin interacting with antigen during the initial phase of an immune response.[11] The pentameric structure is held together by the J chain. IgM participates in the immune response by binding to multiple antigen sites on the surface of a cell, which, in turn, activates the complement cascade, leading to phagocytosis and lysis of the cell.[12]

IgD is present only in minute amounts in serum (less than 1%). The

TABLE 9.1 Physical and Biological Properties of Immunoglobulins*

Characteristic	IgG	IgA	IgM	IgD	IgE
Molecular form	Monomer	Monomer, dimer	Pentamer	Monomer	Monomer
Ig domains	5	4	5	4	5
Total immunoglobulins (%)	8.5%	10%	5%	<1%	<0.01%
Molecular weight (daltons)	150,000	160,000	950,000	175,000	190,000
Carbohydrate (%)	3	7	1	9	13
Hinge region	+	+	−	+	−
Associated chains		J chain Secretory piece	J chain		
Subclasses	$IgG_{1(\gamma1)}$ $IgG_{2(\gamma2)}$ $IgG_{3(\gamma3)}$ $IgG_{4(\gamma4)}$	$IgA_{1(\alpha1)}$ $IgA_{2(\alpha2)}$	−	−	−
Allotypes (heavy chain)	Gm	Am	Mm	−	−
Serum level (mg/dL)	679–1537 (total) IgG_1 = 430–1300 IgG_2 = 115–750 IgG_3 = 20–130 IgG_4 = 2–165	39–358	33–229	0–15	0–0.09
Half-life (days)	23.0	5.8	5.1	2.8	2.5
Complement fixation (classic pathway)	IgG_1, IgG_3, IgG_2	−	+	−	−
Placental transfer	+	−	−	−	−
Other properties	Secondary response	Mucous secretions	Primary response rheumatoid factor	Class switching	Allergy
Cells bound	Macrophages, neutrophils	None	None	None	Mast cells, basophils

*Five heavy-chain isotypes have been described. Because the H chain of an antibody is responsible for effector function, immunoglobulins are named by their heavy-chain isotype: IgA (Alpha chain), IgD (delta chain), IgE (epsilon chain), IgG (gamma chain), and IgM (mu chain). Each of these immunoglobulins has distinct physical and biological properties.

(Adapted from Jerke DJ, Capra JD: Immunoglobulins: structure and function. In: Fundamental immunology. Paul WE, ed. New York, Raven Press, 1984.)

exact function of IgD has not been elucidated, but it is found to be co-expressed with IgM on the surface of B cells and may be important in signaling class switching to the B lymphocytes.[13]

IgE is found in extremely low concentrations in serum (less than 0.01%, 10–500 ng/mL), but is elevated (can be more than 25,000 ng/mL) in atopic

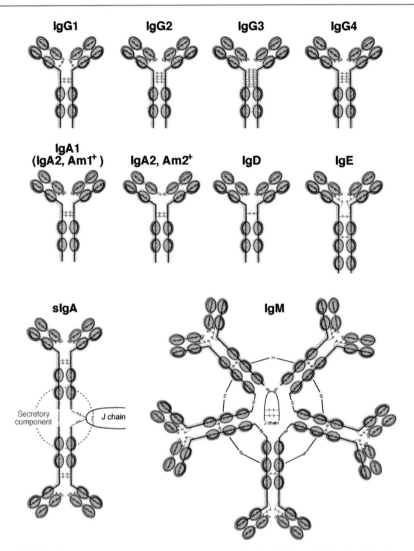

FIGURE 9.3 Schematic diagram of human immunoglobulin. Immunoglobulin A (IgA) comprises approximately 10% of serum immunoglobulins and is found in secretions of mucosal surfaces. IgA exists in both monomeric and dimeric forms, which are coupled by the J chain and are stabilized by a protein component (secretory piece). (From Mostov KE, Kraehenbuhl J, Blobel G. Receptor-mediated transcellular transport of immunoglobulin: synthesis of secretory component as multiple and large transmembrane forms. Proc Natl Acad Sci U S A 77:7257, 1980.)

persons and in persons with parasitic infections.[14] A "hyper IgE" syndrome has been described in young children with recurrent skin and respiratory infections.[15] Therefore, although elevated serum concentrations of IgE are indicative of atopic conditions, they are not, by either their sole presence or absence, pathognomonic of such conditions.

IgE has the unique property of binding to mast cells and basophils via its Fc receptor and is responsible for immediate-type hypersensitivity reactions. Locally produced IgE binds initially to local mast cells. Subsequently, as additional IgE enters circulation, binding occurs to both circulating basophils and tissue-fixed mast cells throughout the body. IgE can also bind to low-affinity receptors on eosinophils, macrophages, and platelets. Eosinophils activated by IgE antibodies are quite effective at killing parasites.

Both T-helper (T_H) cells and T-suppressor (T_S) cells can influence B-cell production of IgE via IgE-binding factors (IgE-BF). T_H cells produce IgE-potentiating factor (IgE-PF), whereas T_S cells produce IgE-suppressor factor (IgE-SF). These factors are differentiated in the post-translational glycosylation of the IgE-BF. The relative amounts produced of these factors are controlled by other antigen-specific T-cell–produced factors. Although the mechanisms behind the regulation of IgE production are not fully understood, the IgE-BFs presumably interact with surface-IgE positive B cells to either stimulate or inhibit IgE production. Interleukin 4 can also stimulate IgE production.[16]

Hypersensitivity to specific allergens may be transferred via IgE-containing serum from an individual with an existing hypersensitivity. Passive sensitization of mast cells via serum transfer can last up to 12 days despite an IgE serum half-life of 2.5 days.

ANTIBODY-ANTIGEN INTERACTION

Within the variable regions of the H chain are areas of hypervariability in amino acid sequence known as complementarity determining regions or idiotypes. These areas account for the highest rate of contact with the antigen.[17] The Fab unit of the antibody binds to the antigen via hydrogen bonds, van der Waals interactions, and ionic bonds.[18]

The surface of circulating B lymphocytes is coated by antibodies. All the antibodies coating a single B cell are identical in structure and thus are capable of recognizing only one antigenic determinant. Once an antigen is presented to an antibody-bearing B cell, the B cell proliferates. This results in the creation of plasma cells, which secrete antibodies directed specifically against the stimulating antigen. B-cell differentiation into memory B lymphocytes for future immune responses also occurs.

Antibodies initially bind antigens in a process called neutralization. Once binding has been accomplished, the antigen may be handled in several ways, depending on the immunoglobulin isotype. When IgM or IgG is involved, fixation of complement occurs, resulting in either phagocytosis or lysis of the antigen. In other cases, the Fc receptor may facilitate direct lysis of antigens via antibody-dependent cell-mediated cytotoxicity. The Fc portion of IgE molecules attaches to the FcεRI high-affinity receptors found on mast cells and basophils. This triggers release of mast cell granules and the beginning of an allergic response.

ANTIBODY GENE DIVERSITY

In 1965, Dreyer and Bennett proposed a molecular basis for immunoglobulin diversity that stated that only a limited amount of DNA is used in a recombinant process to form the vast number of antibodies present in humans.[19] In 1976, Hozumi and Tonegawa discovered that variable and constant regions of immunoglobulin molecules are encoded by separate and multiple genes that reside far apart in the DNA germ line, but become joined to form a complete Ig molecule in B lymphocytes.[20] Researchers have

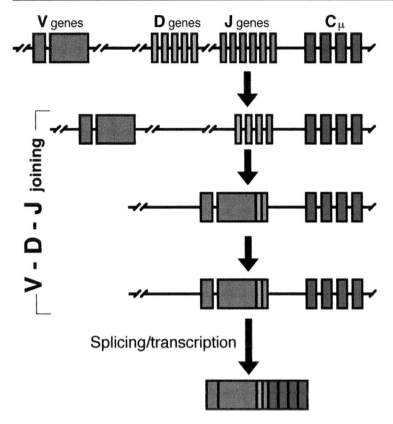

FIGURE 9.4 Assembly of heavy chain. The method of assembly of human immunoglobulin proteins is complex. In this example, the assembly of an immunoglobulin M (IgM) heavy chain from germ line genes on chromosome 14q is depicted. The germ line genes include V (variable) segment, D (diversity) segment, and J (joining) segment genes with intervening areas of peptides.

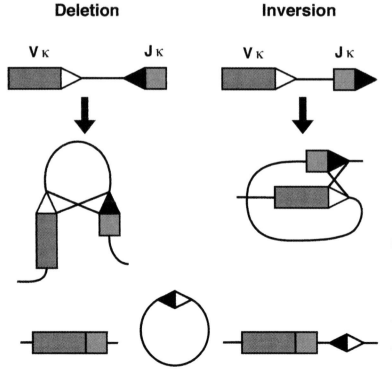

FIGURE 9.5 Gene rearrangement. Four sources of diversity are encountered in forming the vast number of antibodies in the human species: germ line gene diversity, somatic recombination, junctional diversity, and somatic hypermutation. (From Tonegawa S. Somatic generation of antibody diversity. Nature 302:575, 1983.)

shown that the immunoglobulin protein genes are located in three chromosomal regions. The heavy-chain gene locus has been located on chromosome 14q, whereas the kappa light-chain gene locus has been found on chromosome 2p, and the lambda light-chain gene is located on chromosome 22q.[21-23]

The method of assembly of human immunoglobulin proteins is complex and is depicted in Figure 9.4. In this example, the assembly of an IgM heavy chain from germ line genes on chromosome 14q is depicted. The germ line genes include V (variable) segment, D (diversity) segment, and J (joining) segment genes with intervening areas of peptides. Within B-cell lymphocytes, site-specific recombination of the V, D, and J genes is mediated by immunoglobulin recombinase enzymes.

The immunoglobulin diversity that can be formed through recombination of these genes is enormous. Approximately 250 V segment genes, 30 D segment genes, and 6 J segment genes are recognized, all of which can be combined to form the variable segment of an H chain. The variable segment is then combined with the constant segment of different isotypes to form more than 10^{10} different combinations of immunoglobulin heavy chains.[24-27] Similar recombination mechanisms exist for light-chain loci, but D segment genes are absent. In summary, four sources of diversity are encountered in forming the vast number of antibodies in the human species: germ line gene diversity, somatic recombination, junctional diversity, and somatic hypermutation[28] (Fig. 9.5).

IMMUNOGLOBULIN ROLE IN THE OCULAR IMMUNE RESPONSE

The eye and ocular adnexal tissues participate actively in the immune response. The ocular surface contains Langerhans' cells, T and B lymphocytes, mast cells, neutrophils, plasma cells, complement, and immunoglobulins IgG, IgA, and IgM. Chapters and books have been written about the ocular immune response with disease entities occurring in the conjunctiva, cornea, anterior chamber, lens, retina, and choroid. In short, hypersensitivity reactions of types I, II, III, and IV have been well documented to occur in these ocular structures. Immunoglobulins obviously play important roles in ocular allergic disease.

REFERENCES

1. Kabat EA. Getting started 50 years ago: experiences, perspectives and problems of the first 21 years. Annu Rev Immunol 1:1, 1983.
2. Nisonoff A, Hopper JE, Spring SB. The antibody molecule. New York, Academic Press, 1975.
3. Landsteiner K. Die Spezifizitat der Serologischen Reaktionen. Berlin, Springer-Verlag, 1933.
4. Edelman GM. Dissociation of gamma globulin. J Am Chem Soc 81:3155, 1959.
5. Edmundson AB, Ely KR, Abola EE, et al. Conformational isomerism, rotational allomerism, and divergent evolution of domains in immunoglobulin light chains. Fed Proc 35(10):2119, 1976.
6. Wu TT, Kabat EA. An analysis of the sequences of the variable regions of Bence-Jones proteins and myeloma light chains and their implications for antibody complementarity. J Exp Med 132:211, 1970.
7. Porter RR. The hydrolysis of rabbit γ-globulin and antibodies with crystalline papain. Biochem J 73:119, 1959.
8. Gally JA. The structure, genetics, and biological properties of immunoglobulins. In: Immunological diseases. Samter M, ed. Boston, Little, Brown, 1978.
9. Virella G, Silveira Nunes MA, Tamagnini G. Placental transfer of human IgG subclasses. Clin Exp Immunol 10:475, 1972.
10. Mostov KE, Kraehenbuhl J, Blobel G. Receptor-mediated transcellular transport of immunoglobulin: synthesis of secretory component as multiple and large transmembrane forms. Proc Natl Acad Sci U S A 77:7257, 1980.

11. Nossal GJV. The molecular and cellular basis of affinity maturation in the antibody response. Cell 68:1, 1992.

12. Borsos T, Chapuis RM, Langone JJ. Distinction between fixation of C1 and the activation of complement by natural IgM anti-hapten antibody: effects of cell surface hapten density. Mol Immunol 18:863, 1981.

13. Pollock RR, Mescher MF. Murine cell surface immunoglobulin: two native IgD structures. J Immunol 124:1608, 1980.

14. Jefferis R, Pound JD. Immunoglobulins. In: Inflammation: basic principles and clinical correlates. 2nd ed. Gallin JI, Goldstein IM, Snyderman R, eds. New York, Raven Press, 1992.

15. Donabedian H, Gallin J. The hyperimmunoglobulin E recurrent infection (Job's) syndrome: a review of the NIH experience and literature. Medicine (Baltimore) 62:195, 1983.

16. Ishizaka K. Regulation of IgE synthesis. In: 20 years with IgE—new prospects. Debelic M, ed. Surrey, UK, Medicom, 1987.

17. Amit AG, Mariuzza RA, Phillips SE, Poljak RJ. The three dimensional structure of an antigen-antibody complex at 6A resolution. Nature 133: 156, 1985.

18. Alzari PM, Lascombe M-B, Poljak RJ. Three-dimensional structure of antibodies. Annu Rev Immunol 6:555, 1988.

19. Dreyer WF, Bennett JC. The molecular basis of antibody formation: a paradox. Proc Natl Acad Sci U S A 54:864, 1965.

20. Hozumi N, Tonegawa S. Evidence for somatic rearrangement of immunoglobulin genes coding for variable and constant regions. Proc Natl Acad Sci U S A 73:3628, 1976.

21. Anderson ML, Szajnert MF, Kaplan JC, et al. The isolation of a human IgVl gene from a recombinant library of chromosome 22 and estimation of the copy number. Nucleic Acids Res 12: 6647, 1984.

22. Cox DW, Markovic VD, Teshima IE. Genes for immunoglobulin heavy chains and for a 1-antitrypsin are localized to specific regions of chromosome 14q. Nature 297:428, 1982.

23. Meindl A, Klobeck HG, Ohnheiser R, Zachau HG. The V kappa gene repertoire in the human germ line. Eur J Immunol 20:1855, 1990.

24. Berman JE, Mellis SJ, Pollock R, et al. Content and organization of the human IgVh locus: definition of three new Vh families and linkage to the IgCh locus. EMBO J 7:727, 1988.

25. Ichihara Y, Matsuoka H, Kurosawa Y. Organization of human immunoglobulin heavy chain diversity gene loci. EMBO J 7:4140, 1988.

26. Ravetch JV, Siebenlist U, Korsmeyer S, et al. Structure of the human immunoglobulin mu locus: characterization of embryonic and rearranged J and D genes. Cell 27:583, 1981.

27. Schroeder HW Jr, Walter MA, Hofker MH, et al. Physical linkage of a human immunoglobulin heavy chain variable region gene segment to diversity and joining segments. Proc Natl Acad Sci U S A 85:8196, 1988.

28. Tonegawa S. Somatic generation of antibody diversity. Nature 302:575, 1983.

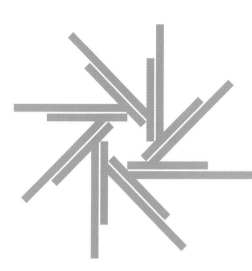

CHAPTER **10**

Cytokines in the Ocular Environment

MARK B. ABELSON ■ **PAULO J. GOMES** ■ **CLYDE SCHULTZ**

Cytokines are a heterogeneous group of noncomplex proteins that serve as communication conduits between the various groups of immune cells. These proteins have a molecular weight in most cases of less than 30 kd and are transiently produced by proinflammatory stimuli. The range of actions of individual cytokines is generally broad. Much of the cytokine research conducted to date has targeted various systemic diseases. This chapter focuses on cytokine function in the ocular environment.

HISTORY OF CYTOKINE RESEARCH

The history of cytokine research is rooted in the work on interferons (IFNs) by Isaacs and Lindenmann.[1] IFNs were originally described as antiviral agents because of their ability to prevent viral replication. In the mid-1960s, the term "lymphokine" came into use with the discovery of macrophage-inhibition factor.[2] These two molecules and those discovered after 1969 were recognized as lymphokines produced by activated T lymphocytes. Lymphokines were originally defined as cell-free soluble extracts that could produce some biological effect on target cells. This field of research expanded during the 1970s with the realization that IFN and other lymphokines had more than one function. Data generated from various laboratories during that decade indicated that antigen-activated thymus-derived T lymphocytes were responsible for the production of lymphokines. IFN could act as a growth promoter as well as preventing viral replication. The term "cytokine" was proposed in the mid-1970s to correct the misconception that secreted proteins were produced solely by lymphocytes. The term "interleukin" was introduced in 1979, based on a protein's ability to act as a communication bridge between different populations of leukocytes. Many cytokines are termed interleukin; however, some are still known by their original names (e.g., tumor necrosis factor [TNF]).

CYTOKINE STRUCTURE

Cytokines are produced by cells in response to extracellular stimuli. This production is controlled at the transcription level, although the regulation is not completely understood. The use of cDNA for various translation products predicts protein chains of 80 to 200 amino acids. Amino acid analysis has shown cysteine residues in a number of the cytokines, which contribute to the tertiary structure. Post-translational modifications of interleukin-1 (IL-1) have shown that pre-translation modified products are biologically active.[3] When cleavage occurs, then the smaller IL-1 protein has a greater degree of activity than the unmodified protein.[4]

NOMENCLATURE

The historical labeling of cytokines has left us with names that no longer fully describe the activity of these proteins. The action of TNF (also called cachectin) has more to do with the initial stimulation of inflammation than with causing tissue damage. The term "interleukin" applies to some, but not all, of the molecules referred to as cytokines. Terms such as "monokine" and "lymphokine" (mentioned earlier) can still be found in the older literature. Many of these terms stemmed from the original identified source or target of the soluble agent. For example, the biomolecule now known as IL-1 was originally named lymphocyte-activating factor because the first studies isolating the molecule revealed this mechanism of action. The term "cytokine" now refers to a heterogeneous group of soluble factors that affect immune cells.

Characteristic features of cytokines as a group include the transient nature of their production and their high binding affinity to cell-surface receptors. The range of cytokine action is great, and target cells are not limited to hematopoietic cells. Cytokines can be distinguished from hormones by the redundancy of cytokine action and by the finding that an individual cytokine may exert multiple actions on different cells and tissue types. Furthermore, cytokines tend to be produced by less specialized cells than are hormones.

MECHANISM OF ACTION

Cytokines may be produced by one or more cell types (Table 10.1).[5] For example, IL-2 and IL-7 are produced by T cells. Other cytokines, such as IL-8 and TNF, are produced by multiple cell types. The biological activities of unrelated cytokines often overlap or complement each other. Thus, cytokines may work together in a synergistic fashion, as do TNF and IL-1 in the inflammatory response.[6] Cytokines exert their effects through cell-surface

TABLE 10.1 Cytokines in Ocular Inflammation*

Cytokine	Source	Activity
Interleukin-1 (IL-1)	Monocytes, macrophages, B cells, resident corneal cells	Mediates acute-phase response, chemotaxis, activation of inflammatory and antigen-presenting cells, and stimulation of neovascularization
Tumor necrosis factor (TNF)	Macrophages, mast cells, T-helper (T_H) and cytotoxic (T_C), natural killer (NK) cells, polymorphonucleocytes, endothelial cells	Mediates acute-phase response; acts on fibroblasts and endothelial cells to induce coagulation and an increase in vascular permeability; induces increased expression of adhesion molecules on vascular endothelial cells; induces production of IL-8; activates macrophages and neutrophils
Interleukin-2 (IL-2)	T_H cells	Stimulates proliferation of T_C and T_H cells; enhances activity of NK and T_C cells; presents with sympathetic ophthalmia
Interleukin-6 (IL-6)	Monocytes, macrophages, T_H cells, fibroblasts, endothelial cells	Mediates acute-phase response; increases secretion of antibodies by plasma cells; co-stimulates (with IL-1) T-cell activation; associated with uveitis
Interleukin-8 (IL-8)	Macrophages, fibroblasts, corneal keratinocytes, retinal pigment epithelial cells	Potent chemoattractant for neutrophils; enhances corneal neovascularization
Interferon-gamma (INF-gamma)	T_H and T_C cells	Enhances activity of macrophages, T_C, TDTH, and NK cells; increases expression of MHC molecules; inhibits cell proliferation and collagen synthesis
Transforming growth factor-beta (TGF-beta)	Platelets, macrophages, lymphocytes	Chemoattractant for monocytes and macrophages; limits inflammatory response and promotes wound healing; induces increased production of macrophages; inhibits proliferation of epithelial, endothelial, and hematopoietic cells; regulator of TNF; inhibitor of lymphocyte production

TDTH, = delayed-type hypersensitivity.

receptors. Most of these cellular receptors are expressed at low density (100–1,000 receptors per cell) in a resting state cell. Receptor expression increases when cells are activated. Cytokine receptors exist in both soluble and membrane-bound forms in association with cellular protein. These proteins may be involved in signal transduction or in the production of functional high-affinity ligand-binding domains. Cytokines may also antagonize the effects of one another. IFN-gamma inhibits TNF-stimulated IL-8 synthesis at the transcriptional level. However, IL-8 stimulation by IFN at the post-transcriptional level has also been reported.

Cytokine release may be stimulated by the action of complement. Complement can activate pathways of the cytokine network involved in inflammation. C3a may cause the release of IL-1, IL-6, and IL-8 by monocytes. Conversely, an increase in the TNF level may cause complement component C3 cleavage to C3a and C3b.[7] Increases in the level of IFN-gamma can cause stimulation of C4 and C2.[7]

CYTOKINES IN OCULAR INFLAMMATION

Interleukin-1

IL-1 is produced by macrophages, epithelial cells, keratinocytes, B cells, and polymorphonuclear leukocytes (PMNs). IL-1 is an endogenous pyrogen and a cofactor for thymocyte proliferation. This cytokine also activates PMNs and induces growth factor responsiveness in Th2 clones. Fibroblasts are also activated and proliferate in response to IL-1. The IL-1 induces the expression of adhesion molecules.

The role of cytokines in ocular disease has received increased attention in recent years. Much evidence links the action of cytokines with the onset of inflammation in the uvea and the anterior and posterior segments. Lipopolysaccharide (LPS) has been shown to cause uveitis or corneal ulcers in rabbits.[8, 9] In addition, IL-1 was measured in the tear film of rabbits in concentrations in excess of 100 pg/mL following exposure to LPS. When IL-1 was topically applied in concentrations of 100 pg/mL or greater, corneal infiltrates and ulcers developed.[10] IL-1 concentrations of only 1 pg/mL injected into the cornea led to infiltrate and ulcer formation within 2 hours. IL-1 injected intravitreally led to the development of uveitis.[11] IL-1 has also been reported as an angiogenic factor that can cause neovascular proliferation.[12] IL-1 blockers have been shown to be potent anti-uveitis drugs.[12a]

Tumor Necrosis Factor

TNF is one of the earliest cytokines produced in response to an inflammatory stimulus such as LPS. Systemically, anti-TNF therapy has been used in animals and is being studied in humans to control life-threatening increases in TNF serum levels caused by LPS stimulation.[13] Evidence indicates that increased protein concentration in aqueous humor correlates with increased serum TNF levels. However, at this point, no evidence suggests TNF involvement in patients with uveitis.

TNF is produced by monocytes, macrophages, T cells, and B cells. It is responsible for MHC expression on leukocytes. T cells are activated in the presence of this cytokine. TNF induces angiogenesis and adhesion molecule expression in the vascular endothelium. TNF also up-regulates conjunctival mast cell surface receptors (ICAM-1) and cell-bound IgE. Elevated levels of TNF-alpha are found in tears after antigen challenge. This cytokine is an early mediator of allergy after conjunctival challenge. Mice lacking the genes encoding TNF receptors (TNFR p55 and TNFR p75) experienced milder endotoxin-induced uveitis than control animals. TNF-alpha is also important for Langerhans cell migration in the cornea.[13a–13d]

Interleukin-2

IL-2 is produced by T cells. It is a growth factor for T, B, and NK cells. IL-1 induces the production of IL-2. IL-2 levels were elevated in the aqueous humor of uveitis patients.[14a]

IL-2 has been demonstrated in patients with sympathetic ophthalmia.[14] In addition, increased IL-2 receptor levels have been shown in patients with various types of ocular inflammatory conditions.[15] Because other cytokines such as TNF and IL-1 have been shown to contribute to ocular disease, IL-2 is probably involved as well.

Interleukin-6

IL-6 is produced by macrophages, T cells, epithelia, mast cells, vascular endothelia, and fibroblasts.

The expression of IL-6 is induced by a variety of stimuli, including TNF and IL-1. Increased levels of intraocular IL-6 were correlated with an increase in the severity of anterior chamber reaction in young rats.[16] However, in adult animals, the levels were not affected. Injection of IL-6 in rats produced uveitis.[17] IL-6 is implicated in herpes simplex virus neuronal reactivation.[17a]

Interleukin-8

IL-8 is produced by macrophages, T cells, PMNs, fibroblasts, vascular endothelia, and keratinocytes.

IL-8 has been shown to be a potent chemoattractant for neutrophils.[18] Concentrations of IL-8 in excess of 100 pg/mL measured in vitreous fluid have been shown to be chemoattractant for neutrophils.[19] IL-8 release may be stimulated from corneal keratinocytes by increased levels of TNF or IL-1.[20] In addition, one report suggests that IL-8, in doses of 1 to 40 ng/cornea, may enhance corneal neovascularization.[21] IL-8 mediates neutrophil chemotaxis at the early phase of HSV-1 corneal infection.[21a]

Interferon-Gamma

IFN-gamma is produced by antigen-stimulated T cells or natural killer cells.

IFN-gamma is a cytokine that inhibits cell proliferation and collagen synthesis. It has been shown in vitro to inhibit proliferation of both normal and keratoconus fibroblast cells equally. Vitreal injection of high concentrations of IFN-gamma produces a significant inflammatory infiltrate, consisting of PMNs and monocytes.[21b]

Transforming Growth Factor-Beta

This cytokine has been postulated to be a suppressive cytokine in aqueous humor. It has been proposed as a regulator of TNF and an inhibitor of lymphocyte production.[22] TGF-beta exists in the aqueous humor of some of the most common mammals used in medical research and in humans.

The inhibitory effect of aqueous humor on endothelial cell growth and angiogenesis is mediated by TGF-beta 2. The inhibitory effect is abolished when anti-TGF-beta 2 is added.[22a] TGF-beta predisposes ocular antigen presenting–cells to secrete IL-10 during antigen processing. IL-10 suppresses a delayed-type hypersensitivity and downregulates Th1 immune responses.[22b] TFG-beta is also found in elevated levels in ocular cicatrical pemphigoid—a systemic autoimmune disease characterized by conjunctival scarring.[22c]

ASSAYS TO DETECT CYTOKINES

Various methods have been used to detect cytokines in serum and in the ocular environment. Enzyme-linked immunoassay (ELISA) and radioimmunoassay have been used to detect cytokine levels in body fluids or supernatant fluids from cell cultures. These methods can be performed quickly and reliably, but even with purification of the cell populations, one cannot ensure that no contaminating cell types may secrete other cytokines. The ELISPOT method can be used to detect certain cytokines released by single cells and thus to quantitate the number of cells secreting cytokine at a given time.[23] The reverse hemolytic plaque assay can be used to quantify the amount of cytokine produced by single cells and the number of secreting cells present.[24, 25]

Other techniques that can be used to detect biologically inactive cytokine are polyacrylamide gel electrophoresis and Western blot or immunoblot assays. These assays detect the denatured protein product based on molecular weight and reactivity with specific antibody. Another technique used to detect cytokine activity associated with ocular tissue is the polymerase chain reaction. This technique involves amplification of a small piece of nucleic acid followed by gel electrophoresis and can be used to detect extremely small amounts of nucleic acid.

Bioassays can be used to detect cytokine release from specific cells in growth and proliferation assays. The advantage of such assays is that they measure biological activity. The disadvantage is that they are laborious and may be less specific than ELISA or immunoblot.

INTRACELLULAR ADHESION MOLECULES

The inflammation associated with ocular allergic disease is caused by an infiltration of inflammatory cells, such as monocytes and lymphocytes, including basophils, neutrophils, and eosinophils into the ocular surface. These inflammatory cells arrive in the ocular tissue via diffusion from the vascular endothelium of the cornea and conjunctiva and through the tear film. The diffusion of the inflammatory cells is enabled and facilitated by cellular adhesion molecules (CAMs), members of the immunoglobin (Ig) superfamily. Cellular adhesion molecules (e.g., ICAM-1, VCAM-1, P and E-selectins) are endothelial membrane-bound glycoproteins that aid in the transportation and recruitment of a number of inflammatory cells. Patients with ocular allergic disease, such as ocular allergic conjunctivitis (AKC) and vernal keratoconjunctivitis (VKC), show increased expression of the adhesion molecules ICAM-1 and VCAM-1.[26] This relationship elucidates the mechanism for inflammation that is clinically associated with ocular allergic disease.

Cellular adhesion molecules are activated by mast cell degranulation in the epithelia via complement-activated Ig-mediated pathways. Allergen crosslinkage in the IgE receptors on the mast cell causes its storage granules to release biochemical proinflammatory mediators into the surrounding tissue. The proinflammatory mediators released include histamine, heparin, and TNF-α that induce production of prostaglandins (PG). The increased concentration of the mast cell–released mediators drive the pathways of expression of CAMs.

In some studies, histamine has been shown to augment the concentration of TNF-α and to regulate CAM expression on vascular endothelium.[27] Increased concentration of TNF-α causes the upregulation of the cytokine IL-1, a potent activator of ICAM-1 (intercellular adhesion molecule).[28] Once activated, ICAM-1 mediates and facilitates the migration of leukocytes across the vascular endothelium into the surrounding ocular tissue.[27]

Histamine release also potentiates increased VCAM-1 (vascular adhesion molecule) and E-selectin expression.[29,30] VCAM-1 is a specific CAM responsible for monocyte migration into the inflamed tissue. E-selectin is another specific transporter of inflammatory cells responsible for movement of neutrophils from the vascular endothelium to the surrounding tissue.[27]

One proposed pathway for prolonged inflammation often involved in allergic disease in the eye is the continued bombardment of CAMs, located on the ocular surface, by leukocytes present in the tear film. Research has shown the presence of leukocytyes in tears.[31] Cams are present on the ocular surface.[32] Once the leukocytes that originate from the tear film bind to CAMs on the ocular surface, they become activated, compounding the inflammatory effect.

REFERENCES

1. Isaacs A, Lindenmann J. Virus interference: I. The interferon. Proc R Soc Lond B Biol Sci 147:258, 1957.
2. Bloom B, Bennett B. Mechanism of reaction in vitro associated with delayed-type hypersensitivity. Science 153:80, 1966.
3. Mosley B, Urdal D, Prickett K, et al. The interleukin-1 receptor binds the human interleukin-1 alpha precursor but not the interleukin-1 beta precursor. J Biol Chem 262:2941, 1987.
4. Fleisher L, Ferrell J, McGahan C. Synergistic uveitic effects of tumor necrosis factor-alpha and interleukin-1 beta. Invest Ophthalmol Vis Sci 33:2120, 1992.
5. Kuby J. Immunology. New York, WH Freeman, 1992, p 252.
6. Fabre E, Bureau J, Pouliquen Y, et al. Binding sites for human interleukin-1 alpha, gamma interferon and tumor necrosis factor on cultured fibroblasts of normal cornea and keratoconus. Curr Eye Res 10:585, 1991.
7. Baldwin W III, Pruitt S, Brauer R, et al. Complement in organ transplantation: contribution to inflammation, injury, and rejection. Transplantation 59:797, 1995.
8. Kulkarni P. Steroidal and nonsteroidal drugs in endotoxin-induced uveitis. J Ocul Pharmacol 10:329, 1994.
9. Schultz CL, Monck DW, McKay S, et al. Lipopolysaccharide induced acute red eye and corneal ulcers. Exp Eye Res 64:3, 1997.
10. Schultz C, George M, Richard K, Abelson MB. Interleukin-1 induced corneal pathology in New Zealand White rabbits. (Submitted.)
11. Chiou GCT, Chen Z, Xuan B, et al. Antagonism of interleukin-1 (IL-1) induced uveitis with synthetic IL-1 blockers. J Ocul Pharmacol Ther 13:427, 1997.
12. BenEzra D, Hemo I, Maftzir G. In vivo angiogenic activity of interleukins. Arch Ophthalmol 108:573, 1990.
12a. Xuan B, Chiou GC, Chen Z, et al. Effective treatment of experimental uveiti with interleukin-1 blockers, CK 123 and CK 124. J Ocul Pharmacol Ther 161:122, 1998.
13. Pennington J. TNF: therapeutic target in patients with sepsis. ASM News 58:479, 1992.
13a. Stahl JL, Cook EB, Graziano FM, Barney NP. Human conjunctival mast cells: expression of Fc epsilon RI, c-kit, ICAM-1, and IgE. Arch Ophthalmol 117:493, 1999.
13b. Vesaluma M, Rosenburg ME, Teppo A, et al. Tumor necrosis factor alpha (TNF alpha) in tears of atopic patients after conjunctival allergen challenge. Clin Exp Allergy 29:537, 1999.
13c. Smith JR, Hart PH, Coster DJ, Wiliams KA. Mice-deficient in tumor necrosis factor receptors p55 and p75, interleukin-4, or inducible nitric oxide synthase are susceptible to endotoxin-induced uveitis. Invest Ophthalmol Vis Sci 39:658, 1998.
13d. Dekaris I, Zhu SN, Dana MR. TNF-alpha regulates corneal Langerhans cell migration. J Immunol 162:4235, 1999.
14. Hooks J, Chan C, Detrick B. Identification of the lymphokines, interferon-gamma and interleukin-2, in inflammatory eye diseases. Invest Ophthalmol Vis Sci 29:1444, 1988.
14a. Murray PI, Caly CD, Mappin C, Salmon M. Molecular analysis of resolving immune responses in uveitis. Clin Exp Immunol 117:455, 1999.
15. Rosenbaum J, Tilden M, Bakke A. Soluble interleukin-2 receptor levels in patients with uveitis. In: Ocular immunology today. Usui M, Ohno S, Aoki K, eds. Amsterdam, Elsevier Science Publishers, 1990, p 77.
16. Hoekzema R, Murray P, van Haren M, et al. Analysis of interleukin-6 in endotoxin-induced uveitis. Invest Ophthalmol Vis Sci 32:88, 1991.
17. Hoekzema R, Verhagen C, van Haren M, et al. Endotoxin-induced uveitis in the rat: the significance of intraocular interleukin-6. Invest Ophthalmol Vis Sci 33:532, 1992.
17a. Kriesel JD, Ricigliano J, Spruance SL, et al. Neuronal reactivation of herpes simplex virus may involve interleukin-6. J Neurovirol 3:441, 1997.
18. Elner V, Strieter R, Pavilack M, et al. Human corneal interleukin-8: IL-1 and TNF-induced gene expression and secretion. Am J Pathol 139:977, 1991.

19. de Boer J, Hack C, Verhoven A, et al. Chemoat-tractant and neutrophil degranulation activities related to interleukin-8 in vitreous fluid in uvei-tis and vitreoretinal disorders. Invest Ophthal-mol Vis Sci 34:3376, 1993.

20. Cubitt C, Tang Q, Monteiro C, et al. IL-8 gene expression in cultures of human corneal epithe-lial cells and keratocytes. Invest Ophthalmol Vis Sci 34:3199, 1993.

21. Strieter R, Kunkel S, Elner V, et al. Interleukin-8: a corneal factor that induces neovasculariza-tion. Am J Pathol 141:1279, 1992.

21a. Miyazaki D, Inoue Y, Araki-Sasaki K, et al. Neutrophil chemotaxis induced by corneal epi-thelial cells after herpes simplex virus type 1 infection. Curr Eye Res 17:687, 1998.

21b. Kusuda M, Gaspari AA, Chan CC, et al. Ex-pression of Ia antigen by ocular tissues of mice treated with interferon-gamma. Invest Ophthal-mol Vis Sci 30:764, 1989.

22. Streilein J, Cousins S. Aqueous humor factors and their effect on the immune response in the anterior chamber. Curr Eye Res 9:175, 1990.

22a. Hayasaka K, Oikawa S, Hashizume E, et al. Anti-angiogenic effect of TGF-beta in aqueous humor. Life Sci 63:1089, 1998.

22b. D'Orazio TJ, Niederkorn JY. A novel role for TGF-beta and IL-10 in the induction of immune privilege. J Immunol 160:2089, 1998.

22c. Elder MJ, Dart JK, Lightman S. Conjunctival fibrosis in ocular cicatricial pemphigoid—the role of cytokines. Exp Eye Res 65:165, 1997.

23. Czerkinsky C, Anderson G, Ekre H-P, et al. Re-verse ELISPOT assay for clonal analysis of cyto-kine production. I. Enumeration of gamma-inter-feron–secreting cells. J Immunol Methods 111:29, 1988.

24. Neill J, Smith P, Luque E, et al. Detection and measurement of hormone secretion from individ-ual pituitary cells. Recent Prog Horm Res 43:175, 1987.

25. Smith P, Luque E, Neill J. Detection and meas-urement of secretion from individual neuroendo-crine cells using a reverse hemolytic plaque as-say. Methods Enzymol 124:443, 1986.

26. Uchio E, et al. Serum levels of soluble intercellu-lar adhesion molecule-1, vascular adhesion mole-cule-1, and interleukin-2 receptor in patients with vernal keratoconjunctivitis and allergic con-junctivitis. Allergy 54:135, 1999.

27. Tonnel AB, Gosset P, Molet S, et al. Interactions between endothelial cells and effector cells in al-lergic inflammation. Ann N Y Acad Sci 796:9, 1996.

28. Kuby J. Immunology, 3rd ed. WH Freeman, New York, 1997.

29. Saito H, Shimizu H, Mita H, et al. Histamine augments VCAM-1 expression on IL-4 and TNF-α stimulated human umbilical vein endothelial cells. Intern Arch Allergy Immunol 111:126, 1996.

30. Van Haaster CM, Derhaag JG, Engels W, et al. Mast cell–mediated induction of ICAM-1, VCAM-1 and E-selectin in endothelial cells in vitro: constitutive release of inducing mediators but no effect of degranulation. Pflugers Arch 435:137, 1997.

31. Sakata M, Sack RA, Sathe S, et al. Polymorpho-nuclear leukocyte cells and elastase in tears. Curr Eye Res 16:810, 1997.

32. Baudouin C, Brignole F, Pisella PJ, et al. Immu-nophenotyping of human dendriform cells from the conjunctival epithelium. Curr Eye Res 16:475, 1997.

CHAPTER 11

Platelet-Activating Factor

MARK B. ABELSON ■ **ERIKA SCHWARTZ** ■ **MICHELLE GEORGE**

Platelet-activating factor (PAF) is a phospholipase A_2-sensitive phospholipid,[1] identified as 1-alkyl-2(R)-acetyl-glycerol-3-phosphorylcholine.[2] PAF is produced by many different kinds of stimulated cells (e.g., basophils, neutrophils, monocytes, macrophages, mast cells, endothelial cells) from phospholipids mobilized from cell membranes by phospholipase A_2. It is not preformed in storage granules. PAF was partially synthesized in 1979,[1] and total synthesis was achieved in 1980.[3] Several structural analogs have been developed, permitting an extensive establishment of the structural requirements for biological activity (Fig. 11.1).[4]

Since PAF was first recovered in vivo, this release has been reported from a wide range of cells when stimulated in vitro with immunoglobulin E, a calcium ionophore, or zymosan particles. PAF has been shown to be released in response to antigen from sensitized guinea pig lung when the lung is challenged intratracheally,[5] but the cellular origin is not yet certain.

PATHOPHYSIOLOGY

PAF is a potent bronchoconstrictor in several species, including guinea pig,[6] rabbit,[7] baboon,[8] and human.[9–11] Additionally, PAF is able to induce a prolonged increase in bronchial responsiveness in animals, such as guinea pig,[12] dog,[13] and monkey.[14] Because PAF is rapidly inactivated by PAF

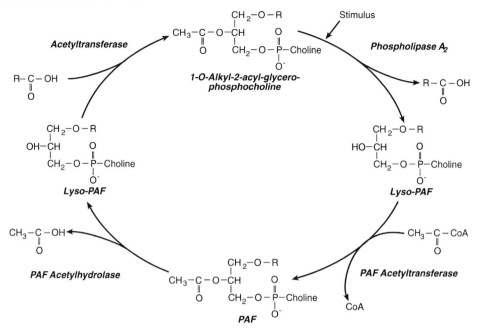

FIGURE 11.1 Platelet-activating factor (PAF) is characterized as a phospholipase A₂–sensitive phospholipid, and has been identified as 1-alkyl-2(R)-acetyl-glycero-3-phosphorylcholine. The formation of PAF from phosphorylcholine is mediated by the enzymes phospholipase A₂ and acetyltransferase.

acetylhydrolases, some of the effects of PAF may be induced through a series of secondary events.[15]

PAF induces microvascular leakage in several tissues at doses approximately 1,000 times lower than those of histamine.[16–18] PAF is able to activate a wide range of inflammatory cells in vitro, including platelets,[19] neutrophils,[20] macrophages,[21] monocytes,[22] and eosinophils.[23] In fact, PAF is approximately 100 times more potent than eosinophilic chemotactic factor or leukotriene B₄ in eliciting eosinophils.[24]

In vivo PAF-induced cellular activity is reflected by the recruitment of various inflammatory cells into tissues after either systemic or local administration.[25–28] Of particular interest is the ability of PAF to induce an eosinophil-rich infiltrate into the lungs of various experimental animals[29, 30] after both local and systemic administration. PAF has also been implicated in the interaction between the major effector cells in the pathogenesis of allergic diseases: mast cells and eosinophils. Evidence exists that PAF elicits a rise in the cytosolic free calcium concentration in human eosinophils leading to degranulation and cationic protein release.[31a]

Following local administration of PAF into the skin of normal healthy volunteers, one sees a substantial infiltration of eosinophils.[25] Four hours after intradermal injection of PAF into human skin, neutrophils predominate, whereas at 24 hours, the cellular infiltrate contains both neutrophils and mononuclear cells.[27] In contrast, in atopic volunteers, PAF results in a selective eosinophil infiltration, reminiscent of that induced with antigen.[25] Thus, the effects of PAF may vary with the inflammatory "phenotype" in humans—that is, different effects in different diseases.[15]

Using mass spectrometry, PAF has been found in psoriatic scale[31] and in blister fluid from a patient with bullous mastocytosis.[32] Additionally, PAF or PAF-like activity has been reported in cerebrospinal fluid from children with meningitis,[33] in pleural fluid from subjects with eosinophilic or neutro-

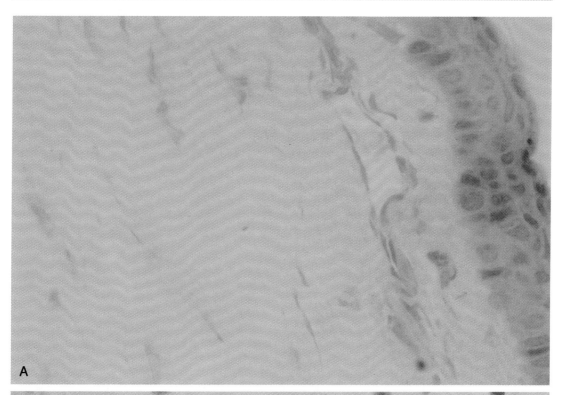

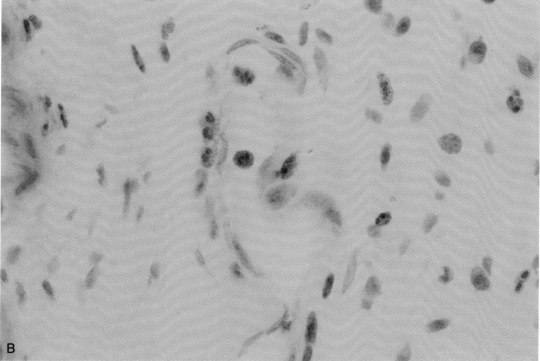

FIGURE 11.2 In a dose-response study that involved topical challenge with platelet-activating factor (PAF) to rabbit eyes, PAF was found to be chemotactic for neutrophils and eosinophils in the conjunctiva. *A,* The conjunctiva of a rabbit eye administered saline did not manifest a chemotactic response. *B,* The conjunctiva of a rabbit eye treated with PAF exhibited a chemotactic response.

philic lung inflammation,[34] in colonic biopsy specimens from patients with active ulcerative colitis,[35] in inflammatory joint fluid,[36] and in urine from infants with hemolytic uremic syndrome.[37]

Inhalation of PAF causes accumulation of neutrophils in human airways.[38] In addition, PAF-like bioactivity has been reported to be released by alveolar macrophages obtained from asthmatic patients,[39] and it has been found in airway fluids of patients with asthma.[40]

OCULAR EFFECTS

Few studies are currently available on the role of PAF in the eye. Intravenous injection of PAF-acether in rabbits resulted in increased microvascular permeability of the retina, characterized by intense ischemia and marked plasma leakage.[41] A PAF-like factor detected in inflamed iris and ciliary body tissues of rabbits has been shown to synthesize another PAF-like factor that induces platelet aggregation, resembles an ether lipid, and is inhibited by the PAF-receptor antagonist SRI 66-441.[42]

The role of PAF as a chemical mediator in external ocular inflammation was examined in a dose-response study that involved topical challenge with PAF to rabbit and human eyes. Clinically significant hyperemia and chemosis, similar in appearance to allergic conjunctivitis, were noted at all doses and all times. Histologically, PAF was found to be chemotactic for neutrophils and eosinophils in the conjunctiva of both species (Fig. 11.2).[43] A useful representative in vitro model system to study the physiological and pathological aspects of the human corneal epithelium has been developed. Primary and SV40 virus–immortalized human corneal epithelial cells were found to express functional PAF receptors. PAF stimulated the mRNA for metalloproteinase-1.[44]

To date, studies suggest that PAF may play an important role in allergic diseases. However, further work is necessary to elucidate this role. Oxatomide (a PAF antagonist) was shown to cause a dose-dependent inhibition of intra- and extracellular PAF activity from asthmatic and nonasthmatic neutrophils.[45] Another PAF antagonist, Y-24180, was shown to inhibit PAF, IL-4, and IL-5 in ovalbumin-challenged mice skin. This inhibition suppressed the allergic cutaneous eosinophilia found in challenged untreated mice.[46] The evaluation of PAF antagonists may provide additional information regarding PAF's role in allergy, and it may play a part in the future management of certain allergic disorders.

REFERENCES

1. Benveniste J, Tence M, Varenne P, et al. Semi-synthesis and proposed structure of platelet activating factor (PAF): PAF-acether an alkyl ether analog of lipophosphatidylcholine. C R Seances Acad Sci D 289:1037, 1979.
2. Damopoulos CA, Pinckard RN, Hanahan DJ. Platelet-activating factor: evidence for 1-0-alkyl-2-acetyl-sn-glyceryl-3-phosphorylcholine as the active component (a new class of lipid chemical mediators). J Biol Chem 254:9355, 1979.
3. Godfroid JJ, Heymans F, Michel E, et al. Platelet-activating factor (PAF-acether): total synthesis of 1-0-acetyl-sn-glycero-3-phosphorylcholine. FEBS Lett 116:161, 1980.
4. Braquet P, Godfroid JJ. Platelet-activating factor (PAF-acether) specific binding sites. II. Design of specific antagonists. Trends Pharmacol Sci 7:397, 1986.
5. Fitzgerald MF, Moncada S, Parente L. The aphylactic phase of platelet-activating factor from perfused guinea pig lungs. Br J Pharmacol 88:149, 1986.
6. Vargaftig BB, Lefort J, Chignard M, et al. Platelet-activating factor induces a platelet-dependent bronchoconstriction unrelated to the formation of prostaglandin derivatives. Eur J Pharmacol 141:185, 1980.
7. Halonen M, Palmer JD, Lohman IC, et al. Respi-

ratory and circulatory alterations induced by acetyl glyceryl ether phosphorylcholine, a mediator of IgE anaphylaxis in the rabbit. Am Rev Respir Dis 122:915, 1980.

8. Denjean A, Arnoux B, Masse R, et al. Acute effects of intratracheal administration of platelet-activating factor in baboons. J Appl Physiol 55:799, 1983.

9. Cuss FM, Dixon CMS, Barnes PJ. Effects of inhaled platelet-activating factor on pulmonary function and bronchial responsiveness in man. Lancet 2:189, 1986.

10. Rubin AE, Smith LJ, Patterson R. The bronchoconstricting properties of platelet-activating factor in humans. Am Rev Respir Dis 136:1145, 1987.

11. Gateau O, Arnoux B, Deriaz H, et al. Acute effects of intratracheal administration of PAF-acether (platelet-activating factor) in humans. Am Rev Respir Dis 133:129A, 1984.

12. Mazzoni L, Morley J, Page CP, et al. Induction of airway hyperreactivity by platelet-activating factor in the guinea pig. J Physiol (Lond) 365:107P, 1985.

13. Chung KF, Aizawa H, Leikauf GD, et al. Airway hyperresponsiveness induced by platelet-activating factor: role of thromboxane generation. J Pharmacol Exp Ther 236:580, 1986.

14. Patterson R, Bernstein PR, Harris KE, et al. Airway responses to sequential challenges with platelet-activating factor and leukotriene D_4 in rhesus monkeys. J Lab Clin Med 104:340, 1984.

15. Barnes PJ, Chung KF, Page CP. Platelet-activating factor as a mediator of allergic disease. J Allergy Clin Immunol 81:919, 1988.

16. Morley J, Page CP, Paul W. Inflammatory actions of PAF-acether in guinea pig skin. Br J Pharmacol 80:503, 1987.

17. Bjork J, Smedegard G. Acute microvascular effects of PAF-acether, as studied by intravital microscopy. Eur J Pharmacol 96:87, 1983.

18. Evans TW, Chung K, Rogers DF, et al. Effect of platelet-activating factor on airway vascular permeability: possible mechanisms. J Appl Physiol 63:479, 1987.

19. Benveniste J, Henson PM, Cochrane CG. Leucocyte dependent histamine release from rabbit platelets: the role of IgE, basophils, and a platelet-activating factor. J Exp Med 136:1356, 1972.

20. Shaw JO, Pinckard RN, Ferrigni KS, et al. Activation of human neutrophils with 1-0-hexadecyl-2-acetyl-sn-phosphorylcholine (platelet-activating factor). J Immunol 127:1250, 1981.

21. Hartung HP, Parnham MJ, Winkleman J, et al. Platelet-activating factor (PAF) induces the oxidative burst in macrophages. Int J Immunopharmacol 5:115, 1983.

22. Yasaka T, Boxer LA, Baehner RL. Monocyte aggregation and superoxide anion response to formyl-methionyl-leucyl-phenylalanine (FMLP) and platelet activating factor (PAF). J Immunol 128:1939, 1982.

23. Lee TC, Lenihan DJ, Malone B, et al. Increased biosynthesis of platelet-activating factor in activated human eosinophils. J Biol Chem 259:5526, 1984.

24. Tamura N, Agrawal D, Suliman FA, et al. Effects of platelet-activating factor on the chemotaxis of normodense eosinophils from normal subjects. Biochem Biophys Res Commun 142:638, 1986.

25. Henocq E, Vargaftig BB. Accumulation of eosinophils in response to intracutaneous PAF-acether and allergens in man. Lancet 1:1378, 1986.

26. Dewar A, Archer CB, Paul W, et al. Cutaneous and pulmonary histopathological response to platelet-activating factor (PAF-acether) in the guinea pig. J Pathol 44:25, 1984.

27. Archer CB, Page CP, Morley J, et al. Accumulation of inflammatory cells in response to intracutaneous platelet-activating factor (PAF acether) in man. Br J Dermatol 112:285, 1985.

28. Archer SB, Page CP, Paul W, et al. Inflammatory characteristics of platelet-activating factor (PAF-acether) in human skin. Br J Dermatol 110:45, 1984.

29. Arnoux B, Denjean A, Page CP, et al. Pulmonary effects of platelet-activating factor in a primate are inhibited by ketotifen. Am Rev Respir Dis 131:2A, 1985.

30. Lellouch-Tubiana A, Lefort J, Pirotzky E, et al. Ultrastructural evidence for extravascular platelet recruitment in the lung upon intravenous injection of platelet-activating factor (PAF-acether) to guinea pigs. Br J Exp Pathol 66:345, 1985.

31. Mallet AI, Cunningham FM. Structural identification of platelet-activating factor in psoriatic scale. Biochem Biophys Res Commun 126:192, 1985.

31a. Takafuji S, Tadokoro K, et al. Release of granule proteins from human eosinophils stimulated with mast-cell mediators. Allergy 53:951, 1998.

32. McPherson JL, Kemp A, Rogers M, et al. Occurrence of platelet-activating factor (PAF) and an endogenous inhibitor of platelet aggregation in diffuse cutaneous mastocytosis. Clin Exp Immunol 77:391, 1990.

33. Arditi M, Manoque KR, Caplan M, et al. Cerebrospinal fluid cachectin/tumor necrosis factor-alpha and platelet-activating factor concentrations and severity of bacterial meningitis in children. J Infect Dis 162:139, 1990.

34. Oda M, Satduchi K, Ikeda I, et al. The presence of Platelet-activating factor associated with eosinophil and/or neutrophil accumulations in pleural fluid. Am Rev Respir Dis 141:1469, 1991.

35. Eliakim R, Karmeli F, Razin E, et al. Role of platelet-activating factor in ulcerative colitis: enhanced production during active disease and inhibition by sulfasalazine and prednisolone. Gastroenterology 95:1167, 1988.

36. Harris ED. Rheumatoid arthritis: pathophysiology and implications for surgery. N Engl J Med 322:1277, 1990.

37. Boccardo P, Benigni A, Noris M, et al. Urinary excretion of platelet activating factor (U-PAF) in the hemolytic uremic syndrome (HUS). J Am Soc Nephrol 1:329A, 1990.

38. Wardlaw AJ, Chung KF, Moqbel R, et al. Effects of inhaled PAF in humans on circulating and bronchoalveolar lavage fluid neutrophils: relationship to bronchoconstriction and changes in airway responsiveness. Am Rev Respir Dis 141:386, 1990.

39. Arnoux B, Joseph M, Simoses MH, et al. Antigenic release of PAF-acether and -glucuronidase from alveolar macrophages of asthmatics. Bull Eur Physiopathol Respir 23:119, 1987.

40. Stenton SC, Court EN, Kingston WP, et al. Platelet-activating factor in bronchoalveolar lavage fluid from asthmatic subjects. Eur Respir J 3:408, 1990.

41. Braquet P, Vidal RF, Braquet M, et al. Involvement of leukotrienes and PAF-acether in the increased microvascular permeability of the rabbit retina. Agents Actions 15:82, 1984.

42. Rosenbaum JT, Boney RS, Samples JR, et al. Synthesis of platelet activating factor by ocular tissue from inflamed eyes. Arch Ophthalmol 109: 410, 1991.

43. George MA, Smith LM, Berdy GJ, et al. Platelet activating factor induced inflammation following topical ocular challenge (abstract). Invest Ophthalmol Vis Sci 31 Suppl:63, 1990.

44. Shariff NA, Wiernas TK, Howe WE, et al. Human corneal epithelial cell functional responses to inflammatory agents and their antagonists. Invest Ophthalmol Vis Sci 39:2562, 1998.

45. Shindo K, Fukumura M. Oxatomide inhibits synthesis and release of platelet-activating factor in human neutrophils. Prostaglandins Leukot Essent Fatty Acids 58:99, 1998.

46. Yamaguchi S, Tomomatsu N, Kagoshima M, et al. Effects of Y-24180, a receptor antagonist to platelet-activating factor, on allergic cutaneous eosinophilia in mice. Life Sci 64:PL 139, 1999.

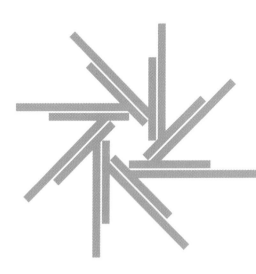

Leukotrienes

MARK B. ABELSON ■ **KELLY K. GRANT** ■ **MATTHEW J. CHAPIN**

Both leukotrienes and prostaglandins are synthesized from arachidonic acid, a normal constituent of the plasma membrane, and are liberated by the action of phospholipases in response to tissue damage or mast cell degranulation. Many investigators have proposed that prostaglandin synthesis is the primary pathway activated in normal tissues and that leukotriene synthesis is activated only in chronic inflammatory conditions.[1, 2] However, various leukotrienes have been identified in tear fluids following topical ocular allergen challenge, a finding suggesting that they may play a role in human allergic disease (Fig. 12.1).[3]

LEUKOTRIENE FORMATION

The iron-containing enzyme 5-lipoxygenase, which consists of 673 amino acids, is dependent on calcium (Ca^{2+}), adenosine triphosphate, and several co-factors for maximal activity.[4] 5-Lipoxygenase translocates from the cytsol to the nuclear cell membrane to initiate leukotriene biosynthesis. The action of this complex forms 5-hydroxyperoxyeicosatetraenoic acid (5-HPETE), an unstable intermediate. 5-Lipoxygenase binds to lipoxygenase-activating protein, a nuclear protein, to make a stable complex.[5] 5-HPETE is then converted to one of two mediators. 5-HPETE can be converted by peroxidase to form 5-hydroxyeicosatetraenoic acid (5-HETE). The 5-HPETE can undergo further processing by 5-lipoxygenase to form leukotriene A_4 (LTA$_4$) through a second stereospecific removal of [10]C hydrogen, followed by radical migration and epoxide formation.[6]

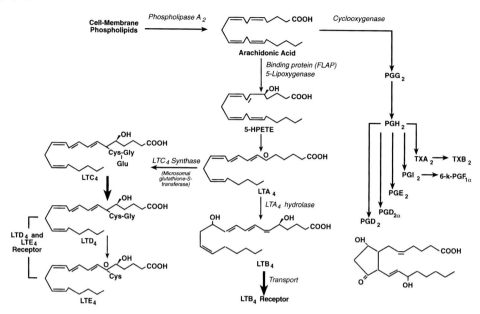

FIGURE 12.1 Arachidonic acid is metabolized by lipoxygenase and cyclooxygenase. The products of the cyclooxygenase pathway are prostaglandins (PGD, PGE, PGF, PGG, PGH, PGI), and the products of the lipoxygenase pathway are leukotrienes (LTA, LTC, LTD, LTE). 5-HPETE, 5-hydroxyperoxyeicosotetranoic acid; TXA_2, thromboxane A_2; TXB_2, thromboxane B_2.

LEUKOTRIENES

LTA_4 is the pivotal intermediate from which all other leukotrienes are synthesized. LTA_4 hydrolase is a zinc-containing cytosolic metalloproteinase possessing aminopeptidase activity.[7] It is also considerably homologous to the aminopeptidase N family of enzymes. LTA_4 is unstable and is hydrolyzed by LTA_4 hydrolase to the dihydroxyacid LTB_4. Alternatively, the enzyme LTC_4 synthase incorporates glutathione to form the peptidoleukotriene LTC_4. LTC_4 synthase has been recognized as an 18-kd integral microsomal membrane protein.

LTC_4 and its metabolites LTD_4 and LTE_4 were previously known as slow-reacting substance of anaphylaxis (SRS-A) because of their ability to induce slow, antihistamine-resistant contractile activity in nonvascular smooth muscle. The subsequent conversion of LTC_4 to LTD_4, a cysteinyl glycinyl derivative, occurs through the action of alpha-glutamyl transpeptidase. LTD_4 is further metabolized to the cysteinyl derivative, LTE_4, by the action of a dipeptidase.

Leukotrienes are rapidly metabolized and removed from the circulation. Peptidoleukotrienes undergo oxidation, resulting in biliary and urinary elimination of biologically less active and inactive metabolites. LTE_4 is an important urinary metabolite that can be used to monitor the production of leukotrienes in humans.[8, 9]

The location of leukotriene synthesis is determined by the cellular distribution of the enzymes that control each step of the pathway. For instance, the distribution of 5-lipoxygenase is limited to myeloid cells, including neutrophils, eosinophils, monocytes, macrophages, mast cells, and basophils. LTC_4 synthase has been identified not only in mast cells and eosinophils, but also in endothelial cells and platelets. LTA_4 hydrolase has been found in human plasma, human erythrocytes, inflammatory cells, bronchoalveolar lavage fluid, and airway epithelial cells.

Because these enzymes are distributed among different cell types, various inflammatory cells, in conjunction with noninflammatory cells, such as endothelial cells or epithelial cells, can participate in the transcellular synthesis of leukotrienes.[10, 11] Monocytes and macrophages release both LTB_4 and LTD_4 after stimulation, whereas most other cells produce significant quantities of either LTB_4 or LTC_4, but not both. LTB_4 is produced mainly by eosinophils and basophils, but also by neutrophils, macrophages, and monocytes. Cellular sources of cysteinyl leukotrienes include mast cells, macrophages, and eosinophils. The predominant products of eosinophils are LTC_4 and cytokines such as interleukin-3, interleukin-5, and granulocyte-macrophage–colony-stimulating factor. These cytokines have been localized in asthmatic airways and are capable of enhancing LTC_4 synthesis.[12, 13]

LTB_4 is probably the most closely studied leukotriene in the eye, and it has been shown to be produced in ocular tissues.[14] LTB_4 has been identified as the lipoxygenase product responsible for the transient aggregation of human polymorphonuclear leukocytes that is induced in vivo by arachidonic acid.[15, 16] Thus, LTB_4 acts as a potent neutrophil chemotactic agent and has platelet-aggregating activity in vivo. In addition, LTB_4 produces both leukocyte chemokinesis and chemotaxis. In fact, LTB_4 appears to be the most potent arachidonic acid metabolite with respect to the in vitro effects on leukocyte aggregation and motility.[17]

Both prostaglandin E_2 (PGE_2) and PGD_2 act synergistically with LTB_4 to enhance vascular permeability, edema formation, and subsequent neutrophil infiltration. The inhibition of the cyclooxygenase pathway leads to increased levels of mediators formed through the 5-lipoxygenase pathway.[12, 13] Thus, the inhibition of the cyclooxygenase pathway by nonsteroidal anti-inflammatory drugs could be beneficial or detrimental, depending on the altered profile of the arachidonic metabolites.

LEUKOTRIENES IN THE EYE

The conjunctiva and iris of a number of animal species are capable of forming lipoxygenase products.[18] High performance chromatography[3] and immunoassays[19] have demonstrated the presence of LTC_4, LTD_4, and LTE_4 in tear fluids following conjunctival allergen challenge.[3, 19–21] LTC_4 was found to reach peak levels between 5 and 10 minutes following ocular allergen challenge. It decreased to baseline levels by 30 minutes.[20] Topical application of LTB_4 to hamster conjunctiva did not cause changes in the conjunctival vascular permeability,[22] although it did cause primary eosinophil and secondary neutrophil chemotaxis in the guinea pig[23] and rat.[24] In rabbits, LTB_4 elicited chemosis, vasodilation, and leukocytic infiltrate in the conjunctiva. These effects peaked at three hours. When PGD_2 was concomitantly administered with LTB_4, an additive effect on the leukocyte infiltration occurred and cell degranulation was apparent.[25] In another study, topical administration of LTB_4, LTD_4, and LTC_4 resulted in eosinophil chemotaxis in guinea pig conjunctiva.[26] One study, however, did not detect LTB_4 in tears of patients with giant papillary conjunctivitis (GPC) secondary to contact lenses.[27] Other studies found elevated LTB_4 and LTC_4 levels in tears of ocular prosthesis–associated GPC[28] and contact lens–associated inflammatory disease.[29] In this study, the mast cell stabilizer lodoxamide significantly reduced LTB_4 and LTC_4 tear levels in those so-affected patients.[28]

LTB$_4$ and other leukotrienes are present in conjunctival smears[30] and tears[31] of patients with chronic conjunctivitis. The role of leukotrienes in allergic conjunctivitis appears to be limited, because topical application of LTB$_4$ to the human conjunctiva did not produce vasodilation. Biopsy revealed dense polymorphonuclear leukocyte infiltration (unpublished observation). Further topical ocular application of LTC$_4$ elicited no observable effect in rabbits or humans.[32] These results suggest that LTB$_4$ and LTC$_4$ may have little role in producing ocular allergies. They may play a role, however, in potentiating mechanisms that have already started. More research is required to determine the contribution of LTC$_4$, LTD$_4$, and LTE$_4$ and ocular immediate hypersensitivity.

The conjunctiva and iris of a number of animal species are capable of forming lipoxygenase products.[32] LTC$_4$, LTD$_4$, and LTE$_4$ have been identified in tears after allergen challenge.[3] Because topical application of LTC$_4$ elicited no effect in rabbits or humans,[32] more research is required to determine the contribution of these mediators to immediate hypersensitivity in the eye.

SYSTEMIC EFFECTS

In humans, a subcutaneous injection of LTB$_4$ causes a wheal and flare response followed 2 to 3 hours later by a tender, indurated lesion consisting of a dermal infiltrate of mainly neutrophils. The systein-containing leukotrienes LTC$_4$, LTD$_4$, and LTE$_4$ are potent bronchoconstrictors in the peripheral airways of animal and humans.[33, 34] They also increase the vascular permeability of postcapillary venules and stimulate mucus secretion in the lung and thus are implicated in asthma. Anaphylactic contraction of bronchi from atopic patients who were sensitive to birch pollen was inhibited by lipoxygenase inhibitors, but not by antihistamine or cyclooxygenase inhibitors.[35] LTD$_4$ causes smooth muscle contraction and increases vascular permeability. LTC$_4$ and LTD$_4$ are powerful depressants of myocardial contractile force, and marked negative inotropic effects are evident when they are administered in picogram to nanogram amounts.[36, 37] Both LTC$_4$ and histamine increase tracheal insufflation pressure in anesthetized and artificially ventilated guinea pigs, but LTC$_4$ is at least 100 times more potent than histamine and causes a longer-lasting increase.[38, 39] These studies implicate these leukotrienes as major mediators of anaphylaxis in the lung. LTE$_4$ has several systemic effects that include vasodilation and potentiating increased vascular permeability produced by histamine and bradykinin. LTD$_4$ has been implicated in seasonal allergic rhinitis. An LTD$_4$ antagonist has been shown to reduce nasal symptoms in a seasonal allergic rhinitis study. Another rhinitis study followed the rise and fall of inflammatory mediators during a nasal allergen challenge. It found no link among clinical symptoms, drug efficacy, and LTC$_4$ release.

The profound biological effects of leukotrienes, as well as the existence of leukotrienes in biological fluids, suggest a role in allergic disease. LTC$_4$, LTD$_4$, and LTE$_4$ are present in the serum and/or urine of patients with asthma. LTB$_4$ is found in the rectal secretions of patients with inflammatory bowel disease and in the joint fluid of patients with rheumatoid arthritis. LTB$_4$, LTC$_4$, LTD$_4$, and LTE$_4$ have been identified in nasal secretions of patients with allergic rhinitis. Observations that leukotriene receptor antagonists and pharmacological agents that inhibit 5-lipoxygenase activity ameliorate the signs and symptoms of many diseases strongly support the involvement of leukotrienes in their pathogenesis.

HYDROPEROXY-EICOSATETRAENOIC AND HYDROXY-EICOSATETRAENOIC ACIDS

The lipoxygenase pathway of arachidonic acid metabolism also produces hydroperoxy-eicosatetraenoic acid (HPETE) and hydroxy-eicosatetraenoic acid (HETE). Studies involving inflammation of the eye, including a hypoxia model[40] and an alkali burn model,[41] have detected HETE in the cornea. The role of HPETE and HETE in ocular allergic conditions remains undefined. Topical application of 5-HETE and 12-HETE on the conjunctiva of rabbits and humans had no effect (author's unpublished data). HETEs are known to be potent mucus-stimulating mediators in the lung,[42] and it is possible that such a role may exist in the eye. Elevated HETE1 and HETE2 levels were identified in the tears of patients with keratoconjunctivitis[43]; therefore, their role in ocular inflammation seems probable.

Lipoxygenase products of arachidonic acid appear to have three important roles in inflammation: (1) as effector molecules (such as chemotaxins and stimulants of end-organ responses), (2) as essential intracellular biochemical intermediates in the cellular mechanisms of mediator release, and (3) as local hormones (autocoids) that deregulate an inflammatory response.

REFERENCES

1. Bhattacherjee P. The role of arachidonate metabolism in ocular inflammation. Prog Clin Biol Res 312:211, 1989.
2. Kliman G, Butrus SI, Weston JH, et al. Modulation of arachidonic acid metabolism in the rabbit conjunctiva (abstract). Invest Ophthalmol Vis Sci 24 Suppl:200, 1983.
3. Bisgaard H, Ford-Hutchinson AW, Charleson S, Tauderf E. Production of leukotrienes in human skin and conjunctival mucosa after specific allergen challenge. Allergy 40:417, 1985.
4. Rouzer CA, Samuelsson B. On the nature of the 5-lipoxygenase reaction in human leukocytes: enzyme purification and requirement for multiple stimulatory factors. Proc Natl Acad Sci USA 82:6040, 1985.
5. Miller DK, Gillard JW, Vickers PJ, et al. Identification and isolation of a membrane protein necessary for leukotriene production. Nature 343:278, 1990.
6. Rouzer CA, Matsumoto T, Samuelsson B. Single protein from human leukocytes possesses 5-lipoxygenase and leukotriene A synthase activities. Proc Natl Acad Sci USA 83:857, 1986.
7. Haeggstrom JZ, Wetterholm A, Vallee BL, Samuelsson B. Leukotriene A$_4$ hydrolase: an epoxide hydrolase with peptidase activity. Biochem Biophys Res Commun 173:431, 1990.
8. Sala A, Voelkel N, Maclouf J, Murphy RC. Leukotriene E$_4$ elimination and metabolism in normal human subjects. J Biol Chem 265:21771, 1990.
9. Maltby NH, Taylor GW, Ritter JM, et al. Leukotriene C$_4$ elimination and metabolism in man. J Allergy Clin Immunol 85:3, 1990.

10. Feinmark SJ, Cannon PJ. Endothelial cell leukotriene C$_4$ synthesis results from intercellular transfer of leukotriene A$_4$ synthesized by polymorphonuclear leukocytes. J Biol Chem 261:16466, 1986.
11. Bigby TD, Lee DM, Meslier N, Gruenert DC. Leukotriene A$_4$ hydrolase activity of human airway epithelial cells. Biochem Biophys Res Commun 164:1, 1989.
12. Silberstein DS, Owen WF, Gasson JC, et al. Enhancement of human eosinophil cytotoxicity and leukotriene synthesis by biosynthetic (recombinant) granulocyte-macrophage colony-stimulating factor. J Immunol 137:3290, 1986.
13. Takafuji S, Bischoff SC, DeWeck AL, Dahinden CA. IL-3 and IL-5 prime normal human eosinophils to produce leukotriene C$_4$ in response to soluble agonists. J Immunol 147:3855, 1991.
14. Kulkarni PS, Srinivasan BD, Kaufman P. Comparison of cyclooxygenase and lipoxygenase pathways in rabbit and monkey ocular tissues (abstract). Invest Ophthalmol Vis Sci 26 Suppl:191, 1985.
15. O'Flaherty JT, Showell HJ, Becker EL, et al. Neutrophil aggregation and degranulation: effect of arachidonic acid. Am J Pathol 95:433, 1979.
16. O'Flaherty JT, Showell HJ, Becker EL, et al. Role of arachidonic acid derivatives in neutrophil aggregation: a hypothesis. Prostaglandins 17:915, 1979.
17. Smith MJH. Biological activities of leukotriene B$_4$ (isomer III). Adv Prostaglandin Thromboxane Leukot Res 9:283, 1982.
18. Williams RN, Bhattacherjee P, Eakins KE. Biosynthesis of lipoxygenase products by ocular tissues. Exp Eye Res 36:397, 1983.

19. Aichane A, Campbell AM, Chanal I, et al. Precision of conjunctival provocation tests in right and left eyes. J Allergy Clin Immunol 92:49, 1993.

20. Mita H, Sakuma Y, Shida T, Akiyama K. Release of chemical mediators in the conjunctival lavage fluids after eye provocation with allergen or compound 48/80. Arerugi 43:800, 1994.

21. Proud D, Sweet J, Stein P, et al. Inflammatory mediator release on conjunctival provocation of allergic subjects with allergen. J Allergy Clin Immunol 85:896, 1990.

22. Woodward DF, Ledgard SE. Comparison of leukotrienes as conjunctival microvascular permeability factors. Ophthalmic Res 17:318, 1985.

23. Spada CS, Woodward DF, Hawley SB, Nieves AL. Leukotrienes cause eosinophil emigration into conjunctival tissue. Prostaglandins 31:795, 1986.

24. Trocme SD, Gilbert CM, Allansmith MR, et al. Characteristics of the cellular response of the rat conjunctiva to topically applied leukotriene B_4. Ophthalmic Res 21:297, 1989.

25. Butrus SI, Corey EJ, Weston JH, Abelson MB. The effect of leukotriene B_4 in rabbit and guinea pig eyes (abstract). Invest Ophthalmol Vis Sci 25 Suppl:109, 1984.

26. Woodward DR, Krauss AH, Nieves AL, et al. Studies on leukotrienes D_4 as an eosinophil chemoattractant. Drugs Exp Clin Res 17:543, 1991.

27. Elgebaly SA, Donshik PC, Rahhal F, Williams W. Neutrophil chemotactic factors in the tears of giant papillary conjunctivitis patients. Invest Ophthalmol Vis Sci 32:208, 1991.

28. Akman A, Irkec M, Orhan M, et al. Effect of lodoxamide on tear leukotriene levels in giant papillary conjunctivitis associated with ocular prosthesis. Ocul Immunol Inflamm 6:179, 1998.

29. Thakur A, Willcox MD. Cytokine and lipid inflammatory mediator profile of human tears during contact lens associated inflammatory disease. Exp Eye Res 67:9, 1998.

30. Abelson MB. Lipoxygenase products in ocular inflammation (abstract). Invest Ophthalmol Vis Sci 25 Suppl:42, 1984.

31. Nathan H, Naveh H, Meyer E. Levels of prostaglandin E_2 and leukotriene B_4 in tears of vernal conjunctivitis patients during a therapeutic trial

with indomethacin. Doc Ophthalmol 85:247, 1994.

32. Weston JH, Abelson MB. Leukotriene C_4 in rabbit and human eyes (abstract). Invest Ophthalmol Vis Sci 26 Suppl:191, 1985.

33. Smedegard G, Heqvist P, Dahlen SE, et al. Leukotriene C_4 affects pulmonary and cardiovascular dynamics in monkey. Nature 295:327, 1982.

34. Weiss JW, Drazen JM, Coles N, et al. Bronchoconstrictor effects of leukotriene C in humans. Science 216:196, 1982.

35. Hansson G, Bjorck T, Dahlen SE, et al. Specific allergen induces contraction of bronchi and formation of leukotrienes C_4, D_4, and E_4 in human asthmatic lung. Adv Prostaglandin Thromboxane Leukotriene Res 12:153, 1983.

36. Burke JA, Levi R, Corey EJ. Cardiovascular effects of pure synthetic leukotrienes C and D. Fed Proc 40:1015, 1981.

37. Levi R, Burke JA, Corey EJ. SRS-A, leukotrienes and immediate hypersensitivity reactions of the heart. Adv Prostaglandin Thromboxane Leukot Res 9:215, 1982.

38. Drazen JM, Austen KF, Lewis RA, et al. Comparative airway and vascular activities of leukotrienes C_1 and D in vivo and in vitro. Proc Natl Acad Sci USA 77:4354, 1980.

39. Hedquist P, Dahlen SE, Gustafsson L, et al. Biological profile of leukotrienes C_4 and D_4. Acta Physiol Scand 110:331, 1980.

40. Vafeas C, Mieyal PA, Urbano F, et al. Hypoxia stimulates the synthesis of cytochrome P450–derived inflammatory eicosanoids in rabbit corneal epithelium. J Pharmacol Exp Ther 287:903, 1998.

41. Conners MS, Urbano F, Vafeas C, et al. Alkali burn–induced synthesis of inflammatory eicosanoids in rabbit corneal epithelium. Invest Ophthalmol Vis Sci 38:1963, 1997.

42. Lundgren JD, Shelhamer JH, Kaliner MA. The role of eicosanoids in respiratory mucus hypersecretion. Ann Allergy 55:5, 1985.

43. Horak F, Toth J, Hirschwehr R, et al. Effect of continuous allergen challenge on clinical symptoms and mediator release in dust mite–allergic patients. Allergy 53:68, 1998.

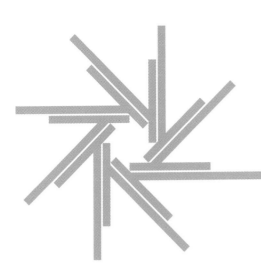

CHAPTER 13

Prostaglandins

MARK B. ABELSON ■ **KELLY K. GRANT** ■ **MATTHEW J. CHAPIN**

The prostaglandins are a complex group of oxygenated fatty acids that have been detected in virtually all mammalian species. Prostaglandins include some of the most potent natural substances known and are important both as bioregulators and as participants in pathological states. They are released in small amounts in conjunction with normal physiological processes such as neuromuscular events or synaptic transmission. Much larger amounts are released from tissues in connection with pathophysiological and pathological processes, such as overstimulation, tissue damage, or phagocytosis. Prostaglandins are not stored by tissue, but rather, they are synthesized as a result of membrane disturbances that cause the release of free fatty acids, generally arachidonic acid, from esterified lipid sources. On its release from the plasma membrane, arachidonic acid is broken down by a process known as the arachidonic acid cascade. Free arachidonic acid acts as a substrate for cyclooxygenase, the first enzyme in the pathway of prostaglandin synthesis. Cyclooxygenase oxygenates arachidonic acid to the endoperoxide intermediate, prostaglandin G_2 (PGG_2), which is then converted to other biologically active products, the nature of which is determined by the enzyme content of the tissue under consideration. PGG_2 is converted into PGH_2, which may be converted into PGI_2 by prostacyclin synthetase, PGF_2 by reductase, PGD_2 by isomerase, or PGE_2 by isomerase as well.

Prostaglandins contribute to the signs and symptoms of diseases ranging from rheumatoid arthritis to acute allergic disorders. The original discovery of the biological activity of prostaglandins was based on the identification of smooth muscle contraction and vasodilator activity present in human semen. The term "prostaglandin" resulted from the erroneous conclusion that the prostate gland was the primary source of these lipid-soluble acids.

SYSTEMIC EFFECTS

Although prostaglandins alone do not cause pain, they do sensitize pain receptors to other mediators. The subdermal injection of prostaglandins in humans results in an increase in pain sensitivity to chemical and mechanical stimulation. These effects are cumulative and depend not only on the amount of prostaglandin administered, but also on the duration of exposure.[1]

Fever can be induced by injection of small amounts of PGE_1 or PGE_2 into the central nervous system of cats,[2] where the substance acts at the thermoregulatory center in the pre-optic area of the hypothalamus. Fever is also induced by $PGF_{2\alpha}$ when it is infused into women for the purpose of inducing abortion.[3]

Other effects attributed to prostaglandins include bronchospasm ($PGF_{2\alpha}$, PGD_2),[4, 5, 5a] pulmonary vasodilation and inhibition of platelet aggregation (PGI_2),[6] inhibition of macrophage spreading and surface adherence (PGE_2),[7] bronchodilation,[8] vasodilation,[9] and erythema (PGE_1 and PGE_2).[10] PGE_2 has been reported to prevent allergen-induced bronchoconstrictor responses. Inhaled PGE_2 attenuated allergen-induced early decline in forced expiratory volume, hyperresponsiveness, and inflammation.[10a, 10b]

OCULAR EFFECTS

The earliest studies on prostaglandins in the eye revealed that these substances were released in response to ocular injury, and they mediated inflammatory events such as breakdown of the anterior segment blood-aqueous barrier. Later experiments demonstrated the proinflammatory effects of prostaglandins in the eye. Importantly, because the basic cell membrane is impermeable to prostaglandins and because prostaglandins are not effectively metabolized by ocular tissues, the carrier-mediated active transport processes play a primary role in terminating the effects of locally produced prostaglandins by preventing their accumulation in intraocular tissues and fluid compartments. Active transmembrane transport is demonstrated by the concentrated accumulation of prostaglandins by tissues of the anterior uvea and choroid plexus.[11] Prostaglandin biosynthesis has been found to occur in the iris, in the conjunctival tissue, in the ciliary body, and, to a lesser degree, in the corneal and retinal tissues. PGE_1, PGE_2, $PGF_{2\alpha}$, and PGD_2 have all been isolated from the ocular tissue and aqueous humor.[12]

In experimentally induced uveitis, the transport mechanism across the ciliary processes that normally eliminates PGE_2 from the eye rapidly no longer functions adequately. Although prostaglandins do not have direct effects on vascular permeability, PGE_2 markedly enhances edema formation by promoting blood flow in the inflamed region. However, PGEs inhibit the participation of lymphocytes in delayed hypersensitivity reactions. They also inhibit the release of hydrolases and lysosomal enzymes from human neutrophils as well as from mouse peritoneal macrophages.

PGD_2 is the primary prostaglandin produced by the mast cell in type I hypersensitivity reactions. When topically applied to guinea pig or human eyes, PGD_2 causes redness, conjunctival chemosis, a discharge of tenacious mucus, and an eosinophilic infiltrate. Similar signs are seen in patients with ocular allergic disorders.[13]

Topical application of PGJ_2, a metabolite of PGD_2, to the eyes of guinea pigs resulted in eosinophil infiltration into the conjunctival epithelium[14] and goblet cell discharge with resultant mucus hypersecretion.[15] Similar challenge with PGE_2 produced an itch-scratch response that was more dramatic than that observed with either PGD_2 or $PGF_{2\alpha}$. Although prostaglandins enhance sensitivity to pain, much of the pain and itching associated with an inflammatory response may be caused by lipoperoxides formed during the synthesis of prostaglandin.

Evidence suggests that PGF may also be involved in allergic disease. Elevated tear levels of PGF were detected in patients with chronic trachoma and vernal conjunctivitis.[16] Although $PGF_{2\alpha}$ had a poor pruritogenic effect, it was capable of causing marked ocular surface hyperemia in human volunteers, similar to that seen with PGD_2.[17, 18]

A study of experimental allergic conjunctivitis revealed that tear levels of PGI_2[19] and PGD_2 are substantially elevated following allergic provocation.[20–22] PGD_2 peaked within 2 hours of provocation and was mitigated with oral loratadine.[20] Non–mast cell origins of PGI_2 have been proposed, including infiltrating leukocytes and resident cells such as those associated with the vasculature.[19] Certainly, infiltrating leukocytes, notably eosinophils, are a hallmark of allergic conjunctivitis and are likely to contribute inflammatory mediators in addition to those released from mast cells.[15]

Studies also suggest that certain prostaglandins may have anti-inflammatory actions, participating in the negative feedback system that makes the allergic response self-limiting. PGE_1 and PGE_2 decrease secretion of anaphylactic mediators in a dose-related manner; this action is mirrored by changes in intracellular cyclic adenosine monophosphate. Those prostaglandins that are the most potent stimulators of cyclic adenosine monophosphate are also the most potent inhibitors of histamine release. It has become increasingly evident that prostaglandins not only act as mediators of pathological processes, but also play a significant role as regulators of mediator secretion in allergic reactions.[23]

PROSTAGLANDIN INHIBITION

Many of the common medications used to control pain, fever, and inflammation are primarily effective as a result of inhibition of prostaglandin metabolism. Aspirin, possessing anti-inflammatory activity, irreversibly inhibits cyclooxygenase by acetylation of the enzyme, thereby reducing levels of prostaglandins. Corticosteroids exert their anti-inflammatory actions by blocking the action of phospholipases, thus reducing the availability of arachidonic acid for prostaglandin metabolism. The nonsteroidal anti-inflammatory drugs, such as indomethacin, prevent cyclooxygenase from converting arachidonic acid to the cyclic endoperoxides. Aspirin, steroids, and nonsteroidal anti-inflammatory drugs are nonspecific in their depressive effect on prostaglandin synthesis; thus, they cannot generally be used to inhibit any one of the termination products selectively.[24]

REFERENCES

1. Ferreira SH. Prostaglandins, aspirin-like drugs and analgesia. Nature (New Biol) 240:200, 1972.
2. Milton AS, Wendlandt S. A possible role for prostaglandin E_1 as a modulator for temperature regulation in the central nervous system of the cat. J Physiol (Lond) 207:76P, 1970.
3. Hendricks CH, Brenner WE, Ekbladh L, et al. Efficacy and tolerance of intravenous prostaglandins F_2 and E_2. Am J Obstet Gynecol 111:564, 1971.
4. Wasserman M. Bronchopulmonary responses to prostaglandin F_2 alpha, histamine and acetylcholine in the dog. Eur J Pharmacol 32:146, 1975.
5. Wasserman MA, DuCharme DW, Griffin RL, et

al. Bronchopulmonary and cardiovascular effects of prostaglandin D_2 in the dog. Prostaglandins 13:255, 1977.

5a. Montuschi P, Curro D, Ragazzoni E, et al. Anaphylaxis increases 8-iso-prostaglandin $F_{2\alpha}$ release from guinea-pig lung in vitro. Eur J Pharmacol 365:59–64, 1999.

6. Szczekilk A, Gryglewski RJ, Nizankowska E, et al. Pulmonary and anti-platelet effects of intravenous and inhaled prostacyclin in man. Prostaglandins 16:651, 1978.

7. Cantarow D, Cheung HT, Sundharadas G. Effects of prostaglandins on the spreading, adhesion, and migration of mouse peritoneal macrophages. Prostaglandins 16:39, 1978.

8. Mathe AA, Hedqvist P. Effect of prostaglandins F_2 alpha and E_2 on airway conductance in healthy subjects and asthmatic patients. Am Rev Respir Dis 111:313, 1975.

9. Soloman LM, Juhlin L, Kirschenbaum MB. Prostaglandin on cutaneous vasculature. J Invest Dermatol 51:280, 1968.

10. Crounkhorn P, Willis AL. Interaction between prostaglandins E and F given intradermally in the rat. Br J Pharmacol 41:507, 1971.

10a. Gauvreau GM, Watson RM, O'Byrne PM. Protective effects of inhaled PGE_2 on allergen-induced airway responses and airway inflammation. Am J Respir Crit Care Med 159:31–36, 1999.

10b. Kharitonov SA, Sapienza MA, Barnes PJ, Chung KE. Prostaglandins E_2 and $F_{2\alpha}$ reduce exhaled nitric oxide in normal and asthmatic subjects irrespective of airway caliber changes. Am J Respir Crit Care Med 158:1374–1378, 1998.

11. Bito LZ. Prostaglandins and other eicosanoids: their ocular transport, pharmacokinetics, and therapeutic effects. Trans Ophthalmol Soc U K 105:162, 1986.

12. Leopold IH. Advances in ocular therapy: anti-inflammatory agents. Am J Ophthalmol 78:759, 1074.

13. Abelson MB, Madiwale NA, Weston JH. The role of prostaglandin D_2 in allergic ocular disease. In:

Advances in immunology and immunopathology of the eye. O'Connor GR, Chandler JW, eds. New York, Masson, 1985, p 163.

14. Woodward DF, Hawley SB, Williams LS, et al. Studies on the ocular pharmacology of prostaglandin D_2. Invest Ophthalmol Vis Sci 31:138, 1990.

15. Woodward DF, Nieves AL, Hawley SB, et al. The pruritogenic and inflammatory effects of prostanoids in the conjunctiva. J Ocul Pharmacol Ther 11:339, 1995.

16. Dhir SP, Garg SK, Sharma YR, et al. Prostaglandins in human tears. Am J Ophthalmol 87:403, 1979.

17. Guiffre G. The effects of prostaglandin $F_{2\text{-alpha}}$ in the human eye. Graefes Arch Clin Exp Ophthalmol 222:139, 1985.

18. Nakajima M, Goh Y, Azuma I, et al. Effects of prostaglandin D_2 and its analog, BW 245C, on intraocular pressure in humans. Graefes Arch Clin Exp Ophthalmol 229:411, 1991.

19. Helleboid L, Khatami M, Wei ZG, et al. Histamine and prostacyclin: primary and secondary release in allergic conjunctivitis. Invest Ophthalmol Vis Sci 32:2281, 1991.

20. Horak F, Toth J, Hirschwehr R, et al. Effect of continuous allergen challenge on clinical symptoms and mediator release in dust mite–allergic patients. Allergy 53:68–72, 1998.

21. Aichane A, Campbell AM, Chanal I, et al. Precision of conjunctival provocation tests in right and left eyes. J Allergy Clin Immunol 92:49–55, 1993.

22. Proud D, Sweet J, Stein P, et al. Inflammatory mediator release on conjunctival provocation of allergic subjects with allergen. J Allergy Clin Immunol 85:896–905, 1990.

23. Morley J, Beets JL, Bray MA, et al. Regulation of allergic responses by prostaglandins: a review. J R Soc Med 72:443, 1980.

24. Poole MD, Pillsbury HC. Prostaglandins and other metabolites of arachidonic acid: an overview for the otolaryngologist. Arch Otolaryngol 111:317, 1985.

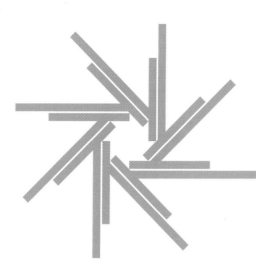

CHAPTER 14

Mast Cell Tryptase: Its Role in Ocular Allergic Inflammation

SALIM BUTRUS ■ **PAULA WUN**

Mast cells in the conjunctiva play an important role in ocular allergic inflammation. Similar to those in the skin and submucosa of the small intestine,[1] conjunctival mast cells are predominantly of the connective tissue type (CT cells). Their granules contain both neutral proteases, chymase, and tryptase.[2, 3] On the other hand, T mast cells, containing only tryptase, are found in lung tissue and small intestinal mucosa. Patients with vernal keratoconjunctivitis (VKC) and giant papillary conjunctivitis (GPC) have a pronounced increase of CT mast cells. However, in patients with VKC, T mast cells are also significantly elevated and are actively recruited.

Activated conjunctival CT mast cells release biologically potent chemical mediators including preformed substances such as biogenic amines (histamine and, in some rodents, serotonin), proteoglycans (heparin and chondroitin sulfates), neutral proteases (tryptase and chymase), acid hydrolases and cytokines, such as interleukin-4 and others.[3] Other mediators are synthesized de novo on appropriate stimulation and include products of arachidonic acid metabolism (e.g., prostaglandin $D_2[PGD_2]$ and leukotriene C_4 $[LTC_4]$), and cytokines such as tumor necrosis factor.

TABLE 14.1 Differences Between Tryptase and Histamine as Mast Cell Products*

	Amount/Mast Cell	Amount/Basophil	Half-life	Types	Immunoassay
Tryptase	10–35 pg	0.04 pg	1.5–2 hr	α, β	Yes $B_{12\alpha,\beta}$ $G_{5\alpha}$
Histamine	1–3 pg	1–3 pg	1–3 min	—	Yes

* Several differences exist between tryptase and histamine as mast cell products. Notably, the half-life of tryptase in circulation is approximately 1.5 to 2 hours[6]; this is much longer than that of histamine, which is 1 to 3 minutes.

PHARMACOLOGICAL VALUE

Tryptase, a neutral serine protease, is concentrated in mast cell secretory granules. Basophils are the only other cell type with detectable but negligible, levels of tryptase, that are several hundredfold lower than in mast cells. Other mediators such as histamine are secreted from basophils[4, 5] whereas PGD_2 and LTC_4 are secreted from both leukocytes and monocytes. The half-life of tryptase in the circulation is approximately 1.5 to 2 hours[6]; this is much longer than that of histamine, which is 1 to 3 minutes (Table 14.1). PGD_2 and LTC_4 are rapidly metabolized, rendering their detection difficult. The two types of recombinant tryptase are termed a and b. Two primary immunoassays are employed to measure tryptase in plasma and in body fluids. The B_{12} assay measures both a and b tryptase, whereas the G_5 assay measures primarily b tryptase. With each immunoassay, comparable levels of tryptase can be measured in serum or plasma during insect sting–induced systemic anaphylaxis, in which levels correlate to the severity of the clinical reaction. Tryptase is not detectable by G_5 immunoassay (less than 1 ng/mL) in serum and plasma obtained from healthy subjects; however, the B_{12} immunoassay reveals that serum and plasma samples actually contain approximately 5 ng/mL of tryptase.

ENZYMATIC ACTIVITY

Tryptase cleaves peptide and ester bonds on the carboxyl side of the basic amino acids, arginine and lysine. The enzyme has a particular affinity for tripeptide substrates with basic amino acid residues at the P1 and P2 positions.[8] Tryptase is a tetrameric protein with an active site at each of the four glycosylated subunits, and it is stabilized in its active tetrameric form by an ionic association with heparin. Once the tryptase is free from heparin, as in plasma, it dissolves into its four subunits, undergoes significant structural change, and is irreversibly inactivated.[9]

We have shown significant elevation of tryptase levels in tears obtained from patients with VKC (60–500 ng/mL; mean, 400), GPC (less than 40–1760 ng/mL; mean, 70), and symptomatic allergic conjunctivitis (less than 40–820 ng/mL; mean, 70). Normal levels (less than or equal to 40 ng/mL) were seen in controls, in patients with nonallergic ocular inflammation,[10] and in those with asymptomatic seasonal allergic conjunctivitis. Furthermore, we were able to demonstrate tryptase release in human tears after provoking the conjunctivae with different allergens, compound 48/80, and knuckle rubbing. Tryptase levels in tears are considered to be sensitive markers to diagnose and follow ocular allergic disease.[11] They can also be used to monitor therapy and to compare different mast cell stabilizing agents.

The role of tryptase in ocular allergy is not fully understood. Several biological activities of the enzyme have been identified, including the following: (1) to degrade fibrinogen[12]; (2) to potentiate the effects of histamine on bronchoconstriction[13]; (3) to hydrolyze neuropeptides that cause bronchodilation[14]; (4) to activate prostromelysin[15]; (5) to degrade fibronectin[16]; (6) to stimulate fibroblast proliferation[17]; (7) to produce $C3_a$ from human $C3$[18]; and (8) to activate mast cells (Table 14.2).[19] It has been shown that tryptase when applied topically to the ocular surface has no biological effect on rabbit eyes.[20]

Although studies on ocular mast cell tryptase are scarce, there is no doubt that tryptase is emerging as an important mediator and target for therapeutic intervention in rhinitis, conjunctivitis, and most notably asthma. Reports exist that tryptase alters the mechanical activity of animal airway smooth muscle and spontaneously sensitized human isolated airways, as well as increases the histamine reactivity of bronchi. These effects of tryptase on histamine-induced contraction were completely abrogated in the presence of the protease inhibitor benzamidine. The physiological changes were accompanied by increases in mast cell numbers in the tryptase-exposed subepithelial tissue and by decreases in the epithelial layer, suggesting that the alterations in bronchial contractile response are mediated by changes in mast cell distribution within the airway walls.[20]

Tryptase has been found to stimulate the release of histamine from mucosal mast cells in vitro, acting as an amplification signal for mast cell activation.[21] The potent granulocyte chemoattractant IL-8 was released in a dose-dependent fashion in response to physiologically relevant doses of tryptase in human umbilical vein endothelial cells. This effect was negated by heat inactivation, suggesting the necessity for an intact catalytic site on tryptase. Up-regulation of IL-8 as well as IL-1 beta was also shown, indicating that the leukocyte chemotaxis stimulated by tryptase may be mediated in part by the selective secretion of IL-8 from vascular endothelial cells.[22]

Further studies have confirmed the specificity and reliability of tryptase measurement as a marker for allergic activation and a parameter that

---

✳ TABLE 14.2 Functions of Tryptase*

Functions of Tryptase	Potential Significance
Degradation of fibrinogen	Prevention of clotting at local sites of mast cell activation
Potentiation of the effects of histamine on bronchoconstriction	Increase in hypersensitivity reactions to histamine and allergens
Hydrolysis of bronchodilatory neuropeptides	Increase in hypersensitivity reactions to histamine and allergens
Activation of prostromelysin	Tissue repair
Degradation of fibronectin	Tissue repair
Stimulation of fibroblast proliferation	Tissue repair and wound healing
Production of C3a	Increase in effects of hypersensitivity reactions
Activation of mast cell	Increase in effects of hypersensitivity reactions

* Although the role of tryptase in ocular allergy is not fully understood, several biological activities have been identified.

reflects the efficacy of therapy. In two studies on the beneficial effects of immunotherapy, nasal tryptase released after allergen provocation was found significantly decreased compared with baseline.[23, 24]

Tryptase inhibitors have potent mast cell–inhibiting properties. The availability of potent and selective tryptase inhibitors has facilitated the evaluation of this protease as a target for pharmacological modulation. Four classes of selective tryptase inhibitors have been isolated and tested in the airways and skin of sheep—three synthetic and one natural in origin: (1) peptidic inhibitors (e.g., APC-366); (2) dibasic inhibitors (e.g., pentamidine-like); (3) Zn^{2+}-mediated inhibitors (e.g., BABIM-like), and (4) heparin antagonists (e.g., lactoferrin). Aerosol administration of each class of tryptase inhibitor 30 minutes, 4 hours, and 24 hours after allergen challenge abolished late phase bronchoconstriction and airway hyperresponsiveness in a dose-dependent manner. Intradermal injection of the first generation tryptase inhibitor, APC-366, was also shown to block the cutaneous response to antigen. Clinical studies are ongoing. In phase II for this novel drug, further evidence was provided of a pathological role of tryptase in allergic disease.[25] The possibility of a topical ocular tryptase inhibitor effective for the broad range of mast cell–mediated ocular allergic diseases is an exciting direction for future studies.

REFERENCES

1. Irani AA, Schechter NM, Craig SS, et al. Two types of human mast cells that have distinct neutral protease compositions. Proc Natl Acad Sci U S A 83:4464, 1986.
2. Irani AA, Butrus SI, Tabbara KF, et al. Human conjunctival mast cells: Distribution of MC_T and MC_{Tc} in vernal conjunctivitis and giant papillary conjunctivitis. J Allergy Clin Immunol 86:34, 1990.
3. Schwartz LB, Irani AA, Roller K, et al. Quantization of histamine, tryptase and chymase in dispersed human T and Tc mast cells. J Immunol 138:2611, 1987.
4. Schwartz LB, Austin KF. The mast cell and mediators of immediate hypersensitivity. In: Immunological diseases. 4th ed. Vol. 1. Sauter M, Talinage DW, Frank MM, et al., eds. Boston, Little, Brown, 1988, p 157.
5. Castell MC, Irani AA, Schwartz LB. Evaluation of human peripheral blood leukocytes for mast cell tryptase. J Immunol 138:2184, 1987.
6. Schwartz LB, Yunginger JW, Miller J, et al. Time course of appearance and disappearance of human mast cell tryptase in the circulation after anaphylaxis. J Clin Invest 83:1551, 1989.
7. Schwartz LB, Sakal K, Bradford TR, et al. The a form of human tryptase is the predominant type present in blood at baseline in normal subjects, and is elevated in those with systemic mastocytosis. J Clin Invest 96:7, 1995.
8. Cromlish JA, Siedah M, Marcinkiewicz J, et al. Human pituitary tryptase: molecular forms, NH_2-terminal sequence, immunocytochemical localization, and specificity with prohormone and fluorogenic substrates. J Biol Chem 262:1363, 1987.
9. Schwartz LB. Laboratory assessment of immediate hypersensitivity and anaphylaxis: use of tryptase as a marker of mast cell-dependent events. Diagn Lab Immunol 14:339, 1994.
10. Butrus SI, Ochsner KI, Abelson MB, et al. The level of tryptase in human tears: an indicator of activation of conjunctival mast cells. Ophthalmology 97:1678, 1990.
11. Butrus SI, Abelson MB. Laboratory evaluation of ocular allergy. Int Ophthalmol Clin 28:324, 1988.
12. Schwartz, LB, Bradford TR, Littman BH, et al. The fibrinogenolytic activity of purified tryptase from human lung mast cells. J Immunol 135: 2762, 1985.
13. Sekizawa K, Caughey GH, Lazarus SC, et al. Mast cell tryptase causes airway smooth muscle hyperresponsiveness in dogs. J Clin Invest 83: 175, 1989.
14. Tom EK, Caughey GH. Degradation of airway neuropeptides by human lung tryptase. Am J Respir Cell Mol Biol 3:27, 1990.
15. Schwartz LB. Tryptase: a mediator of human mast cells. J Allergy Clin Immunol 86:594, 1990.
16. Lohi J, Harvima I, Keski-Oja T. Pericellular substrates of human mast cell tryptase: 72,000 dalton gelatinase and fibronectin. J Cell Biochem 50:337, 1992.
17. Hartmann T, Ruoss SJ, Raymond WW, et al. Human tryptase as a potent, cell-specific mitogen: role of signaling pathways in synergistic responses. Am J Physiol 262:6528, 1992.
18. Schwartz LB, Kawahara MS, Hugli TE, et al. Generation of C3a anaphylatoxin from human C3 by human mast cell tryptase. J Immunol 130: 1891, 1983.
19. Craig SS, Schechter NM, Schwartz LB. Ultrastructural analysis of maturing human T and TC mast cells in situ. Lab Invest 60:147, 1989.
20. Berger P, Compton SJ, Moliard M, et al. Mast

cell tryptase as a mediator of hyperresponsiveness in human isolated bronchi. Clin Exp Allergy 29:804–812, 1999.

21. He S, Gaca MD, Walls AF. A role for tryptase in the activation of human mast cells: modulation of histamine release by tryptase and inhibitors of tryptase. J Pharmacol Exp Ther 286:289–297, 1998.

22. Compton SJ, Cairns JA, Holgate ST, Walls AF. The role of mast cell tryptase in regulating endothelial cell proliferation, cytokine release, and adhesion molecule expression: tryptase induces expression of mRNA for IL-1beta and IL-8 and stimulates the selective release of IL-8 from human umbilical vein endothelial cells. J Immunol 161:1939–1946, 1998.

23. Klimek L, Wolf H, Mewes T, et al. The effect of short-term immunotherapy with molecular standardized grass and rye allergens on eosinophil cationic protein and tryptase in nasal secretions. J Allergy Clin Immunol 103:47–53, 1999.

24. Carlos AG, Carlos ML, Santos MA, et al. Immunotherapy and mast cell activation. Allerg Immunol (Paris) 30(8):257–258, 1998.

25. Rice KD, Tanaka RD, Katz BA, Numerof RP, Moore WR. Inhibitors of tryptase for the treatment of mast cell mediated diseases. Curr Pharm Des 4(5):381–396, 1998.

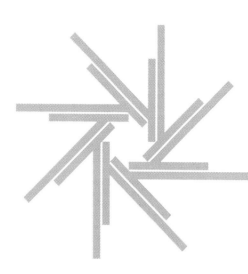

CHAPTER 15

Acute Allergic Conjunctivitis

LOUIS M. T. COLLUM ■ **DARA J. KILMARTIN**

Acute allergic conjunctivitis is the most prevalent allergic disease of the eye. Acute allergic conjunctivitis is usually a 24-hour phenomenon. The clinical course of acute allergic conjunctivitis differs from that of seasonal allergic conjunctivitis (SAC) or hay fever conjunctivitis, but their basic origin and pathogenesis have significant similarities. Acute allergic conjunctivitis is frequently associated with other allergic conditions, such as allergic rhinitis, skin allergies, and asthma. Patients frequently have a positive family history for atopy.

Although acute allergic conjunctivitis is not a sight-threatening condition, it may be associated with significant morbidity in patients and an inability to carry on normal activities. This finding is in contrast to some of the more severe allergic conditions of the eye, such as vernal conjunctivitis and eczematous keratoconjunctivitis, which can be sight-threatening. The management of acute allergic conjunctivitis is usually simple and does not require toxic or systemic medications.

EPIDEMIOLOGY

Atopic disease has been estimated to occur in approximately 20% of the population.[1, 2] Allergies usually begin in childhood and many "burn out" at puberty.[3] The disease can often recur later. A smaller percentage of the population develops allergic disease later in life.

In addition, one frequently notes a strong genetic pattern in the patients who develop atopic disease later in life, who commonly have a positive family history of related allergies.[4] Approximately 70% of patients with asthma and hay fever have positive family histories for allergic disorders.[1] Patients who are homozygous for atopy tend to develop the allergic disease at an earlier age and the allergy tends to be more severe and chronic. Compared with a child with no family history of atopy, a child who has one atopic parent has approximately a 4-fold increased likelihood of developing allergies. A child with both parents having atopy has a 10 times greater likelihood of developing allergies. Apart from allergic conjunctivitis, conditions such as asthma, hay fever, dermatitis, and rhinitis have all been shown to have genetic associations.[4]

Geographical location is a significant factor. Both seasonal and perennial allergens can be involved. Seasonal allergens include those associated with tree pollination, which occurs in the spring, grasses growing in the summer, and ragweed reactions in the late summer and early fall. In addition, outdoor molds such as *Cladosporium* may also be involved. Perennial allergens include house dust mites, various molds, and animal dander. One may note a strong seasonal preponderance for allergens that may otherwise be considered perennial. Seasonal allergic disease is more common than perennial disease. This finding is surprising given that the house dust mite, which is the most common perennial allergen, is present at all times and in many homes. Therefore, some allergens probably affect the conjunctiva more severely than others, or a significant individual variation in response may exist.

The ocular allergic response is initiated when allergen dissolves in the tears and binds with immunoglobulin E (IgE) antibodies, which occupy the Fc receptors on the conjunctival mast cells. The ensuing mast cell degranulation with the release of various mediators produces a myriad of clinical signs and symptoms. Whether the condition is perennial or seasonal depends on the causative agent, the volume of allergen present, and the individual response of patients.

CLINICAL FEATURES

For the purposes of this chapter, we consider acute allergic conjunctivitis and SAC (caused by hay fever and ragweed) as two separate entities.

Acute Allergic Conjunctivitis

Acute allergic conjunctivitis occurs suddenly and rapidly in susceptible patients. It is a local reaction manifested as acute lid and conjunctival edema. The eyes are watery, and the edematous conjunctiva may bulge through the eyelids. The lids may become so swollen that they close completely. The watery discharge may become mucoid or, if secondary infection develops, purulent. The condition lasts approximately 24 hours and clears quickly when the patient is no longer in contact with the allergen. By the time patients seek medical attention, their severe symptoms and clinical signs usually have abated and they are left with a mildly irritated, watery eye.

A diagnostic pathognomonic clinical symptom is itching. Although itching is usually bilateral, one eye may be more severely affected than the other. Because the signs and symptoms are so clearly diagnostic, the condition is unlikely to be confused with anything else.

Seasonal Allergic Conjunctivitis

The signs and symptoms of SAC are less dramatic than those of acute allergic conjunctivitis, although the pathophysiological features are similar. SAC can develop suddenly when the patient comes in contact with an appropriate antigen, such as pollen. However, in most patients, the onset of symptoms develops more gradually. The patient develops a watery discharge from the eye, and itching is a prominent feature. The eye is hyperemic, and the patient may have slight ptosis (Fig. 15.1). SAC is frequently associated with allergic rhinitis.[5] A late-phase–like component may accompany the allergic response. However, whether a true late-phase response (LPR) occurs in ocular allergy is controversial.

The severity of signs and symptoms varies from day to day, often fluctuating with pollen counts. Sensitive persons should monitor the pollen count to reduce the frequency and severity of allergic reactions.

A few entities mimic SAC or hay fever conjunctivitis. Conditions such as tear disease or chronic blepharitis (Fig. 15.2) tend to be more persistent and generally are not associated with true itching. However, patients with tear defects may be more prone to allergic conjunctivitis because of their inability to wash away allergens from the conjunctival sac. A full assessment of tear function and stability should be carried out as part of the differential diagnosis of SAC.

Infectious conjunctivitis should be considered in the differential diagnosis, and appropriate laboratory tests should be conducted to exclude bacterial, chlamydial, and viral infections. The clinical signs, however, should permit the correct diagnosis.

Conditions such as vernal keratoconjunctivitis (VKC), giant papillary conjunctivitis (GPC), and atopic keratoconjunctivitis are unlikely to present a diagnostic dilemma because the signs and symptoms are more aggressive and often different (e.g., cobblestones, Trantas' dots). During seasons of low pollen counts or relative lack of sunshine, the incidence and severity of SAC and hay fever allergic conjunctivitis are significantly reduced.[6]

DIAGNOSIS AND DIAGNOSTIC TOOLS

Systematic and careful examination of the patient usually leads the clinician to the correct diagnosis. In some patients, the clinician may need to resort to laboratory tests, although such tests are generally confirmatory and academic. From a clinical point of view, the classic symptom indicating the presence of an allergic phenomenon is itching. However, patients may complain of watering, irritation, and grittiness, which occurs in other conditions such as tear film disease, lid margin disease, meibomianitis, and atmospheric pollution irritation. The amount of discharge tends to vary, but the classic discharge is watery or slightly mucoid. In addition, 70% of patients provide either a personal or familial allergic history.[5]

In acute and hay fever allergic conjunctivitis, papillae are not a feature, but a follicular reaction with mild conjunctival edema (chemosis) is not uncommon. Nonspecific hyperemia of both the bulbar and palpebral conjunctiva is present. In addition, the patient may have slight lid edema as a result of irritation.

Laboratory tests may be used to confirm a diagnosis or to establish a diagnosis in the few patients who have no classic symptoms and signs at the time of examination. The simplest laboratory test is examination of conjunctival scrapings for eosinophils. Eosinophils are present in scrapings

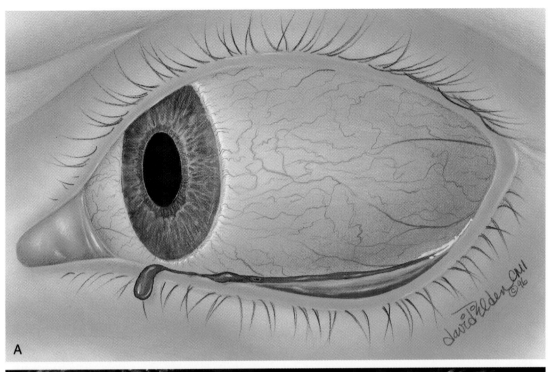

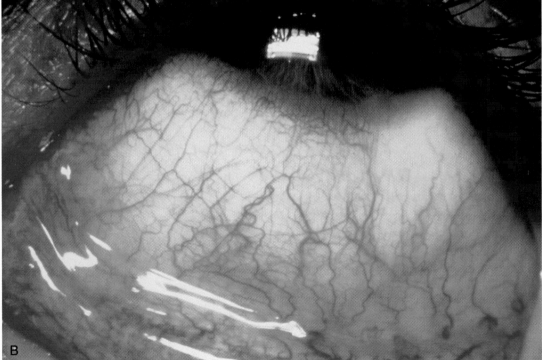

FIGURE 15.1 *A* and *B,* The clinical presentation of seasonal allergic conjunctivitis is similar to that of acute allergic conjunctivitis. Hyperemia, itching, chemosis, and tearing occur in both types of allergic responses.

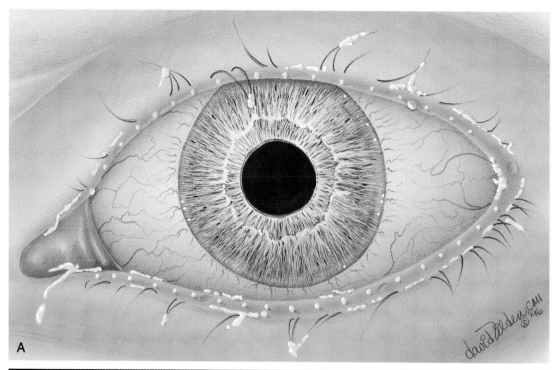

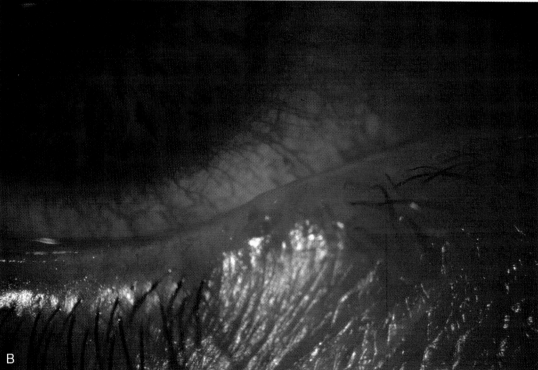

FIGURE 15.2 *A* and *B*, Conditions such as blepharitis may mimic the signs and symptoms of allergic conjunctivitis. These conditions tend to be more persistent, however, and are generally not associated with true itching.

in 20 to 80% of cases of acute allergic conjunctivitis.[7, 8] Abelson and associates[9] found that 45% of their patients with hay fever conjunctivitis had eosinophils in their conjunctival scrapings. A negative scraping does not necessarily rule out the diagnosis of allergic conjunctivitis because the harvesting of these eosinophils depends on the technique and vigor used in taking the scrapings. Eosinophils may be situated deep within the conjunctiva, a finding that may account for negative results.[7]

Tear levels of IgE are elevated in most patients.[10–12] In addition, serum IgE levels are elevated and correlate with tear IgE levels (when tear IgE is greater than 4 IU/mL).[13] The radioallergosorbent test measures specific IgE levels for a specific allergen. However, this test is not as sensitive as skin testing and is really only applicable in patients in whom skin testing is contraindicated.

Skin testing can be performed readily, and various techniques are employed. Severity of antigenic response can be assessed by using different concentrations of the test allergen. In addition, conjunctival provocation tests may be carried out, although some clinicians may find these tests troublesome and probably not applicable to most clinical situations.

Mast cell activity can be estimated by using immunoassays for tryptase. The enzyme is unique to mast cells, but it is detectable only in the early-phase reaction. Histamine levels in the tear film can also be measured. As with tryptase, detection of histamine depends on the amount of time between the initiation of the allergic reaction and the tear collection.

Laboratory testing may be useful for complete documentation and workup of both suspected and well-established cases of acute allergic conjunctivitis. However, in the majority of cases, it is not necessary.

PATHOPHYSIOLOGY

The pathophysiology of acute allergic conjunctivitis is multifaceted. However, all components of the inflammatory response and mediator cascade follow the initial mast cell degranulation. Acute allergic conjunctivitis is traditionally thought to be an immediate (type I) hypersensitivity reaction (Fig. 15.3). Allergenic proteins dissolve in the tear film and bind to IgE antibodies that adhere to the mast or basophil cell membrane and cause cell degranulation. IgE is the principal cytotropic immunoglobulin in humans; however, in experimental animals, both IgE[14] and IgG[15] act as cytotropic antibodies and exhibit different abilities to cause mast cell sensitization.[16]

In sensitized individuals, crosslinking of antigen with IgE antibodies bound to Fc receptors on mast cells causes the receptors to aggregate.[17] This event leads to mast cell degranulation and release of chemical mediators that produce the signs and symptoms of acute allergic conjunctivitis. Preformed mediators from secretory granules are released immediately, and mast cells are stimulated to synthesize and secrete mediators derived from arachidonic acid.

Mast cell degranulation accounts for the immediate reaction in sensitized individuals exposed to antigen. Acute allergic conjunctivitis usually resolves rapidly on removal of the antigen, but immediate hypersensitivity reactions may not be always short-lived. In human skin, the Prausnitz-Kustner wheal-and-flare reaction[18] to intracutaneous antigen injection in a sensitized person is immediate, but it may be followed by a late recurrence of signs and symptoms. This LPR peaks at 6 to 8 hours and may last up to 12 hours.[19] The classic definition of an LPR is a clinical, histological, or chemical response to an antigen that occurs 3 to 12 hours after the initial acute (early-phase) mast cell–mediated allergic reaction[20] (Fig. 15.4).

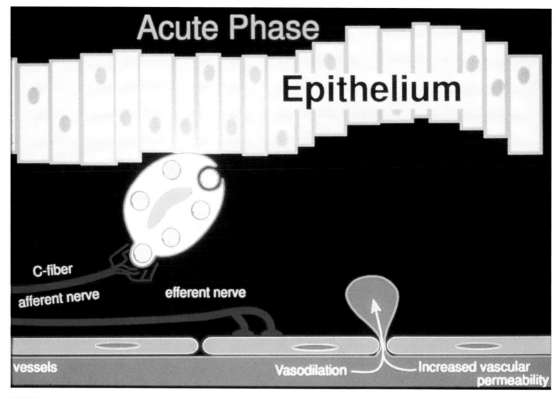

FIGURE 15.3 Histamine and other mediators released during mast cell degranulation lead to hyperemia and itching associated with acute allergic conjunctivitis.

LPRs have been described in bronchial asthma,[21] allergic rhinitis,[22] and cutaneous reactions.[23] A conjunctival LPR has been described in an experimental animal model of ocular type I hypersensitivity[24] and in SAC in human patients.[25] Eosinophils and neutrophils most likely play a role in the LPR in human skin,[26] although the extent of LPR in allergic conjunctivitis is controversial.[27] Bonini and Bonini[5] suggested that the pathophysiology of acute allergic conjunctivitis is multifactorial and is not solely the result of a type I hypersensitivity reaction. Non–IgE-mediated mast cell activation, nonspecific conjunctival hyperactivity, and conjunctival LPR may confound the pathophysiological features.

ACUTE (EARLY-PHASE) REACTION

Mast Cell

In the normal conjunctiva, mast cells are rarely found in the epithelium, with the majority located in the substantia propria. Conjunctival mast cells have been counted and biochemically differentiated in both normal[28] and allergic conjunctivae.[29] Mast cells are of essentially two types, the connective tissue type (MCtc) and the mucosal type (MCt), which differ morphologically and biochemically. This differentiation was first described in the rat by Enerback,[30] who noted a consistent relationship between morphology and function. Befus et al.[31] found similar mast cell subtypes in humans. Mast

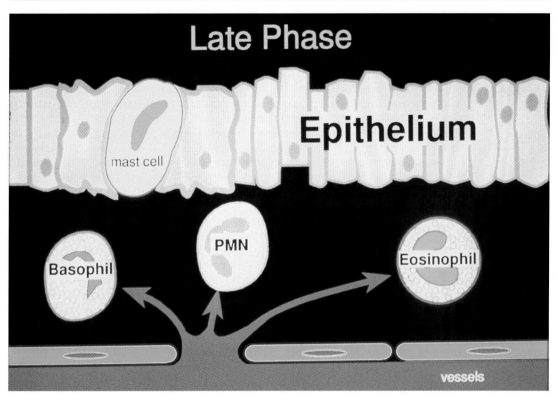

FIGURE 15.4 The late-phase reaction, which occurs 6 to 12 hours following exposure to allergen, may be mediated by basophils, eosinophils, and polymorphonuclear leukocytes (PMN).

cell subtyping is based on neutral protease composition. MCtc cells contain tryptase and chymase in their granules, whereas the second type of mast cell (MCt), which resembles the mucosal type, contains only tryptase.[29] MCtc cells are more numerous than MCt cells, and one sees a marked increase in the number of mast cells (MCtc) in the substantia propria and subepithelial region in acute allergic conjunctivitis, vernal conjunctivitis, and GPC.[32]

Tears can be analyzed to study immunoglobulin and mediator characteristics in allergic eye disease. The level of tryptase in tears is an indicator of mast cell activation (normal tear tryptase is 40 ng/mL or less).[34] Tryptase is elevated in the tears of patients with acute allergic conjunctivitis, vernal conjunctivitis, and GPC.[33] Elevated levels of total tear IgE and pollen-specific tear IgE were found by Dart et al. in allergic conjunctivitis.[20] Usually, a correlation exists between tear and serum IgE levels[13] found when serum IgE is greater than 100 IU/mL and tear IgE is greater than 4 IU/mL. Serum levels of IgE are low in healthy persons (around 1/50,000 the concentration of IgG),[35] a finding that suggests that IgE production is tightly regulated. Extremely small doses of allergenic proteins are required to elicit IgE antibody production in atopic individuals. For example, investigators have estimated that only 1 μg of ragweed pollen antigen is inhaled per person per year in those with ragweed hay fever conjunctivitis.[36]

With allergen-IgE crosslinking and Fc receptor aggregation, mast cells are activated through a number of intracellular steps. A critical serine protease is activated,[36] and rapid influx of calcium ions occurs. Intracellular cyclic adenosine monophosphate (cAMP) levels drop. Granules containing preformed mediators migrate and fuse with the cell-surface membrane, discharging their contents by exocytosis. Preformed mediators include histamine, tryptase, chymase, carboxypeptidase, kininogenase, beta-glucosaminodase, cathepsin G–like protein, heparin, chondroitin sulfate, eosinophilic chemotactic factor, neutrophil chemotactic factor, platelet-activating factor (PAF), interleukin-3 (IL-3), IL-4, IL-5, and IL-6, granulocyte-macrophage–colony-stimulating factor, and tumor necrosis factor. Preformed mediators play a key role in the early-phase response. Mast cell activation also stimulates the synthesis of newly formed mediators derived from arachidonic acid. Membrane phospholipids liberate arachidonic acid through the activation of the enzyme, phospholipase A_2. Subsequent metabolism by cyclooxygenase produces prostaglandins and thromboxanes and, by lipoxygenase, produces leukotrienes, slow-releasing substance of anaphylaxis (leukotrienes C_4 [LTC_4] and LTD_4), hydroxyperoxyeicosatetraenoic acid (HPETE), and hydroxyeicosatetraenoic acid (HETE).

Studies have suggested that non–IgE-mediated activation of mast cells may occur.[5, 37] Possible non-IgE mast cell activators include T_H2 lymphocytes, which have been cloned from the conjunctival epithelium of patients with vernal conjunctivitis.[38] These cells produce IL-3 and IL-5, which have been shown to activate mast cells and eosinophils.[39] Bonini and Bonini[5] suggested that lymphocytes and macrophages in tears of patients with allergic conjunctivitis may release histamine-releasing factors on exposure to allergens and possibly bacterial and viral antigens. Ricci and colleagues[40] suggested that T_H2 lymphocytes are the best candidates to play a central role in acute allergic inflammation. T cells are the only cells that can directly recognize allergen peptides and release cytokines, which directly induce microvasculature changes and influence the migration and activation of inflammatory cells.

Negative feedback mechanisms regulate mast cell activation. As with many other secretory processes, the rate of granule release varies inversely with the levels of intracellular cAMP. Histamine, the main mediator of the early-phase response, interacts with mast cell histamine receptors to increase the levels of cAMP and to inhibit degranulation.[41, 42] Prostaglandins can also inhibit further degranulation by activating adenyl cyclase,[43] which raises cAMP levels. Beta-adrenergic receptor activation has also been shown to inhibit mast cell degranulation. By contrast, alpha-adrenergic receptor stimulation decreases cAMP levels and stimulates mediator release. Pharmacological modulation of cAMP levels provides important therapeutic strategies for inhibiting inflammatory mediator release. Drugs that stimulate adenyl cyclase activity (isoproterenol, epinephrine) or inhibit its metabolism by phosphodiesterase (aminophylline, theophylline) increase cAMP levels and decrease mediator release. Cholinergic stimulation increases cGMP levels and also promotes degranulation.

Basophil

Basophil degranulation takes place by the same IgE-mediated mechanisms as in mast cells, thus resulting in release of histamine and LTC_4.[44] Basophils respond to a wider range of possible activators, including complement components C5a and C3a, formulated bacterial products, cytokines, histamine-releasing factors, and PAF.[45] Basophils have been seen in biopsy specimens of LPRs in the skin.[46] Lichtenstein et al.[47, 48] showed with bronchoalveolar lavage in asthmatic patients that basophils were increased about 30-fold from the acute to the late phase, whereas mast cell numbers were unchanged. Bonini and colleagues[49] showed a marked increase from baseline of basophils (also neutrophils, eosinophils, and epithelial cells) in tears

6 hours after ocular allergen challenge. Therefore, as with eosinophils and polymorphonuclear lymphocytes, the delayed time course of the basophil may play a more important role in conjunctival LPR than the early-phase reaction.

Eosinophil

The eosinophil has a central effector role in allergic eye disease. Its role has been extensively studied using the conjunctival provocation test,[49-51] in which conjunctival eosinophilia[9] and increased numbers of eosinophils in tears[50] have been demonstrated. Conjunctival eosinophilia is characteristic of VKC and GPC.[9] In acute allergic conjunctivitis, eosinophils may be located deeper in the tissue, and their absence in a conjunctival scraping does not preclude the diagnosis.[7] Eosinophils possess membrane receptors for IgG, IgE, IgA, C3b, histamine, glucocorticoids, and PAF, thereby allowing interactions with immunoglobulins and antigens, and possible pharmacological manipulation.[52] These cells release preformed mediators such as major basic protein (MBP), major cationic protein, and eosinophil-derived neurotoxin. They can also release newly synthesized mediators such as prostaglandins, leukotrienes, and PAF. Eosinophil-derived mediators can modulate mast cell responses; histaminase inactivates histamine, phospholipase inactivates PAF, and aryl sulfatase inactivates certain leukotrienes.[53, 54] On the other hand, MBP can promote mast cell degranulation.[55] Eosinophils probably play a more important role in conjunctival LPR because eosinophilic migration does not occur until 1 to 6 hours after antigen challenge.[56]

Neutrophil

Circulating neutrophils are in a resting state and are attracted into the inflamed conjunctiva by chemotactic factors such as LTB_4, PAF, and IL-8.[57, 58] Neutrophils increase in number markedly approximately 6 hours after conjunctival allergen challenge[49] and so play a more important role in those who develop conjunctival LPR.

LATE-PHASE REACTION

Certain tissues in atopic patients, particularly the skin and lung, manifest a second allergic reaction in the absence of additional allergenic stimulus. This response is referred to as the LPR.[19, 59-63] An LPR has been described[64-70] as a dose-dependent inflammatory reaction with inflammatory cells in tears 6 hours after specific ocular challenge in both animals and human patients.[71] A small dose of allergen produces a limited allergic reaction with rapid spontaneous recovery, whereas a large dose produces a progressive response developing to an LPR.[68] The LPR can be biphasic, as in the nose, but more often it is continuous in the eye. Redness, tearing, itchiness, and foreign body sensation increase 4 to 8 hours after challenge and continue for up to 24 hours.[69] The clinical signs include increased numbers of neutrophils, eosinophils, and lymphocytes in tears.[69] However, the true incidence of ocular LPR outside the clinical research setting is controversial.

Eosinophils are the principal cells activated during the LPR, with consequent release of eosinophil-derived mediators.[5] Increased levels of histamine and LTC$_4$ are also found.[69] Lightman[70] indicated that a second histamine peak 6 hours after allergen challenge indicates basophil or mast cell activity. This activity follows a refractory period accompanied by a rise in eosinophilic cationic protein. Bonini and associates[49] showed that tears collected during the conjunctival LPR after allergen challenge can reproduce a cytological picture of the ocular LPR induced by allergen when reintroduced into the eye of the same patient.

MEDIATORS

Mast cell–derived mediators have been categorized into three groups based on their mode of action.[20] The first group binds to specific cell-membrane receptors and includes substances such as histamine and prostaglandins. The second group causes direct tissue damage and are substances of plasma or cell origin such as complement and MBP. The third group includes chemotactic factors that attract inflammatory cells such as eosinophils, neutrophils, and macrophages.[20]

Histamine

Histamine is the cardinal mediator in the early-phase response and is found in granules of mast cells and basophils. Histamine causes vasodilation, vasopermeability, and pruritus. Ash and Schild[72] first identified the histamine receptor subtype, H$_1$, in 1966 by showing that the antihistamine mepyramine eliminated only the vasodilation and vasopermeability responses to histamine. Black et al.[73] later identified a second subtype, H$_2$ receptors, in 1972. In guinea pigs, the vasodilation response to histamine was initiated by H$_1$- and H$_2$-receptor activation, but increased vascular permeability was mediated solely by H$_1$-receptor activation.[74]

Abelson et al.[75] explored the role of histamine in ocular allergy. Topical histamine induces conjunctival redness and itching, the two principal clinical features of acute allergic conjunctivitis, in a dose-dependent manner.[76] H$_1$-receptor stimulation in the conjunctiva produces pruritus,[77] whereas H$_2$-receptor stimulation produces vasodilation.[78] Early studies revealed elevated histamine levels in the tears of patients with vernal conjunctivitis[75] (16 ng/mL compared with 5 ng/mL in normal eyes) and allergic conjunctivitis. Histaminase activity may play an important role in allergic conjunctivitis[79] by limiting the role of histamine in ocular allergy, except in vernal conjunctivitis.

Neutral Proteases

Neutral proteases are the primary protein components of secretory granules in human mast cells and serve as specific markers for the presence of mast cells.[32] The three main neutral proteases are tryptase, chymase, and carboxypeptidase. Their specificity has allowed tear tryptase levels to be used as a marker of mast cell activity.[34] The biological role of these proteases is still not clearly understood.[80] Proposed roles for tryptase include generation of C3a from C3,[81] destruction of high-molecular-weight kininogen[82] and fibrinogen,[83] and activation of synovial latent collagenase.[84] Chymase catalyzes generation of angiotensin II from angiotensin I. Carboxypeptidase converts angiotensin to des-leu10 angiotensin I, which is an inhibitor of angiotensin-converting enzyme.

Eosinophil Chemotactic Factor and Neutrophil Chemotactic Factor

Mast cell–derived products such as histamine metabolites[85] and the acidic tetrapeptides[86] represent a small component of the eosinophilic chemotactic factors involved in anaphylaxis.[57] PAF is, by far, the most potent eosinophil chemotactic factor.[87] LTB$_4$ has also demonstrated potent eosinophil chemotactic activity.[88]

Many neutrophil chemotactic factors have been described, and evidence has suggested that serum neutrophil chemotactic factors seen in the early and late phases may be produced by mononuclear cells.[89] PAF, LTB$_4$, and IL-8 have also been shown to be chemotactic factors for neutrophils.[90–92]

Eosinophil-Derived Enzymes

MBP accounts for approximately half of eosinophil granule protein,[93, 94] it is the main cell product released by activated eosinophils, and it causes mast cell degranulation.[55] MBP may account for prolonged mast cell degranulation in some cases of acute allergic conjunctivitis,[53] and it may be responsible for the corneal and other cellular damage seen in VKC. Eosinophils also release major cationic protein, eosinophil-derived neurotoxin, and eosinophil-derived peroxidase, all of which are directly cytotoxic.[52]

Platelet-Activating Factor

PAF is a phospholipid released by mast cells, basophils, eosinophils, neutrophils, monocytes, and macrophages when they are stimulated by IgE, calcium ionophore, or zymosan particles.[95] PAF produces both eosinophil and neutrophil chemotaxis. It is 100 times more potent than LTB$_4$ as an eosinophilic chemotactic agent,[96] and it leads to eosinophil activation by specific PAF receptors on the eosinophil cell membrane.[97] When applied topically to rabbit and human eyes, PAF was shown to produce dose-dependent conjunctival hyperemia and chemosis similar to that observed in allergic conjunctivitis.[98]

Arachidonic Acid Metabolites

Topical application of arachidonic acid produces conjunctival chemosis in rabbits and conjunctival and episcleral vasodilation in human patients.[99] Arachidonic acid is cleaved from the cell membrane by the action of phospholipase A$_2$ on cell-membrane phospholipids.

Arachidonic acid is metabolized to prostaglandins and thromboxanes by the action of cyclooxygenase. Prostaglandin D$_2$ (PGD$_2$) is the primary prostaglandin produced by the mast cell. In guinea pig or human eyes, topical PGD$_2$ produces conjunctival chemosis, vasodilation, pain, and an eosinophilic infiltrate similar to that found in allergic eye disease.[100] In the skin, topically applied prostaglandins have been found to produce vasodilation,[101] chemosis, and pain.[102] Prostaglandins may have anti-inflammatory actions effected by a negative feedback system that limits the allergic response.[103]

Leukotrienes are derived from arachidonic acid by lipoxygenase. Lipoxygenase may only be activated in chronic inflammation, with cyclooxygenase production of prostaglandins typically being the main pathway in other disease states. LTB_4, an eosinophilic chemotactic agent, has been shown to act with PGE_2 and PGD_2 to increase vasopermeability, conjunctival chemosis, and neutrophil infiltration.[104] Topical LTC_4 has shown no effect in rabbits or humans,[105] but it produced eosinophil chemotaxis in guinea pigs.[106] However, LTC_4, LTD_4, and LTE_4 have been isolated in tears after conjunctival provocation tests.[107] Leukotrienes are believed to play a significant role in conjunctival LPR.

HPETE and HETE are also derived from arachidonic acid by lipoxygenase activity, although their significance in allergic eye disease is unclear. Application of HETEs to the conjunctiva produces no effect, but investigators have hypothesized that these substances stimulate mucus production based on their known activity in the lung.[108]

Interleukins

The role of interleukins in allergy is not well established. Interleukins are lymphocyte-derived cytokines. IL-3 may contribute to mast cell proliferation,[53] and it may be produced when an imbalance exists between helper and suppressor T lymphocytes involved in an allergic response.[109]

Complement

Complement, the name given to a complex series of approximately 20 proteins, produces a rapid, highly amplified response to a trigger stimulus by activation of the classic or alternate pathway. The classic pathway is activated by immune complexes (IgG or IgM) through C1 leading to sequential activation of C4, C2, C3, C5, C6, C8, and C9. The alternate pathway begins by C3 breakdown initiated by IgA, endotoxin, and zymosan. Immune reactions involving complement are classified as type II hypersensitivity reactions. Although complement may not be a classic feature of allergic or type I hypersensitivity, C3 levels in tears are elevated in patients with allergic conjunctivitis.[110] C3a and C5a can also trigger non–IgE-mediated mast cell activation.

TREATMENT

Acute allergic conjunctivitis is self-limiting. By the time the patient seeks medical attention, the clinical signs and symptoms have abated. Therefore, most of these patients do not require any treatment.

The management of the condition, if it occurs frequently, is to identify the allergen in question and to avoid contact. Mast cell stabilizers, such as cromoglycate, lodoxamide, or nedocromil, may be useful for treating patients who have frequent attacks. In addition, antihistamines can also be helpful in alleviating the symptoms in the acute situation. Generally only minimal therapy is required because of the self-limiting nature of the allergic response.

SAC requires treatment. The disease can be debilitating and uncomfortable. Patients are usually aware of when their symptoms are likely to occur, so that the aim of treatment should be to anticipate and prevent the episode.

As indicated in the discussion on pathophysiology, many mediators are involved, most originating in the mast cell. Therefore, treatment should be aimed at targets involving the mediators. Depending on symptoms and severity, the management of hay fever is as follows:

1. Avoidance of the allergen.
2. Modulation of the mast cell and other cell responses.
3. Pharmacological manipulation of the chemical mediators.
4. Immunotherapy.
5. Desensitization.
6. Other immunomodulation.

It may be necessary, and indeed desirable, to use more than one approach, given the number of mediators involved and the difference in response to these mediators in different patients. Selective mediator antagonists may play a role in modulation of the LPR as well as the acute reaction.

Avoidance of Allergen

Identification of the specific allergen and subsequent avoidance are the most effective ways of preventing acute allergic conjunctivitis, but often this is not possible. Patients with SAC may be unable to avoid pollen exposure completely. Therefore, at some stage, many patients require antiallergic medication to prevent and control symptoms (Table 15.1).

TABLE 15.1 Preventive Environmental Measures that Can Significantly Reduce Allergic Symptoms*

Avoidance Measures for Pollens	Avoidance Measures for Mites	Avoidance Measures for Animal Allergens
Limit outdoor activities	Effective barrier cover for mattress and pillows	Eliminate animals from house
Use air conditioning or air filter system	Wash bedding regularly at 60° C (130° F)	Reduce exposure to all reservoirs for allergen (carpets, upholstered furniture, curtains, etc.)
Drive or ride in car with windows closed and with air conditioning or filtering	Remove carpets, upholstered furniture, curtains, books, stuffed animals, and any other reservoirs of dust	
Use protective eyewear when outdoors	Reduce humidity	
	Vacuum and damp dust entire house weekly	

* Identification of the specific allergen and subsequent avoidance are the most effective ways of preventing acute allergic conjunctivitis.

Mast Cell (and Basophil) Stabilizers

Most clinicians agree that the goal of pharmacological treatment for SAC should be directed toward preventing mast cell degranulation.[111] Mast cell stabilizers have greatly improved the clinical management of acute allergic conjunctivitis. Currently, three drugs—sodium cromoglycate, nedocromil sodium, and lodoxamide tromethamine—are used topically as prophylactic agents to prevent mast cell degranulation. Some mast cell stabilizers may also be able to inhibit leukocyte activity directly,[112–114] in addition to inhibiting mediator release from mast cells, basophils, eosinophils, and neutrophils.[114]

Sodium cromoglycate is well tolerated and has a slow onset of action, typically taking 5 to 14 days to achieve full therapeutic effect.[115] The drug must be used before allergen exposure, and maintaining therapy is crucial. Juniper et al.[116] compared the prescribed, scheduled use with "as-needed" use of sodium cromoglycate in the treatment of SAC. These investigators found that prophylactic use is more effective than as-needed use in preventing a clinically relevant deterioration in some quality-of-life parameters. Typically, sodium cromoglycate 2% is used four times daily, a regimen that may limit patient compliance. Collum et al.[117] showed that 4% sodium cromoglycate used twice daily is at least as effective as 2% sodium cromoglycate used four times daily. However, sodium cromoglycate proves ineffective more often than either topical corticosteroids or H_1-receptor antagonists given alone.[118] Ehlers and Donshik suggested that sodium cromoglycate use be preceded by a course of topical antihistamines, adding the sodium cromoglycate and decreasing the antihistamines as the symptoms subside.[119] A major advantage of sodium cromoglycate is that it is well tolerated and nontoxic[120] and can be used even in contact lens wearers.

Lodoxamide tromethamine is more potent than sodium cromoglycate,[121] and is also well tolerated. Lodoxamide 0.1% was found to be more effective than sodium cromoglycate and 25 times more potent than nedocromil sodium in inhibiting rat conjunctival mast cell mediator release.[121] In the United States, lodoxamide is indicated for the treatment of VKC. Lodoxamide was particularly effective in preventing keratitis and shield ulcers associated with VKC. This effect is of particular importance because such changes are typically resistant to treatment. Systemic absorption of lodoxamide appears to be negligible. Transient burning, stinging, and ocular discomfort after instillation were experienced by approximately 15% of patients participating in clinical trials of this drug. Other adverse events occurring in 1 to 5% of patients included itching, hyperemia, blurred vision, tearing, dry eye symptoms, and foreign body sensation. Fahy et al.[122] showed, in a randomized double-blind trial, that lodoxamide 0.1% produced a faster and greater improvement in signs and symptoms of allergic eye disease than did sodium cromoglycate 2%. The lodoxamide-treated group had fewer reported side effects. Lodoxamide 0.1% has also been shown to be significantly superior to placebo in alleviating the signs and symptoms associated with pollen-induced allergic conjunctivitis.[123] Lodoxamide is available as Alomide Ophthalmic Solution 0.1%; the recommended dosage for adults and children older than 2 years of age is one to two drops per affected eye four times per day for up to 3 months (Alomide package insert, Alcon Laboratories).

Nedocromil sodium, a pyraquinoline mast cell stabilizer, has been shown to be effective in ragweed SAC in a double-blind trial.[111] Nedocromil sodium has a more rapid onset of action than sodium cromolyn, is well tolerated, and appears to possess anti-inflammatory properties in addition to mast cell stabilization.[124] Blumenthal et al.[124] found, in a multicenter double-blind trial conducted over an 8-week period, that nedocromil sodium 2% produced significant improvement in SAC-associated pruritus and hyperemia.[125] Leino et al.[125] showed that nedocromil sodium 2% used twice daily was as effective in SAC as sodium cromoglycate 2% administered four times daily. Nedocromil appears to be as effective as the oral antihistamines terfenadine[126] and astemizole in the treatment of acute allergic conjunctivitis.[127]

Antihistamines

Antihistamines form a major component of the medical therapy of acute allergic conjunctivitis.[118] These agents competitively and reversibly block histamine receptors located in the conjunctiva and the lids,[128] thus blocking the action of the main preformed mediator of the mast cell. Antihistamines can be given in both oral and topical form. In the past, oral antihistamines were associated with annoying sedation. However, newer nonsedating oral H_1-receptor antagonists have been developed for the treatment of allergic diseases.[129] Two oral nonsedating antihistamines, astemizole and terfenadine, were found to be equally effective in controlling pollen-induced conjunctivitis.[130] The full effects following oral administration of these drugs may not be achieved for several hours or days.[129] Therefore, they need to be used in a prophylactic manner. Investigators have noted that saturation of the histamine receptors may take as long as 3 hours.[131]

Oral administration of antihistamines is generally not considered the best route of delivery for treatment of allergic conjunctivitis. It is difficult to attain adequate concentrations at the desired target, the conjunctiva, because of systemic metabolism and insufficient absorption. Many oral antihistamines are associated with drying of the mucous membranes, including the conjunctiva, a feature that only exacerbates the ocular condition. It is curious that these effects are not observed with topical application. In addition, the potential for systemic adverse effects and drug interaction exists with oral administration of antihistamines.

Topical antihistamines are available both alone and in combination with vasoconstrictors. The advantages of topical administration compared with oral therapy are a more rapid onset of action, direct application to the diseased site, and reduced potential for systemic side effects.

Levocabastine is a highly specific H_1-receptor antagonist[132] that has been shown to be 15,000 times more potent than chlorpheniramine in the rat model of 48/80-induced mortality.[133] Vasodilation and increased vascular permeability, previously thought to be the domain of H_2 receptors alone, were also reduced.[133] The plasma concentration of levocabastine after topical ocular application is low.[134] The onset of action following topical application is within minutes of administration,[135] and a long duration of action allows for convenient daily dosage.[136] Three double-blind randomized trials comparing therapeutic efficacy of levocabastine 0.05% eye drops with that of oral terfenadine (60 mg twice daily) were performed over an 8-week period during the pollen season.[137–139] Statistically significant differences were reported for therapeutic efficacy in favor of topical levocabastine.[137, 139] This trend was maintained on days of high pollen counts and was associated with more symptom-free days. Topical levocabastine has been reported to be significantly more effective than sodium cromoglycate in the treatment of SAC.[140–143] Symptom severity was consistently lower in the levocabastine-treated group. In one study, 33% of levocabastine-treated patients were symptom-free on high pollen days, compared with only 6% of those treated with sodium cromoglycate and 4% of those in the placebo group.[142, 143] Abelson et al.[144] conducted a study comparing the efficacy of 0.05% levocabastine and 4% sodium cromoglycate in the allergen challenge model. Levocabastine was found to be significantly more effective than sodium cromoglycate in inhibiting itching, hyperemia, lid swelling, chemosis, and tearing after an initial challenge and a 4-hour rechallenge.[144]

Olopatadine (Patanol 0.1%) is the first dual-action allergy therapy to receive approval as both an antihistamine and a mast cell stabilizer. The H_1 selectivity of olopatadine was superior to that of other ocular antihistamines including ketotifen, levocabastine, antazoline, and pheniramine.[145, 146] Olopatadine has been shown in vitro to inhibit histamine, tryptase, and PGD_2 release in a concentration-dependent fashion (IC_{50} = 559 μM) from human conjunctival mast cell preparations.[146, 147] This agent is indicated for the relief of ocular itching, and the recommended dosing regimen is one to two drops two times a day at 6- to 8-hour intervals.

Emedastine is an antiallergic agent with antihistaminic properties that has been shown to inhibit histamine-induced vascular permeability changes in the conjunctiva. Emedastine exhibits high affinity for H_1 receptors, with significantly weaker affinities for H_2 and H_3 receptors.[148] The antihistaminic activity of emedastine has been shown to be comparable to that of ketotifen and significantly more potent than that of chlorpheniramine, levocabastine, pheniramine, and antazoline.[149] Emedastine has been shown in vitro to inhibit histamine release in rat peritoneal mast cells[150] and eosinophil chemotaxis.[151]

Although antihistamines are effective alone, some antihistamine-vasoconstrictor combinations are on the market. Vasoconstrictors can provide symptomatic relief by decreasing conjunctival edema and hyperemia. These drugs activate the postjunctional alpha-adrenergic receptors found on the precapillary and postcapillary blood vessels. Activation of these receptors causes the vessels to constrict. The use of a vasoconstrictor with an antihistamine has been shown to be more effective than the use of either agent alone.[152] Examples of some antihistamine-vasoconstrictor combination products are Naphcon-A (Alcon), Vasocon-A (CIBA Vision), AK-con-A (Akorn), and Opcon-A (Bausch & Lomb). The recommended dosing regimen for combination products is one or two drops to each eye three or four times per day.

Nonsteroidal Anti-inflammatory Drugs

Nonsteroidal anti-inflammatory drugs (NSAIDs) are being investigated for the treatment of allergic conjunctivitis. The therapeutic rationale is to block the effects of newly synthesized cell-membrane phospholipid derivatives from mast cells, basophils, and newly recruited eosinophils and neutrophils. Most NSAIDs block the action of cyclooxygenase, inhibiting the conversion of arachidonic acid to prostaglandins and thromboxanes.[156] Ketorolac tromethamine is a potent analgesic that may inhibit prostaglandin synthetase.[99] Topical ketorolac 0.5% used four times daily for 1 week was found to be significantly more effective than placebo in relieving itching, erythema, edema, and mucous discharge in acute allergic conjunctivitis.[154] Ketorolac is approved in the United States for the treatment of ocular itching.

Although not approved for such use, flurbiprofen and diclofenac have been evaluated for the therapy of allergic conjunctivitis. Topical 0.03% flurbiprofen has also been found to be superior to vehicle control in patients with allergic conjunctivitis and in reducing conjunctival and episcleral hyperemia and ocular itching.[153] Laibovitz et al.[155] reported the results of a randomized clinical trial comparing diclofenac sodium 0.1% to placebo for relief of ocular signs and symptoms in patients with SAC. Diclofenac was statistically and clinically superior in relieving itching and conjunctival injection after 2 weeks of treatment, but 4 patients out of 10 experienced some transient ocular burning and stinging with diclofenac.[155] Suprofen is a topical NSAID that has been shown to be effective in treating VKC.[156] Thus, by blocking the cyclooxygenase pathway and reducing prostaglandin synthesis, NSAIDs are effective in treating acute allergic conjunctivitis. Their use may allow a concomitant increase in leukotriene synthesis, but this effect does not appear to exacerbate the signs and symptoms of allergic conjunctivitis.[153]

Corticosteroids

Corticosteroids inhibit phospholipase A_2, thereby blocking the formation of lipid-derived mediators from arachidonic acid. Corticosteroids markedly suppress the LPR in both clinical and experimental settings;[65, 157] however, they have demonstrated a lesser effect in suppressing the acute-phase response. Topical corticosteroid treatment may partially inhibit mediator release in the nose in vivo.[157] Although steroids provide an excellent means of inhibiting the inflammatory cascade, ocular side effects including glaucoma, cataract, and secondary herpetic or bacterial infections limit their usefulness in acute allergy. Prednisolone has been used as "pulse therapy" in extremely acute and severe cases. Short trials of 0.12% prednisolone two to three times daily resulted in few complications.[158] Thus, only in persistent or extremely severe cases of ocular allergy should mild topical steroids, such as fluorometholone or medrysone,[159, 160] be used, and then only in the short term. Safer alternatives to topical steroid therapy should be used when possible. Systemic or subconjunctival corticosteroids should not be used in acute allergic conjunctivitis.

Loteprednol etabonate, a "soft drug," is a newly formulated steroid that offers the therapeutic benefit of existing steroids, but with minimal side effects. The "soft steroid" undergoes rapid hydrolysis to an inactive derivative after penetrating the cornea.[161] Despite rapid metabolism, loteprednol retains its anti-inflammatory effects in the cornea[162] and has been shown to be effective in treating GPC.[163]

Rimexolone is another "soft steroid" with decreased propensity to raise intraocular pressure.[164] Rimexolone has been shown to reduce the signs and symptoms associated with allergic conjunctivitis.[165] The ocular hypertensive effect of rimexolone 1.0% was comparable to that of fluorometholone alcohol 0.1%, but less than that of dexamethasone phosphate 0.1% or prednisolone acetate 1.0%. The corticosteroid is indicated for the treatment of postoperative inflammation following cataract surgery and for treatment of anterior uveitis. Rimexolone is commercially available in a 1.0% ophthalmic suspension (Vexol, Alcon).

Immunotherapy

Immunotherapy is increasingly being used in the clinical setting and should be considered when acute allergic conjunctivitis is severe or when allergic conjunctivitis is only part of a systemic allergic manifestation. Immunotherapy has been used in allergic disease in which the specific allergen is well established. Small and increasing doses of the specific allergen (as tolerated by the patient) are given as a series of inoculations over time.[166] Cooke et al.[167] first noted the development of non-cytotropic (IgG) antibody as a con-

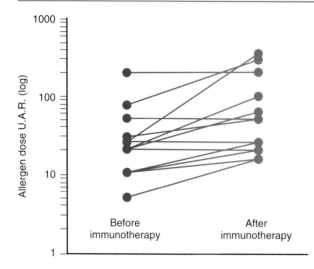

FIGURE 15.5 Conjunctival allergen threshold dose before and after local specific immunotherapy. Although the threshold dose of reaction increased for some patients after immunotherapy, the pattern was not consistent in all recipients. The increase in levels, furthermore, was not dramatic in most cases of upper airway resistance (UAR).

sequence of desensitization. The generation of IgG antibodies can neutralize an antigen and prevent mast cell degranulation.[168] This mechanism appears to be effective immunotherapy for stinging insect venoms, but, in general, little correlation exists between the increase in IgG levels and clinical efficacy for allergic conjunctivitis (Fig. 15.5).

Inhibition of IgE has also been suggested as a possible mechanism of action of immunotherapy.[163] Another allergy-suppressing mechanism of action may be an increase in specific CD8+ T cells.[164, 165] Immunotherapy may also cause a shift in helper T cells. Immunotherapy may induce the activation of the T_H1 cell, which stimulates gamma interferon, and inhibition of IgE synthesis, rather than induce activation of the T_H2 cell, which secretes cytokines that stimulate the production of IgE.[166] The production of histamine-releasing factors by T cells, monocytes, and platelets has also been shown to be reduced with immunotherapy.[173]

Although the specific mechanism explaining the cytological and biochemical basis for immunotherapy is still unclear, its efficacy in allergic conjunctivitis has been well demonstrated. Seasonal allergens, including ragweed pollen, grasses, and mold (e.g., *Cladosporium*),[174–176] have all been used in immunotherapy. Koizumi et al.[169] demonstrated the suppression of allergic conjunctivitis in guinea pigs with oral administration of antigen. Oral administration of ovalbumin and cedar pollen extract significantly reduced conjunctival exudation. Furthermore, the number of inflammatory cells in the conjunctiva of the ovalbumin-fed group was significantly suppressed during the LPR. The investigators also noted that serum levels of anti-ovalbumin IgE and anti-cedar pollen extract IgE were suppressed, and a positive correlation existed between the IgE level and amount of Evans blue dye leakage, which serves as an index of permeability, in the early phase.[169] Oral immunotherapy has also been shown to produce good results in birch pollen–associated rhinoconjunctivitis in children.[177]

Mediator Antagonists and Investigational Drugs

Lipoxygenase inhibitors, which block the synthesis of leukotrienes, are currently being investigated. These agents could potentially be effective at blocking ocular the LPR responsible for the sometimes prolonged course of acute allergic conjunctivitis. Nakagawa et al.[178] showed that ONO-1078, a specific leukotriene receptor antagonist, significantly reduced wheezing and dyspneic attacks in asthmatic patients. ONO-1078 has also been shown to be effective in inhibiting antigen-induced bronchoconstriction in passively sensitized guinea pigs and in human bronchial provocation tests. REV 5901 is a potent lipoxygenase inhibitor that has been shown to reduce lens protein–induced ocular inflammation in rabbits significantly.[179] MK-571 is a selective, potent LTD_4 receptor antagonist that has been shown to block LTD_4-induced bronchoconstriction in several animal models.[179] However, the use of anti-LTD_4 in the eye is questionable because LTD_4 has yet to be identified as an integral mediator in ocular allergy. These compounds are still investigational drugs and have yet to be proven clinically in large, randomized multicenter trials.

Pentigetide is a synthetic peptide derived from the Fc region of human IgE.[180] It has been shown to inhibit cutaneous and systemic IgE-mediated allergic reactions in humans,[181] as well as non–IgE-mediated inflammation in mice.[182] In a randomized, double-blind, parallel 2-week comparison of pentigetide 0.5% and sodium cromoglycate 4%, Kalpaxis and Thayer[180] demonstrated that pentigetide use resulted in greater improvement in the clinical signs and symptoms of acute allergic conjunctivitis than that obtained with sodium cromoglycate.

Deflazacort, an oral derivative of prednisolone, has been shown to reduce LPRs in the conjunctival epithelium significantly.[183] Increased cAMP levels inhibit mast cell degranulation, and pharmacological modulation of cAMP levels may allow important inhibition of inflammatory mediator release. Drugs that stimulate adenylate cyclase, such as isoproterenol, epinephrine, and aminophylline, have been demonstrated to inhibit the breakdown of cAMP, which, in turn, decreases mediator release.[35]

REFERENCES

1. Weeks ER. Epidemiology of hay fever and perennial allergic rhinitis. Monogr Allergy 21:1, 1987.
2. Smith JM. Epidemiology and natural history of asthma, allergic rhinitis and atopic dermatitis (eczema). In: Allergy principles and practice. Vol 2. Middleton E Jr, Reed CE, Ellis E, et al, eds. St. Louis, CV Mosby, 1988, p 891.
3. Wallace W IV. Diseases of the conjunctiva. In: Clinical ocular pharmacology. Barlett JD, Jaanus SD, eds. Boston, Butterworths, 1984, p 533.
4. Allansmith MR, Abelson MB. Ocular allergies. In: The cornea: scientific foundations and clinical practice. Smolin G, Thoft RA, eds. Boston, Little, Brown, 1983.
5. Bonini S, Bonini S. IgE and non-IgE mechanisms in ocular allergy. Ann Allergy 71:296, 1993.
6. Miyamoto T, Takafuji S, Shuji S, et al. Allergy and changing environments: industrial/urban pollution. In: Progress in allergy and clinical immunology. Pichler WJ, ed. Toronto, Hogrefe & Huber, 1989, p 265.
7. Abelson MB, Udel IJ, Weston JH. Conjunctival eosinophils in allergic ocular disease. Arch Ophthalmol 101:631, 1983.
8. Bonini S, Bonini S, Vecchione A, et al. Inflammatory changes in conjunctival scrapings after allergen provocation in humans. J Allergy Clin Immunol 82:462, 1988.
9. Abelson MB, Madiwale NA, Weston JH. Conjunctival eosinophils in allergic ocular disease. Arch Ophthalmol 101:555, 1983.
10. Dart JKG, Buckley RJ, Monnickenda M, et al. Perennial allergic conjunctivitis: definition, clinical characteristics and prevalence. Ophthal Soc U K 105:513, 1986.
11. Allansmith MR, Hann GS, Simon MA. Tissue tear and serum IgE concentrations in vernal conjunctivitis. Am J Ophthalmol 81:506, 1976.
12. Brauninger GE, Centifano YM. Immunoglobulin E in human tears. Am J Ophthalmol 72:558, 1971.
13. Insler MS, Lim JM, Queng JT, et al. Tear and serum IgE concentrations by tandem-R IgE immunoradiometric assay in allergic patients. Ophthalmology 94:945, 1987.
14. Ishizaka K, Ishizaka T, Hornbrook MM. Physiochemical properties of reaginic antibody. V. Correlation of reaginic activity and γE-globulin antibody. J Immunol 97:840, 1966.
15. Ishizaka K, Ishizaka T, Hornbrook MM. Allergen-binding activity of γE, γG and A antibodies in sera from atopic patients: in vitro measurements of reaginic antibody. J Immunol 98:490, 1967.
16. Bryant DH, Burns MW, Lazarus L. Identification of IgG antibody as a carrier of reaginic activity in asthmatic patients. J Allergy Clin Immunol 56:417, 1975.

17. Roitt IM. Clinical immunology hypersensitivity. In: Essential immunology. Oxford, Blackwell Scientific Publications, 1994, p 313.

18. Prausnitz C, Kustner H. Studien uber die Ueberempfindlichkeit. Zentralbl Bakteriol 86:160, 1921.

19. Solley GO, Gleich GJ, Jordon RE, et al. The late phase of the immediate wheal and flare skin reaction: its dependence on IgE antibodies. J Clin Invest 58:408, 1976.

20. Abelson MB, George MA, Garofalo C. Differential diagnosis of ocular allergic disorders. Ann Allergy 70:95, 1993.

21. Killan D, Cockroft DW, Hargreave FE, et al. Factors in allergen-induced asthma: relevance of the intensity of the airway's allergic reaction and nonspecific bronchial reactivity. Clin Allergy 6:219, 1976.

22. Pelikan A. Late and delayed responses of the nasal mucosa to allergen challenge. Ann Allergy 41:37, 1978.

23. Solley GO, Gleich GJ, Jordan RE, et al. The late phase of the immediate wheal and flare skin reaction: its dependence upon IgE antibodies. J Clin Invest 58:408, 1976.

24. Trocme SD, Bonini S, Barney NP, et al. Late phase reaction in topically induced ocular anaphylaxis in the rat. Curr Eye Res 7:437, 1988.

25. Bonini S, Bonini S, Vecchione A, et al. Inflammatory changes in conjunctival scrapings after allergen provocation in humans. J Allergy Clin Immunol 82:462, 1988.

26. Lieferman KM, Fujisawa T, Gray BH, et al. Extracellular deposition of eosinophil and neutrophil granule proteins in the IgE-mediated cutaneous late-phase reaction. Lab Invest 62:579, 1990.

27. Trocme SD, Raizman MB, Bartley GB. Medical therapy for ocular allergy. Mayo Clin Proc 67:557, 1992.

28. Allansmith MR, Greiner JV, Baird RS. Number of inflammatory cells in the normal conjunctiva. Am J Ophthalmol 86:250, 1978.

29. Irani AMA, Butrus SI, Tabbara KF, et al. Human conjunctival mast cells: distribution of Mct and Mctc in vernal conjunctivitis and giant papillary conjunctivitis. J Allergy Clin Immunol 86:34, 1990.

30. Enerback L. Mast cell heterogeneity: the evolution of the concept of a specific mucosal mast cell. In: Mast cell differentiation and heterogeneity. Befus AD, Bienenstock J, Denburg JA, eds. New York, Raven Press, 1986, p 1.

31. Befus D, Goodacre R, Dyck N, et al. Mast cell heterogeneity in man: histologic studies of the intestine. Int Arch Allergy Appl Immunol 76:232, 1985.

32. Schwartz LB. Mediators of human mast cells and human mast cell subtypes. Ann Allergy 58:226, 1987.

33. Wenzel S, Irani AA, Sanders JM, et al. Immunoassay of tryptase from human mast cells. J Immunol Method 86:139, 1986.

34. Friedlander MF. Current concepts in ocular allergy. Ann Allergy 57:5, 1991.

35. Eisen HN. Antibody-mediated (immediate-type) hypersensitivity. In: General immunology. Philadelphia, JB Lippincott, 1990, p 167.

36. Galli SJ. New approaches for the analysis of mast cell maturation, heterogeneity and function. Fed Proc 46:1906, 1987.

37. Bonini S, Bonini S. Studies of allergic conjunctivitis. Chibret Int J 5:12, 1987.

38. Maggi E, Biswas P, Del Prete G, et al. Accumulation of T_H2-like helper T cells in the conjunctiva of patients with vernal conjunctivitis. J Immunol 146:1169, 1991.

39. Peltz G. A role for CD4+ T-cell subsets producing a selective pattern of lymphokines in the pathogenesis of human chronic inflammatory and allergic diseases. Immunol Rev 123:23, 1991.

40. Ricci M, Matucci A, Rossi O. T cells, cytokines, IgE and allergic airways inflammation. J Invest Allergol Clin Immunol 4:214, 1994.

41. Lichtenstein LM. Sequential analysis of the allergic response: cyclic AMP, calcium and histamine. Int Arch Allergy Appl Immunol 49:143, 1975.

42. Bourne HR, Lichtenstein LM, Melmon KL. Modulation of inflammation and immunity by cyclic-AMP. Science 184:19, 1974.

43. Veruloet D, Vellieux P, Charpin J. Potentiation of cutaneous reactivity and blood leukocyte histamine release by deuterium oxide in human beings. Acta Allergol 31:367, 1976.

44. Bochner BS, Schleimer RP, Charlesworth EN, et al. Basophil activation and recruitment in allergic disease. In: Progress in allergy and clinical immunology. Pichler WJ, ed. Toronto, Hogrefe & Huber, 1989, p 12.

45. Cohan VL, Massey WA, Gittlen SD, et al. The heterogeneity of human histamine containing cells. In: Mast cell and basophil differentiation and function in health and disease. Galli SJ, Austen KF, eds. New York, Raven Press, 1989, p 149.

46. Gleich GJ. The late phase of the immunoglobulin E–mediated reaction: a link between anaphylaxis and common allergic disease. J Allergy Clin Immunol 70:160, 1982.

47. Lichtenstein LM, Bochner BS. The role of basophils in asthma. In: Advances in the understanding and treatment of asthma. Poper PJ, Krell RD, eds. Ann NY Acad Sci 629:48, 1991.

48. MacDonald SM, Kagey-Sobotka A, Lichtenstein LM. Mast cells and basophils in asthma. Presented at the Third International Meeting on the Pathophysiology of Pulmonary Cells, Torino, 1993.

49. Bonini S, Centofanti M, Schiavone M, et al. Passive transfer of the ocular late-phase reaction. Ocul Immunol Inflamm 4:323, 1993.

50. Bonini ST, Bonini SE, Todini V, et al. Persistent inflammatory changes in the conjunctival late phase reaction of humans. Invest Ophthalmol Vis Sci 29 Suppl:230, 1988.

51. Bonini S, Tracine SD, Barney NP, et al. Late-phase reaction and tear fluid cytology in the rat ocular anaphylaxis. Curr Eye Res 6:659, 1987.

52. Capron M. Eosinophils in diseases: receptors and mediators. In: Progress in allergy and clinical immunology. Pichler WJ, ed. Toronto, Hogrefe & Huber, 1989, p 6.

53. Abelson MB, Allansmith MR, Udell U, et al. Principles and practice of ophthalmology: the Harvard system. In: Allergic and toxic disorders. Philadelphia, WB Saunders, 1994.

54. Allansmith MR. Immunology of the eye. In: The eye and immunology. St. Louis, CV Mosby, 1982, p 64.
55. Trocme SD, Kephart GM, Allansmith MR, et al. Conjunctival deposition of eosinophil granule major protein in vernal keratoconjunctivitis and contact lens associated giant papillary conjunctivitis. Am J Ophthalmol 108:57, 1989.
56. Bonini S, Centofanti M, Schiavone M, et al. The pattern of the ocular late phase reaction induced by allergen challenge in hay fever conjunctivitis. Ocul Immunol Inflamm 2:191, 1994.
57. Kay AB. Eosinophil and neutrophil chemotactic factors in allergy and asthma. In: Progress in allergy and clinical immunology. Pichler WJ, ed. Toronto, Hogrefe & Huber, 1989, p 39.
58. Baggiolini M, et al. Neutrophil activation and the effects of interleukin-8/neutrophil-activating peptide 1 (IL-8/NAP-1). Cytokines 4:1, 1992.
59. Gleich GJ. The late phase of the immunoglobulin E−mediated reaction: a link between anaphylaxis and common allergic disease? J Allergy Clin Immunol 70:160, 1982.
60. Pelikan Z. Late and delayed responses of the nasal mucosa to allergen challenge. Ann Allergy 41:37, 1978.
61. Dolovich J, Little DC. Correlates of skin test reactions to *Bacillus subtilis* enzyme preparations. J Allergy Clin Immunol 49:43, 1972.
62. Pepys J, Hutchcroft BJ. Bronchial provocation tests in etiologic diagnosis and analysis of asthma. Am Rev Respir Dis 112:829, 1975.
63. Kaliner M. Hypotheses on the contribution of late-phase allergic responses to the understanding and treatment of allergic diseases (editorial). J Allergy Clin Immunol 73:311, 1984.
64. Allansmith MR, Baird RS, Greiner JV, et al. Late phase reaction in ocular anaphylaxis in the rat. J Allergy Clin Immunol 73:49, 1984.
65. Trocme SD, Bonini S, Barney NP, et al. Effects of topical pretreatment with dexamethasone on the immediate and late phase of topically induced ocular anaphylaxis in the rat. Acta Ophthalmol 66:24, 1988.
66. Leonardi A, Bloch KJ, Briggs R, et al. Histology of ocular late-phase reaction in guinea pigs passively sensitized with IgG1 antibodies. Ophthalmic Res 22:209, 1990.
67. Leonardi A, Bloch KJ, Briggs R, et al. Clinical patterns of ocular anaphylaxis in guinea pigs passively sensitized with IgG$_1$ antibody. Ophthalmic Res 22:95, 1990.
68. Bonini S, Bonini S, Buci MG, et al. Allergen dose response and late symptoms in a human model of ocular allergy. J Allergy Clin Immunol 86:869, 1990.
69. Bonini S, Bonini S, Berruto A, et al. Conjunctival provocation test as a model for the study of allergy and inflammation in humans. Int Arch Allergy Appl Immunol 88:144, 1989.
70. Lightman S. Therapeutic considerations: symptoms, cells and mediators. Allergy 50 Suppl 21: 10, 1995.
71. Allansmith MR, Ross RN. Ocular allergy and mast cell stabilizers. Surv Ophthalmol 30:229, 1986.
72. Ash ASG, Schild HO. Receptors mediating some actions of histamine. Br J Pharmacol 27:427, 1966.

73. Black JW, Owen DA, Parsons ME. An analysis of the depressor responses to histamine in the cat and dog: involvement of both H$_1$ and H$_2$ receptors. Br J Pharmacol 54:319, 1975.
74. Owen DAA, Poy E, Woodward DF. Evaluation of the role of histamine H1 and H$_2$ receptors in cutaneous inflammation in the guinea pig produced by histamine and mast cell degranulation. Br J Pharmacol 69:615, 1980.
75. Abelson MB, Baird RS, Allansmith MR. Tear histamine levels in vernal conjunctivitis and ocular inflammations. Ophthalmology 87:812, 1980.
76. Abelson MB, Allansmith MR. Histamine and the eye. In: Immunology and immunopathology of the eye. Silverstein AM, O'Connor GR, eds. New York, Masson, 1979.
77. Weston JH, Udell U, Abelson MR. H$_1$ receptors in the human ocular surface. Invest Ophthalmol Vis Sci 20 Suppl:32, 1981.
78. Abelson MB, Udell U. H$_2$ receptors in the human ocular surface. Arch Ophthalmol 99:203, 1981.
79. Berdy GJ, Levene RB, Bateman ST. Identification of histaminase activity in human tears after conjunctival antigen challenge. Invest Ophthalmol Vis Sci 31 Suppl:65, 1990.
80. Schwartz LB. Human mast cell neutral proteases: markers of mast cell heterogeneity and function. In: Progress in allergy and clinical immunology. Pichler WJ, ed. Toronto, Hogrefe & Huber, 1989, p 1.
81. Schwartz LB, Kawahara MD, Hugli TE, et al. Generation of C3a anaphylatoxin from human C3 by human mast cell tryptase. J Immunol 130:1891, 1983.
82. Maier M, Spragg J, Schwartz LB. Inactivation of human high molecular weight kininogen by human mast cell tryptase. J Immunol 130:2571, 1984.
83. Schwartz LB, Bradford TM, Littman BL, et al. The fibrinolytic activity of purified tryptase from human lung mast cells. J Immunol 135: 2762, 1985.
84. Gruber BL, Schwartz LB, Ramamurthy NS, et al. Activation of latent rheumatoid synovial collagenase by human mast cell tryptase. J Immunol 139:2724, 1988.
85. Turnball LW, Kay AB. Eosinophils and mediators of anaphylaxis: histamine and imidazole acetic acid as chemotactic agents for human eosinophil leukocytes. Immunology 31:797, 1976.
86. Goetzl EJ, Austen KF. Purification and synthesis of eosinophilotactic tetrapeptides of human lung tissue: identification as eosinophil chemotactic factor of anaphylaxis. Proc Natl Acad Sci U S A 72:4112, 1975.
87. Nagy L, Lee TH, Goetzl EJ, et al. Complement receptor enhancement and chemotaxis of human neutrophils and eosinophils by leukotrienes and other lipoxygenase products. Clin Exp Immunol 47:541, 1982.
88. Wardlaw AJ, Moqbel R, Cromwell O, et al. Platelet-activating factor. A potent chemotactic and chemokinetic factor for human eosinophils. J Clin Invest 78:1701, 1986.
89. Baggiolini M. Effects of mediators on leukocytes. In: Progress in allergy and clinical immunology. Pichler WJ, ed. Toronto, Hogrefe & Huber, 1989, p 43.

90. Baggiolini M, Dewald B. The neutrophil. Int Arch Allergy Appl Immunol 76:13, 1985.
91. Baggiolini M, Walz A, Kunkel SL. Neutrophil-activating peptide-1/interleukin 8, a novel cytokine that activates neutrophils. J Clin Invest 84:1945, 1989.
92. Leonard EJ, Yoshimura T. Neutrophil attractant/activation protein-1 (NAP-1 interleukin-8). Am J Respir Cell Mol Biol 2:479, 1990.
93. Archer GT, Hirsch JG. Isolation of granules from eosinophil leukocytes and study of their enzyme content. J Exp Med 118:277, 1963.
94. Gleich GJ, Leogering DA, Maldonado JE. Identification of a major basic protein in guinea pig eosinophil granules. J Exp Med 137:1459, 1973.
95. Braquet P, Toqui L, Shen TY, et al. Perspectives in platelet-activating factor research. Pharmacol Rev 39:97, 1987.
96. Tamura N, Agrawal D, Suliman FA, et al. Effects of platelet-activating factor on the chemotaxis of normodense eosinophils from normal subjects. Biochem Biophys Res Commun 142:638, 1986.
97. Kroegel C, Warner J, Giembycz MA, et al. Dual transmembrane signalling mechanisms in eosinophils: evidence of two functionally distinct receptors for platelet-activating factor. Int Arch Allergy Immunol 99:226, 1992.
98. George MA, Smith LM, Berdy GJ, et al. Platelet activating factor induced inflammation following topical ocular challenge. Invest Ophthalmol Visual Sci 31 Suppl:63, 1990.
99. Rooks WH. Pharmacologic activity of ketorolac tromethamine. Pharmacotherapy 10:308, 1990.
100. Abelson MB, Madiwale NA, Weston JH. The role of prostaglandin D2 in allergic ocular disease. In: Advances in immunology and immunopathology of the eye. O'Connor GR, Chandler JW, eds. New York, Masson, 1985.
101. Solomon LM, Juhlin L, Kirschenbaum MB. Prostaglandin on cutaneous vasculature. J Invest Dermatol 51:280, 1958.
102. Ferreira SH. Prostaglandins, aspirin-like drugs and analgesia. Nature (New Biol) 240:200, 1972.
103. Bhattacherjee P. The role of arachidonate metabolism in ocular inflammation. Prog Clin Biol Res 312:211, 1989.
104. Butrus SI, Corey EJ, Weston JH, et al. The effect of leukotriene B$_4$ in rabbit and guinea pig eyes. Invest Ophthalmol Vis Sci 25 Suppl:109, 1984.
105. Weston JH, Abelson MB. Leukotriene C$_4$ in rabbit and human eyes (abstract). Invest Ophthalmol Vis Sci 26 Suppl:191, 1985.
106. Spada CS, Woodward DF, Hawley SB, et al. Leukotrienes cause eosinophil emigration into conjunctival tissue. Prostaglandins 31:795, 1986.
107. Bisgaard H, Ford-Hutchinson AW, Charleson A, et al. Production of leukotrienes in human skin and conjunctival mucosa after specific allergen challenge. Allergy 40:417, 1985.
108. Lundgren JD, Shelhamer JH, Kaliner MA. The role of eicosanoids in respiratory mucus hypersecretion. Ann Allergy 55:5, 1985.
109. Ihle JN, Pepersack L, Rebar L. Regulation of T cell differentiation: in vitro induction of 30 alpha-hydroxysteroid dehydrogenase in splenic lymphocytes is mediated by a unique lymphokine. J Immunol 126:2184, 1981.
110. Ballow M, Donshik PC, Mendelson L. Complement proteins C3 anaphylatoxin in the tears of patients with conjunctivitis. J Allergy Clin Immunol 76:473, 1985.
111. Melamed J, Schwartz RH, Hirsch SR, et al. Evaluation of nedocromil sodium 2% ophthalmic solution for the treatment of seasonal allergic conjunctivitis. Ann Allergy 73:57, 1994.
112. Rainey DK. Evidence of the antiinflammatory activity of nedocromil sodium. Clin Exp Allergy 22:976, 1992.
113. Brogden RN, Sorkin EM. Nedocromil sodium: an updated review of its pharmacological properties and therapeutic efficacy in asthma. Drugs 45:694, 1993.
114. Berdy GJ, Smith LM, George MA, et al. The effects of disodium cromoglycate in the human model of acute allergic conjunctivitis (abstract). Invest Ophthalmol Vis Sci 30 Suppl:503, 1989.
115. Nizami RM. Treatment of ragweed allergic conjunctivitis with 2% cromolyn solution in unit doses. Ann Allergy 47:5, 1981.
116. Juniper EF, Guyatt GH, Ferrie PJ, et al. Sodium cromoglycate eye drops: regular versus "as needed" use in the treatment of seasonal allergic conjunctivitis. J Allergy Clin Immunol 94:36, 1994.
117. Collum LMT, FitzSimon S, Hillery M, et al. Twice daily 4% sodium cromoglycate vs 2% sodium cromoglycate used four times daily in seasonal (grass pollen) allergic conjunctivitis. Doc Ophthalmol 82:267, 1992.
118. Knight A. The role of levocabastine in the treatment of allergic rhinoconjunctivitis. Br J Clin Pract 48:139, 1994.
119. Elders WH, Donshik PC. Allergic ocular disorders: a spectrum of diseases. CLAO J 2:117, 1992.
120. Collum LMT. The management of ocular allergy. Ocul Immunol Inflamm 1:3, 1993.
121. Yanni JM, Weiner LK, Glaser RL, et al. Effect of lodoxamide on an in vitro and in vivo conjunctival immediate hypersensitivity responses in rats. Int Arch Allergy Immunol 101:102, 1993.
122. Fahy GT, Easty DL, Collum LMT, et al. Randomised double masked trial of lodoxamide and sodium cromoglycate in allergic eye disease: a multicentre study. Eur J Ophthalmol 2:144, 1992.
123. Cerqueti PM, Ricca V, Tosca MA, et al. Lodoxamide treatment of allergic conjunctivitis. Int Arch Allergy Immunol 105:185, 1994.
124. Blumenthal M, Casale T, Dockhorn R, et al. Efficacy and safety of nedocromil sodium ophthalmic solution in the treatment of seasonal allergic conjunctivitis. Am J Ophthalmol 113:56, 1992.
125. Leino M, Ennevaara K, Latvala AL, et al. Double blind group comparative study of 2% nedocromil sodium eye drops with 2% sodium cromoglycate and placebo eye drops in the treatment of seasonal allergic conjunctivitis. Clin Exp Allergy 22:929, 1992.
126. Alexander M. Comparative therapeutic studies with Tilavist. Allergy 50 Suppl 21:23, 1995.
127. Miglior M, Scullica L, Secchi AG, et al. Nedo-

cromil sodium and astemizole alone or combined, in the treatment of seasonal allergic conjunctivitis. Acta Ophthalmol 71:73, 1993.

128. Abelson MB, Weston JH. Antihistamines. In: Clinical ophthalmic pharmacology. Lamberts DW, Potter DE, eds. Boston, Little, Brown, 1987, p 417.

129. Simons FER. H-receptor antagonists: clinical pharmacology and therapeutics. J Allergy Clin Immunol 84:845, 1989.

130. Juniper ER, White J, Dolovich J. Efficacy of continuous treatment with astemizole and terfenadine in ragweed pollen-induced rhinoconjunctivitis. J Allergy Clin Immunol 82:670, 1988.

131. Bain WA, Broadbent JL, Warin RP. Comparison of Anthistan (mepyramine maleate) and Phenergan as histamine antagonists. Lancet 2: 47, 1949.

132. Van Wauwe JP. Animal pharmacology of levocabastine: a new type of H_1-antihistamine well-suited for topical application. In: Rhinoconjunctivitis: new perspectives in topical treatment of seasonal allergic rhinitis. Mygind N, Nacieno RM, eds. Toronto, Hogrefe & Huber, 1989, p 27.

133. Abelson MB, Rombaut N, Vanden Bussche G. Levocabastine: evaluation of human ocular histamine and 48/80 models. Allergol Immunol Clin 2:281, 1987.

134. Dechant KL, Goa KL. Levocabastine: a review of its pharmacological properties and therapeutic potential as a topical antihistamine in allergic rhinitis and conjunctivitis. Drugs 41:202, 1991.

135. Stokes TC, Feinberg G. Rapid onset of action of levocabastine eye drops in histamine-induced conjunctivitis. Clin Exp Allergy 23:791, 1993.

136. Tomiyama S, Ohnishi M, Okuda M. The dose and duration of effect of levocabastine, a new topical H_1-receptor antagonist, on nasal provocation reaction to allergen. Am J Rhinol 7:85, 1993.

137. Bahmer FA, Ruprecht KW. Safety and efficacy of topical levocabastine compared with oral terfenadine. Ann Allergy 72:429, 1994.

138. Frostad AB, Olsen AK. A comparison of topical levocabastine and sodium cromoglycate in treatment of pollen-provoked allergic conjunctivitis. Clin Exp Allergy 23:406, 1993.

139. Livostin Study Group. A comparison of topical levocabastine and oral terfenadine in the treatment of allergic rhinoconjunctivitis. Allergy 48: 530, 1993.

140. Palma-Carlos AG, Chiera C, Conde TA, et al. Double-blind comparison of levocabastine nasal spray with sodium cromoglycate nasal spray in the treatment of seasonal allergic rhinitis. Ann Allergy 57:394, 1991.

141. Schata M, Jorde W, Richarz-Barthauer U. Levocabastine nasal spray better than sodium cromoglycate and placebo in the topical treatment of seasonal allergic rhinitis. J Allergy Clin Immunol 87:873, 1991.

142. Azevedo M, Castel-Branco MG, Ferrex Oliveira J, et al. Double-blind comparison of seasonal allergic conjunctivitis. Clin Exp Allergy 21:689, 1991.

143. David BH, Mullins J. Topical levocabastine is more effective than sodium cromoglycate for the prophylaxis and treatment of seasonal allergic conjunctivitis. Allergy 48:519, 1993.

144. Abelson MB, George MA, Smith LM. Evaluation of 0.05% levocabastine versus 4% sodium cromolyn in the allergen challenge model. Ophthalmology 102:310, 1995.

145. Sharif NA, Xu SX, Yanni JM. Olopatadine (AL-4943A): ligand binding and functional studies on a novel, long acting H_1-selective histamine antagonist and anti-allergic agent for use in allergic conjunctivitis. J Ocul Pharmacol Ther 12: 401, 1996.

146. Sharif NA, Xu SX, Miller ST, et al. Characterization of the ocular antiallergic and antihistaminic effects of olopatadine (AL-4943A), a novel drug for treating ocular allergic diseases. J Pharmacol Exp Ther 278:1252, 1996.

147. Yanni JM, Stephens DJ, Miller ST, et al. The in vitro and in vivo ocular pharmacology of olopatadine (AL-4943A), an effective anti-allergic/antihistaminic agent. J Ocul Pharmacol Ther 12:389, 1996.

148. Sharif NA, Xu SX, Yanni JM. Emedastine: a potent, high affinity histamine H_1-receptor-selective antagonist for ocular use: receptor binding and second messenger studies. J Ocul Pharmacol Ther 10:653, 1994.

149. Yanni JM, Stephens DJ, Parnell DW, et al. Preclinical efficacy of emedastine, a potent, selective histamine H_1 antagonist for topical ocular use. J Ocul Pharmacol Ther 10:665, 1994.

150. Saito T, Hagihara A, Igarashi N, et al. Inhibitory effects of emedastine difumarate on histamine release. Jpn J Pharmacol 62:137, 1993.

151. El-Shazley AE, Masuyama K, Samejima Y, et al. Inhibition of human eosinophil chemotaxis in vitro by the antiallergic agent emedastine difumarate. Immunopharmacol Immunotoxicol 18:587, 1996.

152. Abelson MB, Allansmith MR, Friedlaender MH. Effects of topically applied ocular decongestant and antihistamine. Am J Ophthalmol 90:254, 1980.

153. Bishop K, Abelson MB, Cheetham J, et al. Evaluation of flurbiprofen in the treatment of antigen-induced allergic conjunctivitis. Invest Ophthalmol Vis Sci 31:487, 1990.

154. Tinkelman D, Rupp G, Kaufman H, et al. Ketorolac tromethamine 0.5% ophthalmic solution in the treatment of seasonal allergic conjunctivitis: a placebo-controlled clinical trial. Surv Ophthalmol 38 Suppl:33, 141–148, 1993.

155. Laibovitz RA, Koester J, Schaich L, et al. Safety and efficacy of diclofenac sodium 0.1% ophthalmic solution in acute seasonal allergic conjunctivitis. J Ocul Pharmacol Ther 11:361, 1995.

156. Buckley DC, Caldwell DR, Reaves TA. Treatment of vernal conjunctivitis with suprofen, a topical non-steroidal anti-inflammatory agent. Invest Ophthalmol Vis Sci 27 Suppl:29, 1986.

157. Schleimer RP. Effects of glucocorticosteroids on inflammatory cells relevant to their therapeutic applications in asthma. Am Rev Respir Dis 141: S59, 1990.

158. Allansmith MR. Vernal conjunctivitis. In: Clinical ophthalmology 4. Rev. ed. Duane TD, Jaeger EA, eds. Philadelphia, Harper & Row, 1991.

159. Abelson MB, Smith LM. Levocabastine: evaluation in the histamine and compound 48/80 models of ocular allergy in humans. Ophthalmology 95:1494, 1988.

160. Becker B, Kolker AE. Intraocular pressure response to topical corticosteroids. In: Ocular therapy: complications and management. Leopold IH, ed. St. Louis, CV Mosby, 1967, p 79.

161. Druzgala PD, Wu WM, Winwood D, et al. Ocular absorption and distribution of loteprednol etabonate: a "soft" steroid. Invest Ophthalmol Vis Sci 32 Suppl:735, 1991.

162. Leibowitz HM, Kupferman A, Ryan WJ, et al. Corneal anti-inflammatory steroidal "soft drug." Invest Ophthamol Vis Sci 32 Suppl:735, 1991.

163. Leibowitz RA, Ghormley NR, Insler MS, et al. Treatment of giant papillary conjunctivitis with loteprednol etabonate, a novel corticosteroid. Invest Ophthalmol Vis Sci 32 Suppl:734, 1991.

164. Leibowitz HM, Rich R, Crabb JL, et al. Intraocular pressure raising potentials of rimexolone 1.0% in steroid responders. Invest Ophthalmol Vis Sci 35 Suppl:735, 1991.

165. Abelson MB, George M, Drake M, et al. Evaluation of rimexolone ophthalmic suspension in the antigen challenge model of allergic conjunctivitis. Invest Opthalmol Vis Sci 33 Suppl:2094, 1994.

166. Sale S. Immunotherapy. In: Allergy: theory and practice. 2nd ed. Korenblat P, Wedner HJ, eds. Philadelphia, WB Saunders, 1992, p 279.

167. Cooke RA, Barnard JH, Helbald S, et al. Serological evidence of immunity and coexisting sensitization in a type of human allergy (hay fever). J Exp Med 62:733, 1935.

168. Loveless MH. Immunological studies of pollinosis. IV. The relationship between thermostable antibody in the circulation and clinical immunity. J Immunol 47:165, 1943.

169. Koizumi T, Abe T, Sakuragi S. Suppression of experimental allergic conjunctivitis in guinea pigs by oral administration of antigen. Ocul Immunol Inflamm 3:113, 1995.

170. Miller SD, Hanson DG. Inhibition of specific responses by feeding protein antigen. IV. Evidence of tolerance and specific active suppression of cell-mediated immune responses to ovalbumin. J Immunol 123:2344, 1979.

171. Lider O, Santos LMB, Lee CSY, et al. Suppression of experimental autoimmune encephalomyelitis by oral administration of myelin basic protein. II. Suppression of disease and in vitro immune response is mediated by antigen-specific CD8+ T lymphocytes. J Immunol 142:748, 1989.

172. Hoyne GF, Callow MG, Kuhlman J, et al. T-cell lymphokine response to orally administered proteins during priming and unresponsiveness. Immunology 78:534, 1993.

173. Bousquet J, Michel FB. Advances in specific immunotherapy. Clin Exp Allergy 22: 889, 1992.

174. Bousquet J, Hejjaoui A, Soussana M, et al. Double-blind, placebo-controlled immunotherapy and mixed grass-pollen allergoids. J Allergy Clin Immunol 85:490, 1990.

175. Bousquet J, Maasch H, Hejjaoui A, et al. Double blind, placebo-controlled immunotherapy and mixed grass pollen allergoids. III. Comparison with an unfractioned allergoid, a fractionated allergoid and a standardized orchard grass pollen in rhinitis, conjunctivitis and asthma. J Allergy Clin Immunol 84:546, 1989.

176. Karlsson R, Agrell B, Dreborg S, et al. A double-blind, multi-center immunotherapy trial in children, using a purified and standardized *Cladosporium herbarum* preparation. II. In vitro results. Allergy 41:141, 1986.

177. Moller C, Dreborg S, Lanner A, et al. Oral immunotherapy of children with rhinoconjunctivitis due to birch pollen allergy. Allergy 41:271, 1986.

178. Nakagawa T, Yamashita N, Mizushima Y, et al. Inhibition of allergic bronchoconstriction in guinea pigs and in asthmatics by the leukotriene antagonist ONO-1078. Int Arch Allergy Immunol 99:490, 1992.

179. Ford-Hutchinson AW. Lipoxygenase inhibitors as future anti-allergy drugs? In: New approaches to the treatment of allergic diseases: an update on anti-allergy drugs. Boston, ACAI, 1989, p 43.

180. Kalpaxis JG, Thayer TO. Double-blind trial of pentigetide ophthalmic solution 0.5% compared with cromolyn sodium 4% ophthalmic solution for allergic conjunctivitis. Ann Allergy 66:393, 1991.

181. Hamburger RN. Recent studies with human IgE pentapeptide (HEPP). In: New trends in allergy. Ring J, Burg G, eds. Berlin, Springer-Verlag, 1981, p 311.

182. Hahn GS, McClurg MR, Plummer JM. Subcutaneous pentigetide (IgE pentapeptide) suppresses substance p-induced inflammation in mice (abstract 48). Ann Allergy 62:250, 1989.

183. Ciprandi G, Buscaglia S, Pesce G, et al. Allergic subjects express intercellular adhesion molecule-1 (ICAM-1 or CD54) on epithelial cells of conjunctiva after allergen challenge. J Allergy Clin Immunol 91:783, 1993.

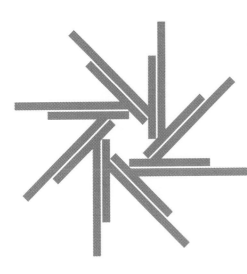

CHAPTER 16

Atopic Keratoconjunctivitis

RICHARD CASEY

DESCRIPTION

Atopy is a hereditary condition that manifests in ocular disease, skin abnormalities, and respiratory tract dysfunction. Atopy occurs in 5 to 20% of the general population. Atopic keratoconjunctivitis (AKC) is a term used to describe one of the most severe forms of allergic disease in the eye. However, this term is misleading. Although the ocular surface disease may be the most prominent feature, the disease typically involves the lids, as well as intraocular and non-ocular structures.

HISTORY

Atopy, as defined by Cocoa and Cooke,[1] originally referred to the inability of serum from asthma patients to fix complement. The intravascular entity responsible for this phenomenon remained elusive until Prausnitz[2] showed that a fish allergy could be transferred from a patient (Kustner) to himself by the simple transfer of serum. Subsequent exposure to the offending antigen resulted in the classic wheal-and-flare skin response, known as the Prausnitz-Kustner reaction. Ishizaka and Ishizaka[3] later determined that immunoglobulin E (IgE) was the serum agent mediating this response.

Since that time, IgE has been implicated as a major component of the pathological mechanism observed in atopic disorders.

EPIDEMIOLOGY

In 1953, Hogan[4] reported a unique form of keratoconjunctivitis in five male patients with atopic dermatitis. This disorder, AKC, is now well recognized and is known to occur in up to 25% of patients with atopic dermatitis.[5] These patients possess an inherited predisposition for hypersensitivity to specific allergens. A review of family history frequently reveals the presence of other atopic diseases such as asthma, hay fever, and urticaria. AKC occurs most frequently in men. Symptoms of the disorder typically begin in the late teens or early twenties, and they persist until the fourth or fifth decade of life. The peak incidence of AKC occurs between the ages of 30 and 50 years.[6] In many affected patients, clinical signs of the disease generally improve with age and may totally regress. However, patients with severe cases do not follow this trend. AKC is often worse in the winter, but it usually has a perennial pattern of occurrence.

CLINICAL FEATURES

The most frequently reported symptom of AKC is bilateral itching. Tearing is also common. The associated ocular discharge is characteristically stringy or rope-like because of the accumulation of cellular debris, fibrin, and mucin. Burning, photophobia, and blurred vision are frequent complaints as well.

Atopic blepharitis is typically characterized by tylosis, a thickening of the eyelid margins, and eyelid swelling associated with a scaly, indurated, and wrinkled appearance of the periocular skin.[7] With profound swelling, a Dennie-Morgan fold or "Dennie line" is seen. Chronic inflammation can produce upper eyelid ptosis. Fissures frequently develop at the lateral canthus, owing to excessive eye rubbing. An absence of lateral eyebrows, or Hertoghe's sign, is seen in severe forms of atopic lid disease. Marginal blepharitis caused by staphylococcal infection is common.

A hallmark of AKC is chronic ocular surface inflammation. The conjunctiva becomes hyperemic and edematous. Tarsal conjunctival papillary hypertrophy is a common finding. Limbal papillae frequently give the appearance of gelatinous nodules adjacent to the cornea.[8] Trantas' dots have been seen in association with these lesions. Chronic disease can result in conjunctival cicatrization and symblepharon, most commonly in the inferior fornix (Fig. 16.1).

Corneal involvement may include punctate erosions and keratitis. Intraepithelial microcysts have also been reported. Patients with AKC are at risk to develop both infectious and noninfectious corneal ulcers. In the case of the latter, the lesion is usually horizontally oval, in a paracentral location with irregular borders. Peripheral micropannus is common in chronic AKC. Neovascularization can extend to the central cornea, thereby contributing to visual impairment. All forms of corneal ectasia including keratoconus, pellucid marginal degeneration, and keratoglobus have been reported in patients with AKC. Keratoconus has been reported in as many as 16% of patients with AKC and in approximately 25% of patients with atopic dermatitis overall.

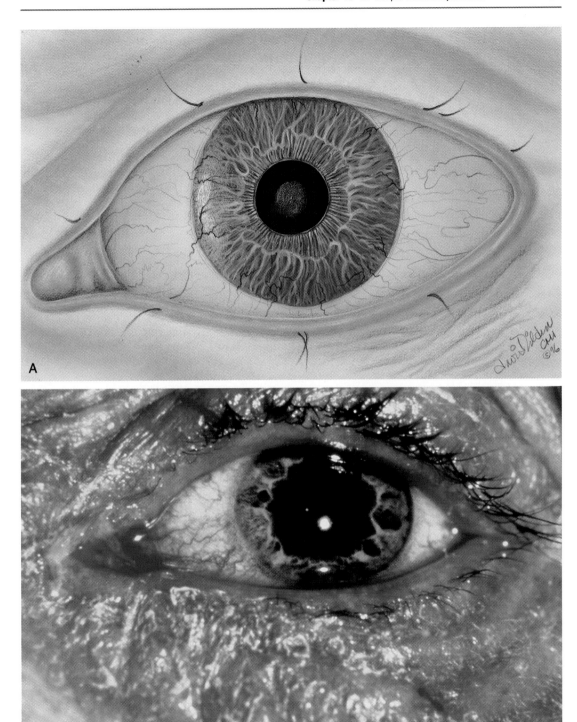

FIGURE 16.1 *A* and *B*, A hallmark of atopic keratoconjunctivitis is chronic ocular surface inflammation. The conjunctiva becomes hyperemic and edematous. Tarsal conjunctival papillary hypertrophy is a common finding. Limbal papillae frequently give the appearance of gelatinous nodules adjacent to the cornea.

Visual deterioration may be compounded by the development of cataracts.[9] The classic AKC-related cataract occurs in the anterior subcapsular region and is often described as a "shield cataract." Lenticular opacities frequently form in the posterior subcapsular region, and long-term corticosteroid use may accelerate the development of these opacities.

Retinal detachments, the cause of which is not entirely understood, are infrequently seen in patients with atopic dermatitis. Several theories have been proposed, including long-term eye rubbing and degenerative vitreous changes. However, none of these theories has been proven.

Systemic disorders associated with AKC can be divided into two groups, major and minor atopies. The major atopies include hay fever, bronchial asthma, and atopic dermatitis. Food allergies, urticaria, and nonhereditary angioedema comprise the minor atopies. One study of patients with AKC revealed that 87% had concomitant asthma and 95% had concomitant eczema.

The dermatitis seen in atopic patients warrants additional mention. Atopic dermatitis (eczema) is a chronic, pruritic inflammation of the skin. The lesions can involve the entire body, but more frequently they are seen on the forehead, cheeks, and flexor surfaces of the arms and legs. Unlike ocular disease, skin manifestations usually begin during childhood. The itching and scratching experienced by patients with atopic dermatitis can be so intense that the skin becomes erythematous, excoriated, lichenified, and hypopigmented. Cutaneous infections compound the atopic dermatitis in these patients.

ETIOLOGY AND HISTOPATHOLOGY

Although the exact origin of AKC is unclear, evidence suggests that both type I hypersensitivity and type IV delayed hypersensitivity responses may be involved. Elevated levels of tear and serum IgE are characteristic of exacerbated AKC. During remissions, serum IgE levels typically decline. Interestingly, although allergen exposure can worsen symptoms of the disease, allergen-specific IgE levels do not increase in the tears of AKC patients compared with non-atopic controls.

During acute attacks of AKC, B-cell levels are elevated, whereas levels of T cells are depressed. Because suppresser T cells play a role in regulating IgE production, the depressed T-cell activity may contribute to the increased IgE levels, thus enhancing the disease by triggering mast cell degranulation.

Reports have shown that approximately 50 million mast cells can be found in the ocular and adnexal tissues. Conjunctival scrapings obtained during acute episodes of the disease also show an excess of eosinophils. The release of mediators such as histamine, prostaglandins, eosinophil major basic protein, complement, neutrophil and eosinophil chemotactic factors, platelet-activating factor, and other arachidonic acid metabolites reliably produces the characteristic features of ocular allergy.

Notable distinctions and similarities exist between the histopathogenesis of AKC and that of atopic dermatitis. Chronic lesions of atopic dermatitis demonstrate an increased number of mast cells and Langerhans' cells (LCs). The LC plays a major role in the immune response because of its antigen-presenting function. The LC possesses numerous surface receptors for a variety of molecules, including cytokines, such as interleukin-2, the Fc fragment of IgG, and complement (C3). Studies show that the LCs of atopic patients have excessive expression of receptors for IgE. Allergen binding to IgE on epidermal LCs results in T-lymphocyte proliferation (resulting from antigen presentation) or eosinophil infiltration and activation induced by eosinophil chemotactic factor. The role of peripheral corneal and limbal LCs in AKC is poorly understood; however, one could speculate that similarities with epidermal LC activation may explain the limbal and peripheral corneal inflammation, scarring, and neovascularization characteristic of this disease.

Dysfunctional or diminished cell-mediated immunity is common. Patients with AKC frequently show no type IV delayed hypersensitivity response to *Candida*. Furthermore, an increased propensity to develop infections, particularly with fungal and viral pathogens, has been observed.

DIAGNOSIS

A detailed family history regarding atopy is extremely important when evaluating patients with symptoms of ocular allergy. An allergic predisposition is nearly three times more common in atopic families compared with non-atopic families. It is rare to see AKC in a patient with a negative family history and no obvious systemic manifestation of the disease.

Several features distinguish AKC from other forms of ocular allergy. The perennial nature of the ocular inflammation immediately distinguishes it from hay fever (or seasonal allergic conjunctivitis) and vernal keratoconjunctivitis (VKC). Although specific allergens such as molds, animal danders, and some foods may exacerbate the disease, some level of disease activity is nearly always present. Giant papillary conjunctivitis can be superimposed on the conjunctival findings seen in AKC. However, this finding is unusual because most atopic patients are intolerant to contact lens wear.

VKC is typically associated with papillae involving the superior conjunctiva compared with the inferior lid involvement seen in AKC. VKC also tends to begin in younger persons, typically in the second decade of life. Although symptoms of AKC may begin in the late teenage years, they most commonly occur later, such as in the third or fourth decade of life. A major characteristic of AKC that cannot be overemphasized is the severity of symptoms and of tissue destruction that accompanies this disorder.

MANAGEMENT

The goal of therapy of AKC is to maintain visual acuity and to alleviate the symptoms associated with ocular and periocular inflammation. In general, the use of cold compresses and vasoconstrictors to reduce swelling and the avoidance of exacerbating allergens is helpful. Similarly, the patient should be instructed to refrain from eye rubbing. This disrupts the itching cycle by preventing mechanically induced degranulation of mast cells. Further trauma to the eyelid skin and ocular surface is also prevented.

Antihistamines

The systemic manifestations of atopy in patients with AKC should not be overlooked. Co-management of the disease with an internist, dermatologist, or allergist may be required, particularly when symptomatic complaints of itching and clinical signs of inflammation extend beyond the ocular and periocular tissues. In such cases, systemic antihistamines are more likely to be efficacious. Antihistamines competitively and reversibly block histamine receptor activation. Commercially available topical ophthalmic preparations containing H_1 antihistamines include antazoline phosphate, pyrilamine maleate, pheniramine maleate, and levocabastine. The last compound is extremely potent when compared with other agents.[10]

Nonsteroidal Anti-inflammatory Drugs

Thromboxanes and prostaglandins are potent mediators of inflammation that are generated by the activity of cyclooxygenase on arachidonic acid. Inhibition of the cyclooxygenase pathway is achieved through the use of nonsteroidal anti-inflammatory drugs (NSAIDs). Topical ketorolac tromethamine, a potent analgesic, prevents ocular inflammation by inhibiting prostaglandin synthetase.[11] Ketorolac 0.25% and 0.5% demonstrated efficacy against corneal neovascularization. Current studies are under way to establish the role of other cyclooxygenase inhibitors and lipoxygenase inhibitors in AKC.

Mast Cell Stabilizers

Topical mast cell stabilizers are effective agents for long-term control of itching and inflammation. These agents are frequently used in conjunction with topical antihistamines because the former lacks the ability to relieve symptomatic itching immediately. Mast cell stabilizers are purported to exert their effect by preventing mast cell degranulation and mediator release. Cromolyn sodium has been shown to inhibit neutrophil and eosinophil activation.[12] Nedocromil sodium blocks both inflammatory cell activation and mediator release from eosinophils, neutrophils, monocytes, macrophages, and mast cells.[13] Lodoxamide has an effect on both mast cells and eosinophils, thus decreasing the ability of the eosinophil to produce eosinophil major basic protein. Lodoxamide 0.1% was demonstrated in one study to be superior to cromolyn sodium 2% in the relief of symptoms and signs of ocular allergy.[13]

Corticosteroids

Corticosteroids block the formation of arachidonic acid metabolites by inhibiting phospholipase A_2. This effect prevents leukocyte migration, hydrolytic enzyme release, fibroblast growth, and changes in vascular permeability.

Topical corticosteroid therapy is extremely effective in relieving symptoms of itching and in reducing the inflammation associated with most cases of AKC. However, the chronic nature of the disease and the need for long-term therapy substantially increase the likelihood of ocular complications with prolonged steroid use. These complications include infection secondary to local immune suppression, steroid-induced glaucoma, cataracts, and corneal melting. Patients should be advised of these risks. Corticosteroids should be used with extreme caution in these patients. "Pulse" administration with topical prednisolone should be reserved for the treatment of acute exacerbations only. Several newer ophthalmic steroids are effective anti-inflammatory agents with a significantly reduced risk of side effects, although the potential for a serious side effect still exists.

Cyclosporine

Several types of therapy displaying potential in other types of ocular disease are also under consideration for treatment of AKC. Cyclosporine, a cyclic peptide, is a potent immunomodulator that inhibits the action of interleukin-2 on T lymphocytes. Cyclosporine 2% in castor oil has been shown to decrease the signs and symptoms of VKC; however, its efficacy in the treatment of AKC remains unknown.[14]

The chronic nature of AKC and its propensity toward visually disabling complications underscore the care and diligence needed to manage the disease adequately. Strict compliance with medication regimens and examinations is extremely important. Treatment often requires the use of combination drug therapy. Various H_1 antihistamines, mast cell stabilizers, and NSAIDs are now available. Although corticosteroids are effective in the management of acute inflammation, they can also have devastating consequences with indiscriminate or prolonged use. The possible need for a multidisciplinary approach with the assistance of an internist, dermatologist, allergist, or psychiatrist cannot be overemphasized.

AKC is an isolated component of a systemic disease sometimes requiring systemic therapy. Optimal management is only achieved when all sites of disease are appropriately treated.

REFERENCES

1. Cocoa AF, Cooke RA. On the classification of the phenomena of hypersensitiveness J Immunol 8:163, 1923.
2. Prausnitz C, Kustner H. Studien uber die Uberempfindlichkeit. Zentralbl Bakteriol 86:160, 1921.
3. Ishizaka K, Ishizaka T. Identification of gamma E antibodies as a carrier of reaginic activity. J Immunol 99:1187, 1967.
4. Hogan MJ. Atopic keratoconjunctivitis. Am J Ophthalmol 36:937, 1953.
5. Braude LS, Chandler JW. Atopic corneal disease. Int Ophthalmol Clin 24:145, 1984.
6. Donshik PC. Allergic conjunctivitis. Int Ophthalmol Clin 28:294, 1988.
7. Garrity JA, Liesegang TJ. Ocular complications of atopic dermatitis. Can J Ophthalmol 19:21, 1984.
8. Friendlaender MH. Conjunctivitis of allergic origin: clinical presentation and differential diagnosis. Surv Ophthalmol 38:105, 1993.
9. Allansmith MR, Ross RN. Ocular allergy. Clin Allergy 18:1, 1988.
10. Abelson MB, George MA, Smith LM. Evaluation of 0.05% levocabastine versus 4% sodium cromolyn in the allergy challenge model. Ophthalmology 102:310, 1995.
11. Rooks WH. Pharmacologic activity of ketorolac tromethamine. Pharmacotherapy 10:208, 1990.
12. Kulkarni PS, Srinivasan BD, Kaufman P. Comparison of cyclooxygenase and lipoxygenase pathways in rabbit and monkey ocular tissues (abstract). Invest Ophthalmol Vis Sci 26 Suppl:191, 1985.
13. Fahy GT, Easty DL, Collun LM, et al. Randomised double-masked trial of lodoxamide and sodium cromoglycate in allergic eye disease. A multicentre study. Eur J Ophthalmol 2:144–149, 1992.
14. Trocme SD, Raizman MB, Bartley GB. Medical therapy for ocular allergy. Mayo Clin Proc 67:557, 1992.

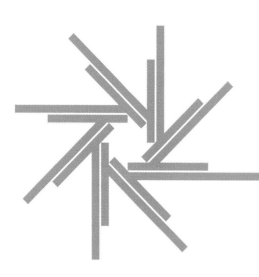

CHAPTER **17**

Giant Papillary Conjunctivitis

JACK V. GREINER

Giant papillary conjunctivitis (GPC) is characterized by the presence of abnormally large papillae (more than 0.3 mm in diameter) on the upper tarsal conjunctiva, conjunctival hyperemia, excess mucus secretion, and foreign body sensation or pruritus. The condition was first reported in 1970 in a patient wearing rigid contact lenses[1] and later in 1974 in patients wearing hydrogel contact lenses.[2] The disease was eventually characterized and named based on observations from a study of rigid and hydrogel contact lens wearers in 1977.[3] GPC has also been reported to result from ocular prostheses,[4–7] exposed suture barbs following anterior segment surgery,[4, 8–15] and the presence of irregularities in the ocular surface. In the last case, such surface abnormalities in the cornea have resulted from foreign bodies,[16] cyanoacrylate glue,[17] and elevated corneal deposits,[18] including band keratopathy.[19] Abnormalities in the remaining tissues of the ocular surface may also present topographical irregularities, such as limbal dermoid,[20] dermolipomas,[21] glaucoma filtering blebs,[19, 22] and extruded scleral buckles.[23]

Although GPC can occur in all the foregoing patient groups, it occurs most often in contact lens wearers, and, as such, most of our knowledge about the condition is from this group. The signs and symptoms in each patient group are similar (Figs. 17.1 and 17.2) and reversible in most cases. Investigators have proposed that the syndrome of papillary hypertrophy, mucus, and itching be recognized as a generalized response to some type of stimulation and not one restricted to any particular disease.[6]

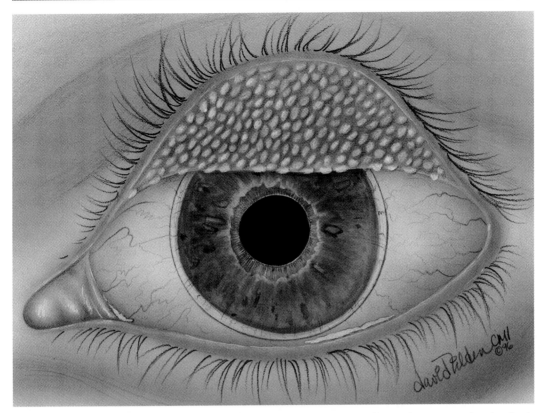

FIGURE 17.1 Giant papillary conjunctivitis. The everted upper eyelid with giant papillae on the upper tarsal conjunctiva is demonstrated.

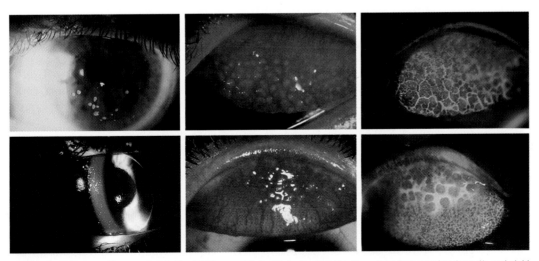

FIGURE 17.2 Giant papillary conjunctivitis (GPC) associated with hydrophilic (soft) contact lens wearing (row 1), and rigid (hard) contact lens wearing (row 2). Ocular surface condition (left column), GPC in white light (middle), fluorescein staining of GPC with cobalt blue light (right column). (Courtesy of Dr. John P. Herman.)

The syndrome of GPC shares some features with vernal conjunctivitis (VC).[24, 25] Both syndromes are characterized by proliferation of subepithelial collagen and development of hyperplastic nodules on the upper tarsal conjunctiva, excess production of mucus, and itching. Such similarities give rise to the possibility that these disorders have similar underlying pathophysiological features. Both GPC and VC involve mechanical trauma. In the case of GPC, the trauma may be due to a prosthetic device, suture, or irregularity in the ocular surface, whereas in VC it is caused by eye rubbing resulting from the presence of antigen. As such, the response of resident mast cells to either eye rubbing, which is known to degranulate mast cells,[26] or the conjunctival trauma induced by the foreign body may be involved in hyperactivity of the tissue. Such hyperactivity can be manifested by release of mast cell mediators, which may result in infiltration of white blood cells, fibroblastic activity, and the consequent formation of conjunctival papillae. A relationship appears to exist between mast cells and inflammatory cells and the proliferation of collagen associated with these diseases.

GPC is an interplay among several factors, which include genetic predisposition, environmental exposure to a provoking agent, duration of exposure to the agent, and the agent's location on the conjunctival surface. As such, the onset of disease appears to be the result of both genetic endowment and exposure.

EPIDEMIOLOGY

GPC appears to be a generalized response to the presence of a foreign body. The most common cause of GPC is the wearing of rigid or hydrogel contact lenses. Contact lens GPC can occur bilaterally or unilaterally.[3] Epidemiological studies demonstrated that the presentation of GPC in hydrogel contact lens wearers is almost exclusively bilateral, with a mean onset time of 31 months after commencing lens wear.[27] Cases of unilateral GPC are rare[28] in the contact lens–wearing population. In GPC associated with sutures, foreign bodies, abnormal growths on the ocular surface, filtering blebs, and scleral buckles, the presentation is more often unilateral.

Retrospective epidemiological studies reveal a strong association of GPC with wearing contact lenses as well as with age. The correlation with age most likely reflects the fact that more younger people wear contact lenses, thus disproportionately representing the contact lens–wearing population.[27] Affected patients range in age from 3 to 60 years.[6] Gender was not found to be an associated factor with the condition.[27]

Investigators have estimated that between 1 and 5% of wearers of rigid gas permeable contact lenses and between 10 and 15% of those wearing hydrogel contact lenses have GPC.[29, 30] A prospective study of 200 wearers of rigid contact lenses revealed a GPC prevalence of 10.5%.[30]

A history of atopy plays a major role in predisposition of GPC.[31, 32] A retrospective study of personal histories of patients with contact lens–associated GPC disclosed a high incidence of atopy.[33] Of further significance is a bi-modal distribution in time of diagnoses of GPC, with peaks in the spring and in late summer to early fall.[33] This study correlated well with the report of increased numbers of patients with GPC diagnosed in March as compared with February.[34] Perhaps GPC occurs more commonly in the spring than in the fall[35] because of the pollen seasons and individual differences in susceptibility. Patients with GPC report a higher incidence of allergy to pollen as well as to medications, including preservatives in contact lens solutions. Pollen and other allergenic substances adhere to contact lenses, especially in patients with dry eye, who have a poor tear film and poor contact lens wetting. No seasonal predilection is reported for non–contact lens–induced GPC. However, report of these cases are so few that such studies have not been performed.

ETIOLOGY

The origin of GPC appears to be a combination of mechanical irritation and allergic factors.[36] In the case of contact lenses, GPC can be observed in both rigid (polymethylmethacrylate) (or gas-permeable) contact lenses as well as hydrogel (soft) lenses, although the incidence is greater in wearers of hydrogel contact lens.[37] Evidence has demonstrated that both chronic mechanical trauma induced by contact lenses on the conjunctiva[29, 38] and intolerance to accumulated lens deposits are important contributing factors in the development of GPC.[3, 30] Moreover, mechanical irritation from the large-diameter soft contact lenses, along with a greater tendency for mucoprotein deposits coating the lenses, increases the potential for development of GPC.[35]

Although increased contact lens coatings may be suspected on lathe-cut lenses, GPC has also been reported to occur in patients wearing ultrathin spin-cast soft contact lenses.[39] In a review of patients wearing hydrogel contact lenses, investigators observed that most of the lenses worn by patients with GPC were large, thin lenses (14.5 mm and greater) with edge thicknesses of 0.06 to 0.21 mm, but not all these lenses were made of the same polymer.[40] The distribution of developing papillae corresponds to the area of the tarsal conjunctiva in contact with the lens periphery or lens edge. The smaller hard contact lens predominantly affects zones 2 and 3 (Fig. 17.3), whereas the relatively larger soft contact lens affects zones 1 and 2. The development of GPC has been reported to be independent of lens polymer type in some studies,[3] but it has also been associated with a high water content of the hydrogel lenses in other studies.[27] Wearing time is a factor because GPC is more prevalent in patients wearing lenses on an extended-wear schedule than in those wearing lenses on a daily-wear basis.

Lens surface deposits appear the same by scanning electron microscopy whether they are from patients with GPC or from contact lens wearers who do not have GPC.[39] This finding suggests that GPC may be more the result of individual susceptibility differences than of differences in lens deposits

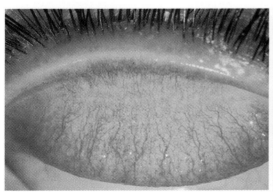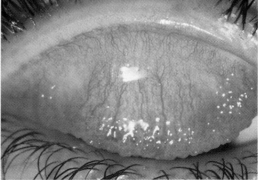

FIGURE 17.3 Unilateral contact lens–associated giant papillary conjunctivitis. The upper tarsal conjunctiva with white light, and the contralateral upper tarsal conjunctiva under the same condition of white light. (Courtesy of Dr. John P. Herman.)

(Fig. 17.4). Investigators have hypothesized that the antigen initiating the hypersensitivity could be found in the deposit on the contact lens as opposed to the antigen being the lens polymer itself. When GPC patients wore a new clean lens of the same composition or an old lens that had protein debris removed, the syndrome improved or disappeared.

A further hypothesis[12] suggests that deposits on the lenses may be the result rather than the cause of the condition. For example, in the case of suture irritation in aphakic patients, excess mucus production occurs. Mucus functions as an important constituent of the preocular tear film, but also it is secreted as a normal response of the eye to rid itself of foreign bodies. With further irritation, mucus produces a papillary response. In the case of contact lens–associated GPC, the edge of the contact lens, rigid or hydrogel, could possibly be traumatizing the upper palpebral conjunctival surface,[41–43] to produce inflammatory cell changes[3, 6] and mucus,[44] thus precipitating the GPC syndrome.

Certainly, trauma could be the initial stage of the disease because all examples to date are associated with foreign bodies and the upper tarsal conjunctiva, except in the case of GPC induced by filtering blebs. The upper eyelid is traumatized in the upper tarsal region of the conjunctiva with each blink of the eyelid. This factor becomes significant when one considers that blinking occurs 16,000 to 19,000 times daily.[45] As the trauma continues, it provides a portal of entry for antigen, whether it is on the contact lens surface or within the tear film. Inducing hypersensitivity in this setting stimulates lymphocytes, mast cells, basophils, and eosinophils to initiate an immune response.

The presence of mast cells in the conjunctival epithelium and of eosinophils and basophils in the epithelium and substantia propria of the conjunctiva reveals a chemotactic response in which these cells react with immunoglobulin E (IgE) and inflammatory mediators.[6] The inflammatory process may also involve type I hypersensitivity. Mast cells can be quantified in the

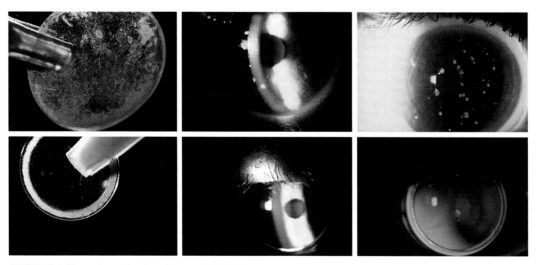

FIGURE 17.4 Film and granular deposits on a hydrophilic (soft) contact lens from a patient with giant papillary conjunctivitis (GPC) (top left), a slit-lamp photograph of a coated soft contact lens (top middle), and a contact lens with "jelly bumps" on the anterior surface in a patient with GPC (top right). Peripheral deposits on a rigid contact lens from a patient with GPC (bottom left); a slit-lamp photograph of a coated rigid contact lens (bottom middle); and the same lens following fluorescein instillation and exposure to cobalt blue light (bottom right). (Courtesy of Dr. John P. Herman.)

epithelium of patients with GPC by routine histological study.[6] In fact, probably more mast cells are present than can be observed by routine histological examination because transmission electron microscopy provides evidence of mast cell degranulation with mast cell remnants that cannot be identified by light microscopy.[46] Mast cells have also been identified in the conjunctival epithelium of monkeys wearing contact lenses from patients with GPC.[47] Data suggest that the development of GPC does not depend on the amount of lens deposition of normal tear proteins IgA, IgG, IgE, lactoferrin, or lysozyme.[48, 49] Statistically significant increases in IgM deposition may reflect an immune response in GPC.[48]

An immune response may be the trigger for the papillary response and papillogenesis. The collection of mucus on the contact lens surface may trap chemicals from the contact lens solutions and other protein that may be in the tear film. Within 8 hours of wear, a contact lens becomes coated with material comprised of mucus, protein, bacteria, cells, cell debris, and airborne pollutants.[50] Even vigorous contact lens hygiene cannot clean a cloudy lens, and cleaning with surfactant and enzymes fails to remove this lens coating completely. Successive days of wear cause a steady increase in lens coating. As time goes by, this contact lens debris (denatured protein) may become a foreign material to the mucous membrane,[3, 30] and patients prone to allergy may develop an antigen-antibody reaction to this foreign protein.

Exposed suture barbs (ends) left after cataract extraction or corneal transplantation also can produce GPC. In these cases, the papillae are usually localized to the region of the upper tarsal conjunctiva opposing the location of suture in the ocular wound. Such observations stress the importance of burying suture knots and ends during cataract[51] and corneal transplantation procedures,[11-15] or during any procedure involving repair of a corneal or conjunctival wound. The GPC response occurs with both 10-0 nylon[12] and Prolene[15] suture material. Following removal of the offending suture, the GPC resolves.

GPC associated with ocular prostheses resolves with discontinuation, refitting or modification, or improved cleaning of the prostheses. The surface coating on the polymethylmethacrylate prostheses and the trauma to the upper tarsal conjunctiva are believed to be associated with the development of GPC.

In the case of irregularities of the ocular surface, GPC resolves when the foreign body or abnormal tissue is removed. In a case of an epibulbar dermolipoma (ectopic hair-bearing skin on the surface of the lesion), marked GPC in the area of the upper tarsal conjunctiva juxtaposed to the dermolipoma has been observed, undoubtedly resulting from the trauma from the surface hairs. Excess mucus secretion was also noted that would obscure vision when it smeared across the visual axis.[21]

In a case of bilateral bleb-related GPC following a filtering procedure for glaucoma, GPC developed 3 years postoperatively. The location of the papillae was related precisely to the site of the bleb in each eye. The blebs had no atypical features, no surface keratinization was present, and no suture material was exposed.[22] That the blebs created an elevation of the normally smooth bulbar conjunctival surface may have been enough of an abnormality to cause GPC.

Dry eye conditions such as meibomian gland dysfunction may also contribute to GPC.[52-56] Investigators have hypothesized that meibomian gland dysfunction contributes to ocular irritation, leading to an increased incidence of GPC. Patients with GPC have been more likely to have meibomian gland dysfunction with gland dropout than patients without GPC.[54] Although a relationship appears to exist between many dry eye conditions and GPC, the mechanism is unclear.

SIGNS AND SYMPTOMS

The earliest signs of GPC may be subtle, consisting of increased mucus in the inner canthus on awakening.[3] With progression of the disease, mucus may be present as a stringy, sheet-like discharge. Patients may complain that the eyelids are "stuck" together on arising in the morning. The predominant diagnostic sign of GPC, the hallmark of the disease, is the appearance of abnormally enlarged papillae (more than 0.3 mm in diameter) on the upper tarsus. These displace the normal-sized papillae,[41, 57] resulting in thickening of the upper tarsal conjunctiva. The number of papillae can vary from hundreds covering the entire tarsal conjunctiva[3, 29, 38] to one papilla. In patients with rigid and hydrogel contact lenses and in patients wearing prosthetic shells, the papillae are raised and have a collagen substructure. A vascular supply is observed radiating from a vessel occupying the central core of each papilla.[3] In patients with hydrogel contact lenses, GPC may start at the upper portion of the lid (see Fig. 17.3). As it progresses, more and more of the lid becomes involved, including the conjunctival tissue subjacent to the lid margin.[37] The progression of papillae to other zones of the conjunctiva may be the result of increased lens movement during disease progression. Signs of GPC can appear after as few as 3 weeks of lens wearing or after as long as 3½ years; the average onset of signs occurs around 18 to 20 months after initiating lens wear.[2, 3, 58, 59]

The papillae associated with rigid (hard) contact lens wear first appear in the central zone of the tarsal plate (see Fig. 17.3).[3, 29] Signs of papillae have been reported to appear even after 9 to 11 years of successful hard contact lens wear.[3, 4] A similar time course occurs in patients wearing ocular prostheses.[7, 60] Papillae associated with suture barbs from 10-0 nylon can occur as early as 6 weeks to as late as 15 months following cataract surgery or keratoplasty.[9, 12]

The second most prevalent sign of GPC is excessive mucus. Although no increase occurs in the number of mucus-secreting goblet cells per unit area of conjunctiva,[61] the overall increase in surface area seen with the development of raised papillae may actually increase the absolute number of goblet cells. Moreover, the mucus vesicles in non-goblet epithelial cells of the conjunctiva (second mucus-secretory system[62]) contribute dramatically to the increase in mucus production (Figs. 17.5 and 17.6).[44, 63, 64] Excess mucus can interfere with vision by coating contact lenses and by being smeared over the visual axis with blinking and eyelid movement. Eversion of the upper eyelid, particularly following fluorescein staining, may reveal strands of mucus streaking over the otherwise smooth upper tarsal conjunctival surface (Fig. 17.7). In severe cases, a milky white discharge covering broad areas of giant papillae may also be present. Patients may report accumulations of mucus in the nasal corner of the eye.

Mild to severe hyperemia of the upper tarsal conjunctiva may also be observed in GPC (Fig. 17.8). The conjunctiva, whether hyperemic or not, remains translucent, but careful observation reveals thickening. With progression and further inflammatory cell infiltration, the conjunctiva begins to lose its transparency. Occasionally, Trantas' dots and limbal inflammation may occur.[65] Ptosis has been associated with GPC[66, 67]; this condition may be secondary to inflammation.

The signs of GPC may be preceded by clinical symptoms, including mild foreign body sensation, intolerance to contact lens wearing, or irritation of the anterior segment resulting from exposed suture barbs or irregularities in the ocular surface. Symptoms range from minimal discomfort with lens insertion or removal to complete contact lens–wearing intolerance.[3] The earliest symptom of GPC is ocular discomfort or itchy, irritated eyes soon

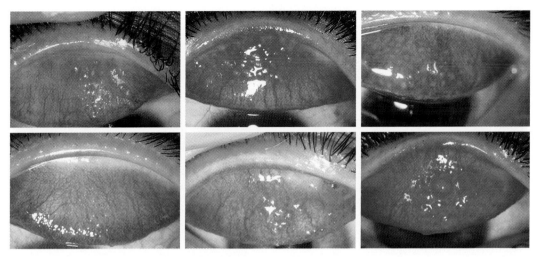

FIGURE 17.5 Zonal distribution of contact lens–associated papillae on the upper tarsal conjunctiva of rigid (hard) contact lens wearers (top row) (left: papillae zone 3 only; center: papillae zones 2 and 3 only; right: papillae in all 3 zones). Zonal; distribution of contact lens–associated papillae in the upper tarsal conjunctiva of soft (hydrophilic) contact lens wearer (bottom row) (left: papillae zone 2 only; center: papillae zones 2 and 3 only; right: papillae in all 3 zones). (Courtesy of John P. Herman.)

after contact lens removal. This complaint usually precedes clinical signs of GPC, and no objective correlates or diagnoses may be made. The severity of GPC can be graded not only by the presence or absence of itching after removal of lenses, but also by how long the itch persists following lens removal. In moderate to severe GPC, itching may persist for several hours after lens removal. If left untreated, the pruritus eventually occurs during lens wear.

When the lens becomes coated with mucus and cellular and environmental debris, the patient complains of irritation and increased lens movement. As a result of both increased mucus and lens coating or displacement, visual clarity varies and may be reduced. When mucus strands are the major sign, patients remark that the vision clears after blinking.

DIAGNOSTIC TOOLS

Obtaining a good history is integral to the proper diagnosis of GPC. Although duration of contact lens wear or daily wear time may not be as important as lens fit and design, patients who have worn lenses for several years may report a recent change in lens type or fitting associated with their symptoms of foreign body sensation and increased mucus secretion. In such cases, the diagnosis of GPC may be excluded. These symptoms coupled with poor lens hygiene, such as not performing daily cleaning or weekly enzymatic cleansing of contact lenses, should prompt suspicion of GPC. Fluctuating vision may provide further suspicion of GPC.

Nevertheless, final diagnosis is made using the simple maneuver of everting the upper eyelid, thus exposing the tarsal conjunctiva. The tarsal surface is examined for papillae with the biomicroscope using white light and 10 and 16 times magnifications. The tarsal conjunctiva should then be examined in more detail with 25 times magnification. Under magnification, papillae are considered to be elevated only when observed to protrude from the surrounding conjunctival surface. Both location and number of papillae

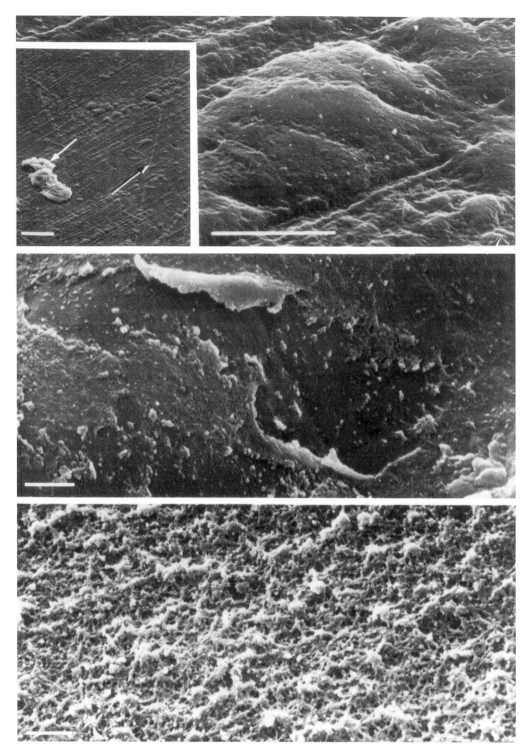

FIGURE 17.6 Scanning electron micrographs of coatings on soft contact lenses from patients with giant papillary conjunctivitis. Deposits may be observed along the lens surface (black on white arrow) as well as what appears to be particulate mucus (arrow, top row). Note peeling of the deposit from the surface of the lens. (From Allansmith MR, Ross RN, Greiner JV. Giant papillary conjunctivitis. In Contact Lenses: The CLAO guide to basic sciences and clinical practice, 2nd edition. Dabezies OH JR (ed). London, Little, Brown, 1989, p. 431.)

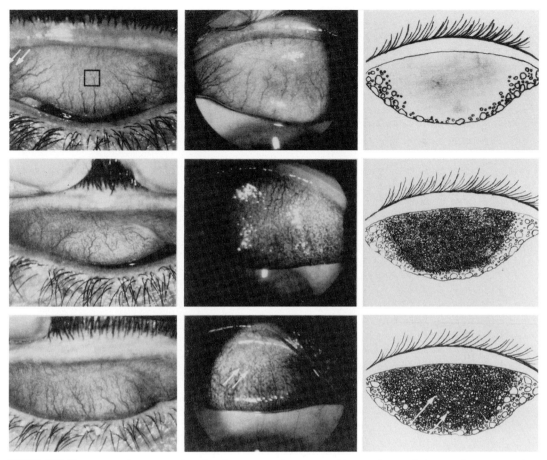

FIGURE 17.7 Three types of upper tarsal conjunctivae as seen in persons with normal eyes. Satin smooth appearance (top row), uniform papillary appearance (middle row), and nonuniform papillary appearance (bottom row). Tarsal conjunctivae with white light (left column) with fluorescein dye and cobalt blue light (middle column), and diagrammatic representation (right column). (From Greiner JV, Covington HI, Allansmith MR. Surface morphology of the human upper tarsal conjunctiva. Am J Ophthalmol 83:892, 1977.)

ranging in diameter from more than 0.3 to 2.0 mm[3, 30] are recorded. The location of papillae is best described by dividing the tarsal plate into three arbitrary zones of equal width (see Fig. 17.8).[3, 29, 38]

Detection of papillae, particularly those less than 0.5 mm diameter, frequently requires examination with cobalt blue light following instillation of fluorescein. The delineation of papillae and also the presence or absence of apical staining can be better visualized with this method. Fluorescein staining occurs with epithelial cell damage and frequently occurs with papillae with apices that are flattened or crater-like. Apical papillary alterations are probably related to the initiating mechanical trauma. The presence of ptosis, especially unilateral ptosis, may be key for suspecting suture-related GPC.

More specialized testing can be employed in the diagnosis of GPC. For example, eosinophils are present in conjunctival smears in 25% of affected patients.[68] However, because of poor yield, smears are not routinely performed. An accurate diagnosis of GPC can almost always be made based on the signs and symptoms alone.

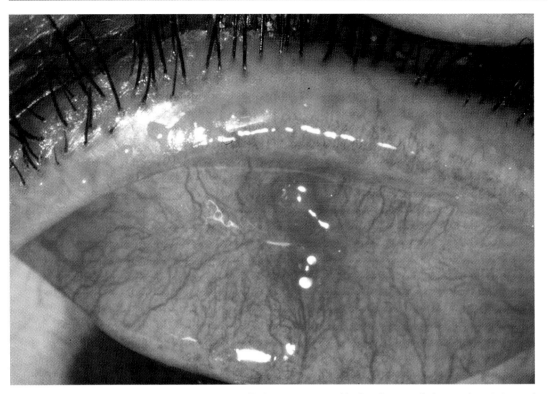

FIGURE 17.8 An enlarged papillae that assumes a follicular appearance with the absence of the usual central vessel characteristic of papillae. (Courtesy of Dr. John P. Herman.)

STAGES

GPC can be classified according to four stages. In stage I, initial symptoms include mucus in the nasal corner of the eye after sleep and mild itching after lens removal. These symptoms are usually elicited only by direct questioning and often are not considered to be relevant by the patient. Stage I is characterized only by symptoms; no signs or papillae are detected despite meticulous examination (Fig. 17.9).

In stage II, the patient has increased severity of mucus and itching and mild blurring of the vision, which occurs after several hours of contact lens wear or toward the end of the usual lens-wearing time. These symptoms are often accompanied by increased awareness of the lens, eliciting a foreign body sensation. Signs include a slight increase in diameter and elevation of papillae. These papillae appear as small, round, light reflexes giving an irregular specular reflection (see Fig. 17.9). The upper tarsal conjunctiva is thickened, edematous, and often hyperemic. These changes obscure the finer vasculature, although the deep conjunctival vasculature over the tarsal plate remains visible. Early demarcation of enlarged "giant" papillae becomes visible with fluorescein instillation and use of cobalt blue light. These "giant" papillae are not the result of enlargement of normal papillae,[41, 57] but rather a substructure from the deep tarsal conjunctiva that is elevating underlying areas of the conjunctiva.

Although papillae can normally occur on the upper tarsal conjunctiva (see Fig. 17.9),[3, 41, 57] conjunctival papillae larger than 0.3 mm in diameter are abnormal. As the giant papillae emerge, they obscure the normal,

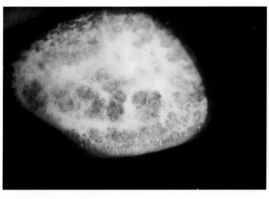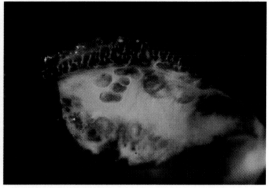

FIGURE 17.9 The fluorescein-stained upper tarsal conjunctive in contact lens–associated giant papillary conjunctivitis with cobalt blue light demonstrating excessive mucus (left) and sheets of mucus (right). (Courtesy of Dr. John P. Herman.)

smaller papillae. In addition, their apices flatten, and one may see conjunctival ulceration.

Stage III is characterized by increased severity of mucus and itching, accompanied by excessive lens movement associated with blinking. The contact lens surface becomes coated with mucus and debris,[3] and patients usually decrease lens-wearing time. Increased numbers of giant papillae enlarged in both diameter and height are present. The apices of the giant papillae may stain with fluorescein (see Fig. 17.9). At this stage, mucus secretion is usually apparent over the conjunctival surface.

Stage IV is characterized by exacerbation of stage III signs and a loss of contact lens–wearing tolerance. The contact lenses can only be worn briefly before foreign body sensation or discomfort forces lens removal. Lenses are coated and cloudy soon after insertion. Mucus secretion is excessive and is present in the form of sheets and strings, which can obscure vision. Flattening of the papillae apices is observed by fluorescein staining (see Fig. 17.9). The contact lens is observed to decenter frequently. One related occurrence has been described as the upper lid "grabbing" the contact lens, pulling it off the cornea, where it remains under the upper lid.[65]

The symptoms associated with each stage do not always parallel the signs,[3] because a high degree of variability exists among patients. The degree of variation is such that some patients have scores of giant papillae covering both tarsal plates, yet they have minimal symptoms and continue uninterrupted lens wearing throughout their waking hours. In contrast, other patients have itching, increased mucus, increased thickness of the conjunctiva, hyperemia, and markedly decreased lens-wearing tolerance, yet few to no giant papillae.

Differences are noted in the clinical presentation of GPC between wearers of rigid and hydrogel contact lenses. The number of papillae is usually less in hard lens wearers. In addition, the apices of papillae have a crater-like morphology in wearers of hard contact lenses, as opposed to the round, flattened morphology of the papillae common in wearers of soft contact lenses. The zonal distribution of papillae also differs.[29, 38] In wearers of hard contact lenses, papillae usually form first in those zones of the tarsal conjunctiva closest to the eyelid margin, whereas in wearers of soft lens contact lenses, papillae usually form first in those zones nearer the tarsal fold. In occasional cases, papillae may develop in a scattered pattern over all tarsal zones. In the fully exacerbated stage of GPC, papillae are found in all three zones of the tarsal conjunctiva in wearers of both rigid and hydrogel lenses. This pattern is nearly indistinguishable from that seen in VC.

DIFFERENTIAL DIAGNOSIS

Ocular diseases that must be differentiated from GPC include VC and trachoma. Unlike VC and GPC, which result from immune hypersensitivities, trachoma is an infectious process caused by *Chlamydia trachomatis.*

VC is a bilateral allergic disease of the palpebral conjunctiva usually occurring in prepubertal patients. Vernal keratoconjunctivitis is rarely seen in adults. The disease may be present for 10 years, with annual recurrences occurring at approximately the same time each year. It is usually associated with atopy. Patients commonly have symptoms of intense itching. Giant papillae occur in the palpebral conjunctiva, accompanied by excessive, stringy mucus discharge. Eosinophils are found in smears of the conjunctival exudate.

Trachoma is the most common ocular disease in the world. It is prevalent in China, India, various developing countries, and in the Southwestern American Indian population. The disease is caused by *Chlamydia* and is spread by direct contact. Major symptoms include mild itching and irritation. Patients have blurring of vision and increased ocular discomfort. Toxins emitted from the chlamydial organisms induce a lymphocytic reaction, which results in cicatrization of the palpebral conjunctiva, particularly over the upper tarsal plate. Follicular and papillary hypertrophy extends to the lid margin of the upper tarsal conjunctiva. The superior limbus and cornea can be involved. In severe cases, the entire cornea may be involved, and vision may be compromised.

Other conditions to consider in the differential diagnosis include allergic conjunctivitis, which may be confused with the early stages of GPC (e.g., stage I). The foreign body sensation, irritation, or mild itch of stage I GPC may be reported by some patients as a corneal or conjunctival foreign body sensation not unlike that associated with dry eye syndrome. Dry eye syndrome may be a predisposing factor in patients with GPC, because investigators have shown that meibomian gland dysfunction may contribute to the pathophysiology of GPC.[52–54]

TEARS

The conjunctiva is protected by an array of nonspecific and specific immune mechanisms. The anatomy of the orbit provides significant protection against mechanical trauma. The tear film bathes the corneal and conjunctival epithelium. The tear film of patients with GPC has a normal concentration of lysozyme, although lactoferrin concentrations are reduced.[69] Lactoferrin is also reduced in patients with the similar conditon of VC. Lactoferrin and lysozyme in the tear film are essential components of the nonspecific immune protection of the external eye. Patients with inactive GPC were found to have normal tear lactoferrin levels.[70] Because lactoferrin has an antibacterial function, perhaps its reduction contributes to increased ocular inflammation or even bacterial contamination of worn contact lenses.[70]

Eosinophils are increased in biopsy specimens of papillae[6] and are present in conjunctival smears in 25% of patients with GPC. However, the concentration of eosinophilic major basic protein in tears does not seem to be increased in all patients.[68] In patients with concurrent atopy and giant papillary conjunctivitis, major basic protein can be found in the affected conjunctiva[71] and in coatings on contact lenses.[72] The eosinophilic granules contain cationic proteins that have cytotoxic effects and could play a major role in the conjunctival inflammatory reaction and subsequent deposition of collagen in GPC.

Other findings indicative of atopy that are found in the tears of patients with GPC include elevated concentrations of IgG and IgE.[73] The elevated immunoglobulin levels may be a response to antigenic coatings on the surface of the worn contact lens. In fact, lenses worn by patients with GPC that were then fitted in the eyes of monkeys induced intense round cell infiltrates at the epithelial stromal junction of the upper tarsal conjunctiva.[47] In one study, tear film IgM levels were measurable in nearly half the patients with GPC, whereas none of the control group patients had detectable amounts of IgM.[73] Studies revealed that local production of immunoglobulin was responsible for the increased tear immunoglobulin levels.[73] Additionally, complement component C3a has been demonstrated in tears of patients with GPC.[73]

Conjunctival mast cells and type I hypersensitivity play key roles in GPC. Thirty percent of conjunctival mast cells are in a state of degranulation in GPC.[74] Immunohistochemical and electron microscopic techniques have demonstrated that most mast cells in GPC are of the connective tissue type, based on their neutral protease content.[75] One also sees an increased level of tryptase, a mast cell–specific product and marker, in tear samples from patients with GPC.[76] Tryptase levels are not detected in patients with blepharitis and other nonallergic ocular inflammatory conditions. Mast cells play a major role in collagen disorders such as cicatricial pemphigoid, in which progressive conjunctival subepithelial fibrosis is closely associated with elevated numbers of mast cells. In this disorder, patients have a significantly higher ratio of connective tissue mast cells to mucosal mast cells.[77] Connective tissue mast cells probably play an important role in the pathogenesis of GPC (e.g., overproduction of collagen, abnormal collagen, or scarring).

Three distinct abnormalities are noted in the inflammatory cell profile in contact lens–associated GPC when compared with normal subjects[78] or contact lens wearers without GPC. Mast cells occur in the epithelium, and both eosinophils and basophils are found in the epithelium and substantia propria.[3, 4] The presence of basophils is suggestive of delayed hypersensitivity, referred to as cutaneous basophil hypersensitivity.[79] The presence of these cells in GPC indicates an immunologic reaction. Unexpectedly, the number of lymphocytes and plasma cells per microscopic field does not increase.[4] However, because the total mass of conjunctiva in GPC is at least double that of normal subjects, the absolute number of these cells does actually increase.[4, 5]

PATHOGENESIS

The common feature of all the conditions associated with GPC is that they inflict trauma to the conjunctival surface during blinking or ocular excursions. The contribution of trauma to the pathogenesis of GPC cannot be ignored. Mechanical trauma caused by rubbing of the contact lens against the tarsal conjunctiva alters the superficial layers of the epithelium (Fig. 17.10).[41–43, 80, 81] Mechanical trauma can result in degranulation of mast cells[26, 72] and disruption of the epithelial surface (Fig. 17.11),[41, 42, 82] which normally acts as a physical barrier to the tear film and the external environment. Studies have demonstrated that physical trauma to the conjunctival epithelium induced by contact lenses stimulates production of neutrophil

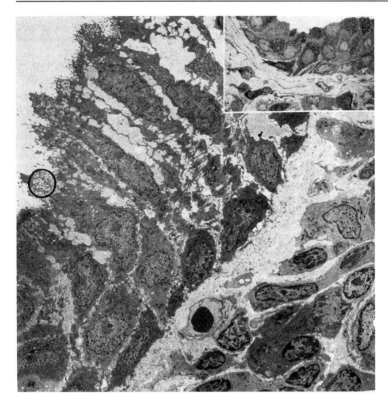

FIGURE 17.10 *Inset* (upper right), light photomicrograph with toluidine blue stain of specimen from the upper tarsal conjunctiva of a patient with contact lens–associated giant papillary conjunctivitis demonstrates metachromatic granules in apical surface of non-goblet epithelial cells. The survey transmission electron micrograph from the corresponding area over the surface of papillae demonstrates what appears to be secretory activity (black circle) from the apices of these epithelial cells. Surface epithelial cells demonstrate numerous vesicular mucus-containing inclusions from non-goblet epithelial cells. (From Greiner JV, Kenyon KR, Henriquez AS, et al. Mucus secreting vesicles in conjunctival epithelial cells of contact lens wearers. Arch Ophthalmol 98:1843, 1980.)

chemotactic factors,[83] inflammatory mediators, and amplification of the response to trauma.

The contact lens type, material, and deposits[84] and lens design have been reviewed and implicated in the pathogenesis of GPC. The coated contact lens or other foreign body serves as a vehicle for the presentation of environmental debris or antigens to the compromised epithelium. The combination of mast cell degranulation with release of inflammatory mediators and the presence of inflammatory cells in the lymphoid conjunctival stroma

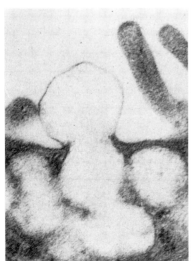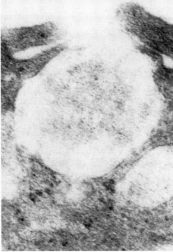

FIGURE 17.11 Transmission electron micrographs demonstrating various stages of discharge of the mucus-secretory granules of non-goblet epithelial cells into the conjunctival sac. (From Greiner JV, Kenyon KR, Henriquez AS, et al. Mucus secreting vesicles in conjunctival epithelial cells of contact lens wearers. Arch Ophthalmol 98:1843, 1980.)

may initiate the changes required for papillogenesis. Increased aggregation of lymphocytes in these foci would result in a concomitant expansion of the stroma and overlying epithelium, as observed clinically. The subsequent papillae enlarge, with development of collagen substructure and increasing numbers of lymphocytes.

Available data indicate that both mechanical trauma and immunologic response are interrelated in the pathogenesis of GPC.[36] The contact lens purportedly serves as an abrasive surface (foreign body) for the development of a compromised epithelium that enhances the immunosensitivity of the conjunctiva to external antigens.

TREATMENT

Treatment of GPC depends on early recognition of the condition. Signs and symptoms will resolve if the patient refrains from wearing contact lenses. However, in some patients although the symptoms resolve and the signs subside, the papillae do not completely resolve. Because the interplay of mechanical and immunological factors in the pathogenesis of GPC is complex, several strategies should be employed in treatment of patients with GPC.

The first strategy should be prevention of GPC. Prevention depends on prescribing the appropriate lens type and edge design and encouraging strict lens hygiene. In the case of suture-induced GPC, burying suture knots is important. In advanced cases, treatment also requires pharmacological therapy to control the conjunctival inflammatory response.

Relief of symptoms may be achieved rapidly with removal of the contact lens, prosthesis, suture, or other surface irregularity from the eye. In fact, the patient is usually totally asymptomatic within 5 days following discontinuation of contact lenses.[3] After discontinuation of contact lens wearing, symptoms dissipate within 48 hours.[3] If the same lenses are reworn, the syndrome will reappear within 5 days.[3, 58] Restarting lens wear with a clean lens or lens of different type or design may be done within days after hyperemia, mucus production, and irritation resolve. For GPC induced by suture, removal causes reduction in inflammation[9, 12] and prompt resolution of foreign body sensation. Within a day or so, excess mucus clears,[9] and the giant papillae disappear within a month.[14]

If discontinuation of contact lens wear is not feasible, changing to a new clean lens can result in decreased symptoms.[3, 85] The use of a new clean lens has led to improvement in itching, even while more mechanically related symptoms such as lens movement, lens awareness, and pain significantly worsened.[86] Changing the type of lens from rigid to hydrogel or vice versa, or even changing from a daily-wear lens to a disposable lens for a period of time, has been shown to be effective in some instances.[85] Additionally, changing lens polymers within the same type of lens may be helpful.[3, 58] Addition of another mode of cleaning such as the use of papain has proven successful in reducing and eliminating symptoms. Patients who wear extended-wear contact lenses may show improvement after switching to daily-wear lenses or disposable lenses. The goal is to eliminate symptoms, not contact lens wear.

For patients with GPC, lens-cleaning agents and saline solution for rinsing and storing lenses should be preservative-free. Clinical experience has shown that daily disinfection with 3% hydrogen peroxide treatment is superior to other methods currently available. Enzymatic cleaning of the lens is essential to minimize the accumulation of lens coatings and to remove built-up environmental antigens that adhere to the lens coating. Finally, lenses should be replaced frequently, at least once yearly in the case of daily-wear or extended-wear lenses. Immunologic components and other proteins from the tear film can form a coating on all lenses that even the best lens care regimen fails to remove completely.[50, 87] Most patients with GPC have coated lenses, whereas many patients without the syndrome have relatively clean lenses despite months of lens wearing.[3]

In cases of patients with severe contact lens coatings, daily use of surfactant cleaner, hydrogen peroxide disinfection, and enzymes prevent buildup of protein deposits and debris accumulating on the lens material. Daily enzymatic cleaning resulted in increased wearing time in the case of rigid contact lenses in patients with keratoconus and GPC;[88] this practice has also been recommended for soft daily-wear lenses.[89]

Clinical observations of unilateral GPC ($n = 14$), although not statistically significant, implicated infrequent lens replacement as an important factor in the development of this asymmetry.[28] Three of the patients had a history of wearing an older lens in the eye that developed GPC. This finding is consistent with the clinical observation of patients who present with a history of having broken a lens and then using an "old spare" lens in the interim for a "few months" until eventually deciding to replace the lens (Fig. 17.12).

Flushing the ocular surface with a stream of saline directed at the conjunctival sac can often provide relief of itching and may decrease the antigen load on the ocular surface. Such irrigation should be performed with unpreserved saline immediately following removal of contact lenses. In more severe cases, irrigation is recommended two to three times daily (Donald Korb, personal communication).

Loteprednol etabonate, a corticosteroid, has been demonstrated to produce significant reduction in GPC-related papillae.[90] Treatment with this agent was safe and did not induce changes in intraocular pressure.[90] Long-term use of corticosteroids is discouraged because such use is fraught with complications, including elevation of the intraocular pressure, formation of posterior subcapsular cataracts, and infection. However, pulse therapy with topically applied dexamethasone or prednisolone 1% four times daily tapering over days to weeks may be effective in patients with severe symptoms that persist after discontinuation of contact lenses.

Because mast cells are involved in the immunopathology of GPC, mast cell stabilizers may be of benefit.[91–93] Mast cell stabilizers include cromolyn sodium, lodoxamide tromethamine, and nedocromil. These agents prevent degranulation of mast cells by inhibiting the transport of calcium across

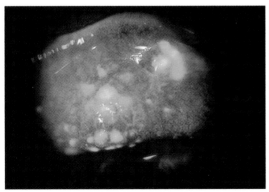 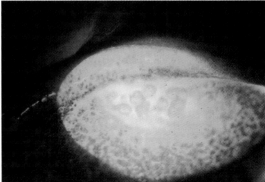

FIGURE 17.12 The upper tarsal conjunctiva in contact lens–associated giant papillary conjunctivitis demonstrates the presence of apical staining in moderate- and large-diameter papillae. (Courtesy of Dr. John P. Herman.)

mast cell membranes, thus stabilizing the membrane and preventing the release of preformed chemical mediators (e.g., histamine, serotonin, slow-reacting substance of anaphylaxis, and eosinophil chemotactic factor). Once such mediators are released, mast cell stabilizers may be of little or no benefit. As such, when GPC occurs, discontinuing contact lens wear so that the eye quiets before mast cell stabilizers are used may be preferable.

Cromolyn sodium 4% ophthalmic solution can be administered four times daily and has been shown to be effective in the treatment of GPC.[91, 94, 95] Topically applied cromolyn sodium can be used without completely discontinuing contact lens wear. It should not be instilled while the patient is wearing contact lenses. The patient should be instructed to remove the lenses before instilling drops and to wait a reasonable amount of time before reinserting the lenses. Minor adverse reactions with cromolyn use include stinging, burning, conjunctival injection, dryness around the eye, puffy eyes, and chalazion formation. Use of cromolyn sodium solution with ocular prostheses resulted in symptomatic resolution within 1 month.[7]

Along with rigorous lens hygiene, a mast cell stabilizer administered four times daily may accelerate resolution of early GPC and may retard its progress. Advanced GPC is more problematic, and mast cell stabilizers are of little benefit. At least one randomized trial of patients with symptomatic GPC, using 6% N-acetyl-aspartyl glutamic acid, indicated that mast cell stabilization in GPC has little effect and treatment should be focused more on inflammatory mediators released because of mechanical stimuli.[96]

Other therapy such as adjuvant therapy of oral aspirin in conjunction with 2% cromoglycate eye drops may provide relief,[97] a method that has been helpful in patients with VC. Topical suprofen has been shown to provide a reduction in signs and symptoms of GPC such as papillae and mucus strands.[98]

Nearly 90% of patients with GPC who comply with treatment can eventually continue wearing contact lenses. Disappearance of hyperemia, mucus, and fluorescein staining on the apices of the papillae are the first signs of improvement and may occur within days of discontinuing lens wearing.[1] Because the papillae may not fully resolve, one does not need to wait until the enlarged papillae regress before restarting contact lens wearing. It may take months or even years for the enlarged papillae to disappear. In some patients, the papillae have not disappeared in more than 20 years, yet these patients remain asymptomatic lens wearers. It is important to focus attention on the lens (eg, design, type, and hygiene) before intervening with potentially unnecessary pharmacotherapy. In the case of other, non–contact lens, causes of GPC, it is best to focus on removal of surface irregularities. If this is not feasible, flushing, lubrication, and possible pharmacotherapy are important. In the absence of signs or symptoms indicating the need for discontinuation of lens wearing, contact lenses may be restarted or reintroduced 3 to 5 days after the hyperemia, excessive mucus production, and itching have been relieved. If the papillae persist and are enlarged enough to induce lens decentration with blinking, they can be surgically removed by shaving them with a scalpel in an attempt to restore the smooth upper tarsal conjunctiva.

REFERENCES

1. Kennedy JR. A mechanism of corneal abrasion. Am J Optom 47:564, 1970.
2. Spring TF. Reaction to hydrophilic lenses. Med J Aust 1:449, 1974.
3. Allansmith MR, Korb DR, Greiner JV, et al. Giant papillary conjunctivitis in contact lens wearers. Am J Ophthalmol 83:697, 1977.
4. Allansmith MR, Korb DR, Greiner JV. Giant

papillary conjunctivitis induced by hard or soft contact lens wear: quantitative histology. Ophthalmology 85:766, 1978.

5. Mackie IA, Wright P. Giant papillary conjunctivitis (secondary vernal) in association with contact lens wear. Trans Ophthalmol Soc U K 98:3, 1978.

6. Srinivasan BD, Takobiec FA, Iwamoto T, et al. Giant papillary conjunctivitis with ocular prostheses. Arch Ophthalmol 97:892, 1979.

7. Meisner DM, Krachmer JH, Goeken JA. An immunologic study of giant papillary conjunctivitis associated with an ocular prosthesis. Am J Ophthalmol 92:368, 1981.

8. Reynolds RMP. Giant papillary conjunctivitis: a mechanical aetiology. Aust J Optom 61:320, 1978.

9. Sugar A, Meyer RF. Giant papillary conjunctivitis after keratoplasty. Am J Ophthalmol 91:239, 1981.

10. Collin HB. Vernal conjunctivitis and giant papillary conjunctivitis. Part II. Suture induced conjunctivitis. Aust J Optom 64:4, 1981.

11. Nirankari VS, Karesh JW, Richards RD. Complications of exposed monofilament sutures. Am J Ophthalmol 95:515, 1983.

12. Jolson AS, Jolson SC. Suture barb giant papillary conjunctivitis. Ophthalmic Surg 15:139, 1984.

13. Friedman T, Friedman Z, Neumann E. Giant papillary conjunctivitis following cataract extraction. Ann Ophthalmol 16:50, 1984.

14. Willie H, Molgaard IL. Giant papillary conjunctivitis in connection with corneoscleral supramid (nylon) suture knots. Acta Ophthalmol 62:75, 1984.

15. Skrypuch OW, Willis NR. Giant papillary conjunctivitis from an exposed prolene suture. Can J Ophthalmol 21:189, 1986.

16. Greiner JV. Papillary conjunctivitis induced by an epithelialized corneal foreign body. Ophthalmologica 196:82, 1988.

17. Carlson AN, Wilhelmuss KR. Giant papillary conjunctivitis associated with cyanoacrylate adhesive. Am J Ophthalmol 104:437, 1987.

18. Dunn JP, Weissman BA, Mondino BJ, et al. Giant papillary conjunctivitis associated with elevated corneal deposits. Cornea 9:357, 1990.

19. Heidemann DG, Dunn SP, Siegal MJ. Unusual causes of giant papillary conjunctivitis. Cornea 12:78, 1993.

20. Friedlander MH. Some unusual nonallergic causes of giant papillary conjunctivitis. Trans Am Ophthalmol Soc 138:343, 1990.

21. Manners RM, Vardy SJ, Rose GE. Localized giant papillary conjunctivitis secondary to a dermolipoma. Eye 9:376, 1995.

22. Francis IC, Lawless MA. Bilateral giant papillary conjunctivitis related to glaucoma drainage surgery blebs. Cornea 13:469, 1994.

23. Robin JB, Regis-Pacheco LF, May WN, et al. Giant papillary conjunctivitis associated with extruded scleral buckle. Arch Ophthalmol 105: 619, 1987.

24. Allansmith MR, Baird RS, Greiner JV. Vernal conjunctivitis and contact lens–associated giant papillary conjunctivitis compared and contrasted. Am J Ophthalmol 87:544, 1979.

25. Allansmith MR, Baird RS, Greiner JV. Contact lens–associated giant papillary conjunctivitis as a model for vernal conjunctivitis. In Immunopathology of the eye. Silverstein A, O'Connor S, eds. New York, Masson, 1979, p 346.

26. Greiner JV, Peace DG, Baird RS, et al. Effects of eye rubbing on the conjunctiva as a model of ocular inflammation. Am J Ophthalmol 100:45, 1985.

27. Hart DE, Schkolnick JA, Bernstein S, et al. Contact lens–induced giant papillary conjunctivitis: a retrospective study. J Am Optom Assoc 60:195, 1989.

28. Palmisano PC, Ehlers WH, Donshik PC. Causative factors in unilateral giant papillary conjunctivitis. CLAO J 19:103, 1993.

29. Korb DR, Allansmith MR, Greiner JV, et al. Biomicroscopy of papillae associated with hard contact lens wearing. Ophthalmology 88:1132, 1981.

30. Korb DR, Allansmith MR, Greiner JV, et al. Prevalence of conjunctival changes in wearers of hard contact lenses. Am J Ophthalmol 90: 336, 1980.

31. Allansmith MR, Ross RN. Ocular allergy and mast cell stabilizers. Surv Ophthalmol 30:229, 1986.

32. Buckley RJ. Pathology and treatment of giant papillary conjunctivitis. II. The British perspective. Clin Ther 9:451, 1987.

33. Begley CG, Riggle A, Tuel JA. Association of giant papillary conjunctivitis with seasonal allergies. Optom Vis Sci 67:192, 1990.

34. Soni PS, Hathcoat G. Complications reported with hydrogel extended wear contact lenses. Am J Optom Physiol Opt 65:545, 1988.

35. Smolin G, O'Connor GR. Ocular immunology. Philadelphia, Lea & Febiger, 1981, p 159.

36. Greiner JV, Korb DR, Allansmith MR. Pathogenesis of contact lens papillary conjunctivitis: a hypothesis. In: Advances in immunology and immunopathology. O'Connor GR, Chandler AW, eds. New York, Masson, 1985, p 302.

37. Key JE. Are hard lenses superior to soft? Arguments in favor of hard lenses. Cornea 9:S9, 1990.

38. Korb DR, Greiner JV, Finnemore VM, et al. Biomicroscopy of papillae associated with soft contact lens wearing. Br J Ophthalmol 67:733, 1983.

39. Fowler SA, Greiner JV, Allansmith MR. Soft contact lenses from patients with giant papillary conjunctivitis. Am J Ophthalmol 88:1056, 1979.

40. Molinari JF. Review: giant papillary conjunctivitis. Aust J Optom 66:59, 1983.

41. Greiner JV, Covington HI, Allansmith MR. Surface morphology of the human upper tarsal conjunctiva. Am J Ophthalmol 83:892, 1977.

42. Greiner JV, Covington HI, Allansmith MR. Surface morphology of giant papillary conjunctivitis in contact lens wearers. Am J Ophthalmol 85: 242, 1978.

43. Greiner JV, Covington HI, Korb DR, Allansmith MR. Conjunctiva in asymptomatic contact lens wearers. Am J Ophthalmol 86:403, 1978.

44. Greiner JV, Allansmith MR. Effect of contact lens wear on the conjunctival mucous system. Ophthalmology 88:821, 1981.

45. Korb DR, Greiner JV, Glonek T, et al. Human and rabbit tear film lipid layer thickness and blink rate. Adv Exp Med Biol 438:305, 1998.
46. Henriquez AS, Baird RS, Korb DR, et al. Histology of hard and soft contact lens–associated giant papillary conjunctivitis. Ann Ophthalmol 12:929, 1980.
47. Ballow M, Donshik PC, Rapacz P, et al. Immune responses in monkeys to lenses from patients with contact lens–induced giant papillary conjunctivitis. CLAO J 15:64, 1989.
48. Richard NR, Anderson JA, Tasevska ZG, et al. Evaluation of tear protein deposits on contact lenses from patients with and without giant papillary conjunctivitis. CLAO J 18:143, 1992.
49. Jones B, Sack R. Immunoglobulin deposition on soft contact lenses: relationship to hydrogel structure and mode of use and giant papillary conjunctivitis. CLAO J 16:43, 1990.
50. Fowler SA, Allansmith MR. Evolution of soft contact lens coatings. Arch Ophthalmol 98:95, 1980.
51. Benvenuto PB. Giant papillary conjunctivitis with resultant keratitis. South J Optom 21:43, 1979.
52. Martin NF, Rubinfield RS, Malley JD, et al. Giant papillary conjunctivitis and meibomian gland dysfunction blepharitis. Ophthalmology 96 Suppl:123, 1989.
53. Martin NF, Rubinfeld RS, Malley JD, et al. Giant papillary conjunctivitis and meibomian gland dysfunction blepharitis. CLAO J 18:165, 1992.
54. Mathers MD, Billborough M. Meibomian gland function and giant papillary conjunctivitis. Am J Ophthalmol 114:188, 1992.
55. Rubinfeld RS, Martin NF. Meibomian gland function and giant papillary conjunctivitis (letter; comment). Am J Ophthalmol 115:120, 1993.
56. Butrus SI, Rabinowitz AI. Meibomian gland function and giant papillary conjunctivitis. [Letter:comment] Am J Ophthalmol 115:120, 1993.
57. Kessing SV. Mucus gland system of the conjunctiva. Acta Ophthalmol 46 Suppl 95:1, 1968.
58. Molinari JF. The clinical management of giant papillary conjunctivitis. Am J Optom Physiol Opt 58:886, 1981.
59. Molinari JF. A case report: a procedure for the clinical management of giant papillary conjunctivitis in a patient wearing contact lenses. Aust J Optom 63:288, 1980.
60. O'Connor RG. The use of disodium cromoglycate in the treatment of vernal keratoconjunctivitis and related disorders. In: Ocular therapeutics. Srinivasan BD, ed. New York, Masson, 1980, p 83.
61. Allansmith MR, Baird RS, Greiner JV. Density of goblet cells in vernal conjunctivitis and contact lens–associated giant papillary conjunctivitis. Arch Ophthalmol 99:884, 1981.
62. Greiner JV, Henriquez AS, Weidman TA, et al. "Second" mucus secretory system of the human conjunctiva. Invest Ophthalmol Vis Sci 18 ARVO Suppl: 123, 1979.
63. Greiner JV, Kenyon KR, Henriquez AS, et al. Mucus secretory vesicles in conjunctival epithelial cells of contact lens wearers. Arch Ophthalmol 98:1843, 1980.
64. Greiner JV, Weidman TA, Korb DR, et al. Histochemical analysis of secretory vesicles in nongoblet conjunctival epithelial cells. Acta Ophthalmol 63:89, 1985.
65. Trocme SD, Raizman MB, Bartley GB. Medical therapy for ocular allergy. Mayo Clin Proc 67:557, 1992.
66. Luxenberg MN. Blepharoptosis associated with giant papillary conjunctivitis. Arch Ophthalmol 104:1706, 1986.
67. Sheldon L, Biedner B, Geltman G, et al. Giant papillary conjunctivitis and ptosis in a contact lens wearer. J Pediatr Ophthalmol Strabismus 16:136, 1979.
68. Udell IJ, Gleich GJ, Allansmith MR, et al. Eosinophil granule major basic protein and Charcot-Leyden crystal protein in human tears. Am J Ophthalmol 92:824, 1981.
69. Rapacz P, Tedesco J, Donshik PC, et al. Tear lysozyme and lactoferrin levels in giant papillary conjunctivitis and vernal conjunctivitis. CLAO J 14:207, 1988.
70. Ballow M, Donshik PC, Rapacz R, et al. Tear lactoferrin levels in patients with external inflammatory ocular disease. Invest Ophthalmol Vis Sci 28:543, 1987.
71. Trocme SD, Kephart GM, Allansmith MR, et al. Conjunctival deposition of eosinophil granule major basic protein in vernal keratoconjunctivitis and contact lens–associated giant papillary conjunctivitis. Am J Ophthalmol 108:57, 1989.
72. Trocme SD, Kephart GM, Bourne WM, et al. Eosinophil granule major basic protein in contact lenses of patients with giant papillary conjunctivitis. CLAO J 16:219, 1990.
73. Donshik PC, Ballow M. Tear immunoglobulins in giant papillary conjunctivitis induced by contact lenses. Am J Ophthalmol 96:460, 1983.
74. Henriquez AS, Kenyon KR, Allansmith MR. Mast cell ultrastructure: comparison in contact lens associated giant papillary conjunctivitis. Arch Ophthalmol 99:1266, 1981.
75. Butrus SI, Laby DM, Zacharia JS, et al. Ultrastructural analysis of conjunctival mast cells in giant papillary conjunctivitis. Invest Ophthalmol Vis Sci 33 ARVO Suppl: 851, 1992.
76. Butrus SI, Ochsner KI, Abelson MB, et al. The level of tryptase in human tears, an indication of activation of conjunctival mast cells. Ophthalmology 97:1678, 1990.
77. Hoang-Xuan T, Foster CS, Raizman MB, et al. Mast cells in conjunctiva affected by cicatricial pemphigoid. Ophthalmology 96:1110, 1989.
78. Allansmith MR, Greiner JV, Baird RS. Number of inflammatory cells in the normal conjunctiva. Am J Ophthalmol 86:250, 1978.
79. Dvorak HF, Dvorak AM, Simpson BA, et al. Cutaneous basophil hypersensitivity: a light and electron microscopic description. J Exp Med 132:558, 1970.
80. Greiner JV, Gladstone L, Covington HI, et al. Branching of microvilli in the human conjunctival epithelium. Arch Ophthalmol 98:1253, 1980.
81. Greiner JV, Covington HI, Fowler SA, et al. Cell surface variations of the human upper tarsal conjunctiva. Ann Ophthalmol 14:288, 1982.
82. Greiner JV, Leahy CD, Welter D, et al. Histopathology of the ocular surface resulting from eye rubbing. Cornea 16:327, 1997.

83. Elgebaly SA, Donshik PC, Rahhal F, et al. Neutrophil chemotactic factors in the tears of giant papillary conjunctivitis patients. Invest Ophthalmol Vis Sci 32:208, 1991.

84. Meisler DM, Keller WB. Contact lens type, material, and deposits and giant papillary conjunctivitis. CLAO J 21:77, 1995.

85. Bucci FA, Lopatynsky MO, Jenkins PL, et al. Comparison of the clinical performance of the Acuvue disposable contact lens and CSI lens in patients with giant papillary conjunctivitis. Am J Ophthalmol 115:454, 1993.

86. Bucci FA, Lopatynsky MD, Jenkins PL, et al. The deposit resistant Hydrocurve Elite soft contact lens and giant papillary conjunctivitis. Invest Ophthalmol Vis Sci 30:256, 1989.

87. Gudmundsson OG, Woodward DF, Fowler SA, et al. Identification of posterior contact lens surface deposits by immunofluorescence microscopy. Arch Ophthalmol 103:196, 1985.

88. Korb DR, Greiner JV, Finnemore VM, et al. Treatment of contact lenses with papain: increase in wearing time in keratoconus patients with papillary conjunctivitis. Arch Ophthalmol 101:48, 1983.

89. Kosmos MA, Gabianelli EB. Daily enzyme cleaning for giant papillary conjunctivitis (letter). Eur J Ophthalmol 2:98, 1992.

90. Bartlett JD, Howes JF, Ghormley NR, et al. Safety and efficacy of loteprednol etabonate for treatment of papillae in contact lens–associated giant papillary conjunctivitis. Curr Eye Res 12: 313, 1993.

91. Donshik PC, Ballow M, Luistro A, et al. Treatment of contact lens–induced giant papillary conjunctivitis. CLAO J 10:346, 1984.

92. Allansmith MR, Ross RN, Greiner JV. Giant papillary conjunctivitis: diagnosis and treatment. In: Contact lenses: the CLAO guide to basic science and clinical practice. 2nd ed. Dabezies OH Jr, ed. Boston, Little, Brown, 1989, p 43.1.

93. Donshik PC. Giant papillary conjunctivitis. Trans Am Ophthalmol Soc 92:587, 1994.

94. Kruger CJ, Ehlers WH, Luistro AE, et al. Treatment of giant papillary conjunctivitis with cromolyn sodium. CLAO J 18:46, 1992.

95. Meisler DM, Berzins UJ, Krachmer JH, et al. Cromolyn treatment of giant papillary conjunctivitis. Arch Ophthalmol 100:1608, 1982.

96. Meijer F, Pogany K, Kok JH, et al. *N*-acetyl-aspartyl glutamic acid (NAAGA) topical eyedrops in the treatment of giant papillary conjunctivitis (GPC). Doc Ophthalmol 85:5, 1993.

97. Srinivas C. Adjuvant therapy of aspirin and cromoglycate 2% eye drops in vernal conjunctivitis. Korean J Ophthalmol 3:42, 1989.

98. Wood TS, Stewart RH, Bowman RW, et al. Suprofen treatment of contact lens–associated giant papillary conjunctivitis. Ophthalmology 95: 822, 1988.

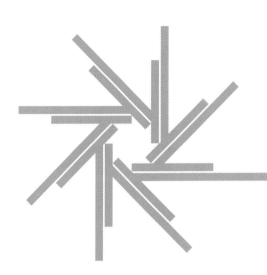

CHAPTER 18

Marginal Infiltrates in the Cornea

MARK B. ABELSON ■ **ANDREW P. SLUGG**

Ocular allergy includes a variety of conditions that share a mutual origin, a hypersensitivity or sensitization to antigens on the ocular surface. Marginal corneal infiltrates appear to be an example of such a condition. Marginal corneal infiltrates, also referred to as peripheral ulcers and catarrhal infiltrates, are most likely the result of a low-grade, epithelial, late-phase allergic reaction associated with two principal conditions, vernal keratoconjunctivitis and bacterial toxins on the ocular surface.[1] Infiltates can also be caused by excessive contact lens wear.[2] Although marginal infiltrates have various pathological origins, they have a shared mechanism of pathogenesis resulting from an acute immune reaction.

CLINICAL FEATURES

Marginal corneal infiltrates typically appear at the 2-, 4-, 8-, and 10-o'clock positions. They are separated from the corneoscleral limbus by about 1 mm of clear cornea.[3] The clear area of cornea between the infiltrate and the limbus is most likely due to the removal of leukocytes or antigens from that region of the corneal epithelium via blood vessels located in the periphery of the cornea.[1] These blood vessels extend only 0.5 mm into the cornea and are derived from the deep episcleral and anterior conjunctival arteries. Marginal corneal infiltrates may appear alone or in groups. They are usually found bilaterally.

Generally, patients with marginal corneal infiltrates present with little or no chemosis; mild, often localized, conjunctival injection; and minimal ocular irritation and normal vision.[2] Although there are no archetypal characteristics in the patient population that experiences marginal corneal infiltrates, the condition has been associated with vernal keratoconjunctivitis, contact lens wear,[4] and compromised corneal epithelium including ocular trauma such as LASIK surgery,[5, 6] recurrent corneal erosion,[7, 8] and corneal graft rejection.[9]

ETIOLOGY

The increased incidence of corneal infiltrates in the periphery of the cornea can be attributed to its unique physiology and anatomy. Comprised of three distinct cell types (epithelium, keratocyte, and endothelium), the cornea is virtually avascular and without lymphatic channels. The cornea's unusual circulatory arrangement causes the majority of its immune reactions to occur in the vascular periphery where there is a larger proportion of inflammatory cells, Langerhans' cells, antibodies, and complement components. The relatively large size of these inflammatory mediators makes their diffusion into the central cornea difficult, concentrating them on the periphery. The peripheral concentration of immune mediators is the best explanation for the increased incidence of hypersensitivity and autoimmune disorders occurring in the periphery of the cornea, such as Mooren's ulcer, collagen vascular disease,[10] and Wegener's granulomatosis.

PATHOGENESIS

Marginal infiltrates are the result of a moderate allergic reaction in which long-term sensitization of an antigen or antigens on the corneal surface initiates a biphasic response. This is believed to consist of type-1 and type-4 hypersensitivity reactions.

The initial presence of antigen in the corneal epithelium increases interleukin-1 (IL-1) concentration, which directly and indirectly induces the migration of mature Langerhans' cells (LC) to the periphery of the cornea.[11] There, LC bind to the antigen. The LC-antigen complex migrates to the vascular limbus where it enters the blood stream via the deep episcleral artery. It is then transported to the homolateral preauricular lymph nodes, ultimately ending in the spleen where the corresponding antibodies and macrophages are synthesized. Once the appropriate antibodies are synthesized, the presenting antigen is recognized by the body's immune system.

After antibodies are manufactured, exposure to the antigen initiates a type-1 hypersensitivity, IgE-mediated immune reaction that leads to mast cell degranulation and histamine release. Extended and/or repeated exposure to the antigen elicits a subsequent late-phase hypersensitivity reaction in which peripheral epithelial cells increase secretion of cytokine IL-1. The increased epithelial concentration of IL-1 initiates the up-regulation of intercellular adhesion molecule-1 (ICAM-1), which aids in the transport of vascular polymorphonuclear leukocytes (usually consisting of T lymphocytes, including helper/inducer cells and B lymphocytes) into the cellular epithelium. Polymorphonuclear leukocyte infiltration of the epithelium is also aided by increased epithelial presence of chemoattractants and increased vascular permeability caused by histamine release during mast cell degranulation in early phase type-1, IgE-mediated response.

Viewed under a slit lamp, infiltration of the corneal epithelium appears as a powder-like outflow of polymorphonuclear leukocytes from limbal blood vessels derived from the anterior conjunctival and deep episcleral arteries. These polymorphonuclear leukocytes later coalesce, forming the focal opaque lesions for which the condition is named.[12]

VERNAL KERATOCONJUNCTIVITIS AND INFILTRATION

Unlike seasonal allergic conjunctivitis, which produces a relatively mild reaction and has no corneal involvement, vernal keratoconjunctivitis (VKC), in more severe cases, produces corneal involvement of the allergic reaction, including the appearance of marginal corneal infiltrates. These must be differentially diagnosed from the Trantas' dots seen mainly in patients with VKC. Trantas' dots are focal aggregates of eosinophils that appear in and on the surface of the corneal epithelium as chalky raised masses.

Studies show that patients with VKC have significantly elevated numbers and abnormal distribution of eosinophils,[13] increased numbers of mast cells, and increased IgE serum levels in tears.[14] Patients with VKC also exhibit higher histamine levels related to lower histaminase levels. These factors predispose VKC patients to intense type-1 and type-4 hypersensitivity reactions that are not seen in non-VKC patients.

Patients with VKC also show significantly higher levels of IL-1 in tears, serum, and IL-1 production from fibroblasts compared with normal subjects.[15] The increased levels of IL-1 combined with the increased concentrations of adhesion molecules, such as ICAM-1,[16] promote the recruitment of polymorphonuclear leukocytes and their transportation into the corneal epithelium, contributing to the pathogenesis of marginal infiltrates in patients with VKC.

BACTERIA ASSOCIATED WITH INFILTRATION

Studies have long shown positive correlations between the presence of bacteria such as *Staphylococcus aureus* on the cornea and marginal infiltrates.[17-19] It is theorized that a bacterial toxin, such as the lipopolysaccharides (LPS) found on the cell walls of gram-negative bacteria, acts as an antigen, eliciting an allergic response in the eye. Late research has refuted this theory, showing the presence of the LPS of gram-negative bacteria to participate in the release of various proinflammatory cytokines, such as IL-1α, IL-1β, and TNF-α.[20, 21] The increase in IL-1α levels, among other regulatory actions, acts as a powerful chemoattractant of neutrophils, aiding in their infiltration of the LPS-exposed tissue. LPS has also been shown to be a potent agonist for the degranulation of neutrophils when compared with several cytokines.[22] In cases of long-term exposure (48 hours) to *S. aureus* endotoxin B (SEB), increased levels of IL-1β have been shown.[23] Long-term exposure to SEB can occur when bacteria invade the palpebral conjunctiva where they may remain for extended periods of time. The constant and direct contact of the antigen on the palpebral conjunctiva with the corneal surface initiates the cascade of events that causes the aforementioned late-phase allergic reaction, leading to marginal corneal infiltration.

CONTACT LENS WEAR AND INFILTRATES

Extended contact lens wear may also provide the opportunity for long-term bacteria exposure to the surface of the cornea, leading to marginal corneal infiltrates. In addition to the increased opportunity for bacterial presence on the ocular surface, continual agitation by extended contact lens wear may induce a mild inflammatory reaction leading to the up-regulation of IL-1 and ultimately the appearance of marginal infiltrates.

DRUG ALLERGY AND INFILTRATION

In addition to bacteria, some drugs, such as the antibiotic gentamicin, may serve as antigens. Upon instillation, they may initiate an allergic response resulting in corneal infiltrates. In such cases, discontinuation of the medication allows the infiltrates to resolve.

TREATMENT

The rate of healing of marginal corneal infiltrates is increased only by the administration of a topical steroid.[24] Unless there is excessive inflammation detected in the anterior segment of the eye, however, steroid treatment is not needed. The infiltrates generally disappear in a week or two without treatment.[25] If steroid use is required, viral infection must be ruled out and steroid treatment initiated cautiously.

In the case of infiltrates associated with contact lens wear, once the lens is removed, the infiltrates totally heal with or without treatment. If the patient is wearing conventional daily-wear lenses, they may experience a reduced occurrence of corneal infiltrates if they wear disposable contact lens.[2] Some experts hypothesize that continual perturbation to the ocular surface by the same set of traditional extended-wear contact lenses over long periods of time has a compound effect. Small regions on the lens continually in contact with the ocular surface may aggravate this highly, immunologically active area, producing the inflammatory reaction and subsequent infiltration as previously described. By the patient's changing lenses daily, the compound aggravating effect of the same lens on the ocular surface is avoided.

Because infiltrates may occur secondary to other ocular infections, they may be treated with a broad-based antibiotic, such as ofloxacin; cefazolin in addition to steroid treatment; or tobramyacin to prevent further exposure and damage to the eye. Ofloxacin has been found to be as effective as tobramyacin and cefazolin, and it has reduced the incidence of ocular toxic effects.[26] If infection persists, a culture should be done to determine the most appropriate therapy. Care should be taken in prescribing an antibiotic if *Pseudomonas* is encountered. In addition to its particularly destructive nature, some literature has shown an emerging resistance to ciprofloxacin in all isolates of *Pseudomonas*.[27]

SUMMARY

Varied in pathological origin, marginal corneal infiltrates offer an interesting example of the immunological reaction in the cornea. The biphasic allergic reaction, resulting in corneal infiltrates, is initiated by the presentation of antigen to the corneal surface. This may occur as a result of a variety of causes including hypersensitivity reactions, excessive contact lens wear, bacterial infection, and drug hypersensitivity. Although these causes offer different methods for antigen presentation, the essential mechanism leading to infiltration is the same.

Because of the variety of antigens that may initiate such a response, the presence of marginal corneal infiltrates should be carefully noted, as it may be a sign of further ocular allergic disease.

REFERENCES

1. Thygeson P. Marginal corneal infiltrates and ulcers. Trans Am Acad Ophthalmol Otol 51:198, 1947.
2. Poggio EC, Abelson MB. Complications and symptoms with disposable daily wear contact lenses and conventional soft daily wear contact lenses. CLAO J 19:95, 1993.
3. Friedlander MH. Allergy and Immunology of the Eye. Hagerstown, MD, Harper and Row Publishers, 1979, p 59.
4. Suckecki JK, Ehlers WH, Donshik PC. Peripheral corneal infiltrates associated with contact lens wear. CLAO J 22:41, 1996.
5. Smith RJ, Maloney RK. Diffuse lamellar keratitis. A new syndrome in lamellar refractive surgery. Ophthalmology 105:1721, 1998.
6. Haw WW, Manche EE. Sterile peripheral keratitis following laser in situ keratomileusis. J Refract Surg 15:61, 1999.
7. Tabery HM. Corneal stromal infiltates in patients with recurrent erosions. Acta Ophthalmol Scand 76:589, 1998.
8. Ionides AC, Tuft SJ, Ferguson VM, et al. Corneal infiltration after recurrent epithelial erosion. Br J Ophthalmol 81:537, 1997.
9. Thoft RA. Cornea, 2nd ed. Boston, Little, Brown, 1987.
10. Craven L. Principles and Practices of Ophthalmology, 2nd ed. 1996.
11. Robinson AB. Ocular Infection and Immunology. WB Saunders, Philadelphia, 1994.
12. Abelson MB, Richard KP. The Mystery of Peripheral Marginal Infiltrates. Review of Ophthalmology. Jan, 1995.
13. Bonini S, Magrini L, Rotiroti G, et al. The eosinophil and the eye. Allergy 52(34 Suppl):44, 1997.
14. Friedlander M. Allergy and Immunology of the Eye. Hagerstown, Harper and Row, 1979, p 185.
15. Leonardi A, Borghesan F, DePaoli M, et al. Procollagens and inflammatory cytokine concentrations in tarsal and limbal vernal keratoconjunctivitis. Exp Eye Res 67:105, 1998.
16. Abu el-Asrar AM, Geboes K, al-Kharashi S, et al. Adhesion molecules in vernal keratoconjunctivitis. Br J Ophthalmol 81:1099, 1997.
17. Mondino BJ. Inflammatory diseases of the peripheral cornea. Ophthalmology 95:463, 1998.
18. Mondino BJ, Adamu SA, Pitchekian-Halabi H. Antibody studies in a rabbit model of corneal phlyctenulosis and catarrhal infiltrates related to *Staphylococcus aureus*. Invest Ophthalmol Vis Sci 32:1854, 1991.
19. Mondino BJ, Lahedi AK, Adamu SA. Ocular immunity to *Staphylococcus aureus*. Invest Ophthalmol Vis Sci 28:560, 1987.
20. Yoshida M, Yoshimura N, Hangai M, et al. Interleukin-1 beta and tumor necrosis factor gene expression in endotoxin-inducing uveitis. Invest Ophthalmol Vis Sci 35:1107, 1994.
21. Planck SR, Huang XN, Robertson JE, et al. Cytokine mRNA levels in rat ocular tissues after systemic endotoxin treatment. Invest Ophthalmol Vis Sci 35:924, 1994.
22. Gill EA, Imaizumi T, Carveth H, et al. Bacterial lipopolysaccharide induces endothelial cells to synthesize a degranulating factor for neutrophils. FASEB J 12:673, 1998.
23. Thakur A, Clegg A, Chauhan A, et al. Modulation of cytokine production from an EpiOcular corneal cell culture model in response to *Staphylococcus aureus* superantigen. Aust NZ J Ophthalmol 25 Suppl 1:S43-S45, 1997.
24. Chignell AH, Easty DL, Chesterton JR, et al. Marginal ulceration of the cornea. Br J Opthalmol 54:433, 1970.
25. Zantos SG. J Am Optom Assoc 55:196, 1984.
26. O'Brien TP, Maguire MG, Fink NE, et al. Efficacy of ofloxacin vs cefazolin and tobramycin in the therapy for bacterial keratitis. Report from the Bacterial Keratitis Study Research Group. Arch Opthalmol 113:1257, 1995.
27. Garg P, Sharma S, Rao GN. Ciprofloxacin-resistant *Pseudomonas* keratitis. Ophthalmology 106:1319, 1999.

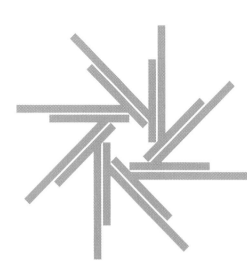

CHAPTER 19

Contact Lens–Induced Allergic Reactions

THOMAS JOHN

A contact lens–induced allergic reaction is similar in appearance to allergic conjunctivitis seen in patients who do not wear contact lenses. Recognition of contact lens–induced allergic reactions is essential, so that patients can be treated appropriately and can gain symptomatic relief.

OCULAR ALLERGIC REACTIONS

Non–Contact Lens–Related Reactions

The hallmark of ocular allergy is "itching."[1] If this symptom is absent, it is difficult to entertain the diagnosis of ocular allergy. Allergic conjunctivitis, which may occur in a contact lens wearer, is associated with environmental allergens and includes hay fever conjunctivitis, atopic keratoconjunctivitis, contact dermatoconjunctivitis, and giant papillary conjunctivitis (GPC; see later). Patients may experience excessive tearing, redness, and increased mucus production. Clinical findings include bulbar conjunctival hyperemia, conjunctival chemosis, and the presence of stringy or ropy mucus in the inferior ocular fornix. Depending on the duration and severity of the allergic conjunctivitis, the upper tarsal conjunctiva may show changes ranging from mild conjunctival hyperemia and fine papillae to giant papillae covering the tarsal conjunctiva. The increased weight of the upper eyelid resulting from cellular infiltration and edema may cause drooping of the upper eyelid or pseudoptosis.

Allergic conjunctivitis may or may not be associated with contact lens wear. In some wearers of soft contact lenses who have allergic conjunctivitis, superficial peripheral corneal opacities similar to Trantas' dots have been reported.[2] In contact lens wearers, this allergic reaction is thought to be secondary to the antigens deposited on the contact lens surface.[3, 4] Rarely, subepithelial, nummular, peripheral corneal opacities may be seen in allergic conjunctivitis. The diagnosis of ocular allergy is usually made clinically, but conjunctival scraping and scratch or prick tests may be used when indicated. If conjunctival scraping yields even one eosinophil or eosinophil granule, a diagnosis of allergic conjunctivitis is favored.[5] However, the absence of eosinophils in the conjunctival scraping does not rule out allergic conjunctivitis. The frequency of eosinophil yield in the conjunctival scrapings varies from 20 to 80%.[5, 6]

Temporary discontinuation of contact lens use is indicated in contact lens wearers with allergic conjunctivitis. Systemic antihistamines may be prescribed to relieve allergic symptoms. Identifying and limiting exposure to the antigen may not always be possible. The vasoconstrictive effect of adrenergic agonists (e.g., phenylephrine hydrochloride [Neo-Synephrine], naphazoline hydrochloride [Naphcon], tetrahydrozoline hydrochloride [Visine], and oxymetazoline hydrochloride [Visine L.R.]) makes them useful as topical ocular decongestants. Topical antihistamines, mast cell stabilizers, and nonsteroidal anti-inflammatory drugs (NSAIDs) may also be useful. Ophthalmic antihistamines include levocabastine hydrochloride (Livostin 0.05%), which selectively blocks the H_1 histamine receptor, and olopatadine. Antihistamine and decongestant combinations are also available for topical ocular use, such as pheniramine maleate 0.3% and naphazoline hydrochloride 0.025% (Naphcon-A, OcuHist). Mast cell stabilizers for ocular use include cromolyn sodium and lodoxamide (Alomide) drops. Ketorolac tromethamine (Acular), an NSAID, is approved for topical use to treat seasonal allergic conjunctivitis. In severe cases of ocular allergy, topical steroids may be used cautiously for short periods with close monitoring of the patient because of the potential for the development of cataract, glaucoma, and infection.[7]

Contact Lens–Related Reactions

GIANT PAPILLARY CONJUNCTIVITIS

To understand this condition better, consider the following:

GPC = allergic conjunctivitis + contact lens changes + ocular changes

resulting from contact lenses. GPC has been associated with both soft and hard contact lenses.[3, 8] Signs and symptoms absent in allergic conjunctivitis, but present in GPC, include increased awareness of the contact lens on the ocular surface, blurred vision because of a mucous coating on the contact lens, and excessive lens movement on blinking, which results from the inflamed upper eyelid pulling on the contact lens.

A contact lens may become coated quickly when worn on the ocular surface.[9, 10] Coatings are a constant feature of GPC.[11] GPC is thought to be due to an immunological response to antigens present in the lens coating.[3]

The term GPC was first used to describe the presence of giant papillae (greater than or equal to 1.0 mm) on the upper tarsal conjunctiva, although currently even papillae 0.3 mm or larger are considered abnormal.[3] GPC is commonly associated with contact lens wear, especially soft lenses. It can also occur with gas-permeable lenses, in the presence of a filtering bleb,[12] an ocular prosthesis,[13] exposed sutures,[14] and scleral buckles.[15] GPC is divided into four stages,[3] although clinically the findings may overlap.

The zonal distribution of papillae associated with wearers of soft and hard contact lenses is different because of the difference in the lens size and the area of contact between the lens and the tarsal conjunctiva. In wearers of soft lenses, papillae first form in the upper margin of the tarsal plate; in wearers of hard lenses, papillae are initially found in the region nearer the lid margin.[11] Papillary shape also differs between soft and hard lens wearers. The apices of the papillae are round in wearers of soft contact lenses and crater-like in wearers of hard contact lenses.[16, 17]

Inflammatory cell infiltrates found in the conjunctiva in GPC are shown in Table 19.1.[3, 18] Other cells present in GPC include lymphocytes and plasma cells. Surface conjunctival changes seen under the scanning electron microscope include variations in epithelial cell size and loss of the normal polygonal cell shape. In addition, the surface microvilli have flattened, branched, and tufted patterns.[19, 20] In GPC, the mast cells are degranulated,[21] with a corresponding increase in tear tryptase levels.[22] Tear samples in GPC have elevated levels of immunoglobulin (IgE) and in some cases IgG and IgM.[23, 24]

The pathogenesis of GPC appears to be a combination of mechanical trauma to the conjunctival surface by the contact lens and an immunological mechanism. The immunological component includes both an immediate hypersensitivity of the IgE-dependent anaphylactic mechanism (type I hypersensitivity) and basophilic hypersensitivity of the conjunctiva that resembles cutaneous basophil hypersensitivity.[11]

In the advanced stages of GPC, the tarsal conjunctival changes may resemble those of vernal conjunctivitis. However, distinct differences exist between GPC and vernal conjunctivitis (Table 19.2).

The goal of treatment is to provide symptomatic relief. However, completely successful treatment for GPC associated with contact lens wear may not exist.[25] Various treatment modalities have been used including tempo-

---

✳ TABLE 19.1 Inflammatory Cellular Infiltrates in the Conjunctiva in Giant Papillary Conjunctivitis*

Cell Type	Epithelium	Substantia Propria
Mast cells	+	
Eosinophils	+	+
Basophils	+	+

* Inflammatory cell infiltrates found in the conjunctiva are associated with giant papillary conjunctivitis.

+, present.

(From Allansmith MR, Korb DR, Greiner JV, et al. Giant papillary conjunctivitis in contact lens wearers. Am J Ophthalmol 83:697, 1977.)

TABLE 19.2 Comparison of Giant Papillary Conjunctivitis with Vernal Conjunctivitis*

Description	Giant Papillary Conjunctivitis	Vernal Conjunctivitis
Eosinophils, basophils, mast cells	Less	More
Eosinophils in conjunctival scraping	<25% of patients	Present routinely
Tear eosinophil major basic protein	No increase	Increase
Tear histamine	No increase	Increase

* Distinct differences exist between giant papillary conjunctivitis and vernal conjunctivitis.

(From Allansmith MR, Korb DR, Greiner JV, et al. Giant papillary conjunctivitis in contact lens wearers. Am J Ophthalmol 83:697, 1977. Data from Abelson MB, Baird RS, Allansmith MR. Tear histamine levels in vernal conjunctivitis and other ocular inflammations. Ophthalmology 87:812, 1980.)

rary discontinuation of the contact lens wear and administration of topical cromolyn sodium and corticosteroids. Apart from cleaning the contact lenses, the patient may need to change the type of lens to disposable daily-wear soft contact lens or gas-permeable lens.

SUPERIOR LIMBIC KERATOCONJUNCTIVITIS

Superior limbic keratoconjunctivitis (SLK) associated with soft contact lens wear has been well described.[26–29] This entity resembles Theodore's idiopathic SLK.[30–32] Patients complain of a foreign body sensation, itching, burning, tearing, and photophobia. Clinically, the superior bulbar conjunctiva displays injection, thickening, and variable staining.[26] Unlike Theodore's SLK, contact lens–induced SLK is not associated with thyroid disease, and filaments are absent. Although thimerosal sensitivity has been implicated,[27] SLK has been noted to occur in the absence of thimerosal.[29] Treatment consists of discontinuation of contact lens wear until the signs and symptoms resolve. Prescribing a brief course of topical steroids may be necessary in some cases. Use of nonpreserved saline solution, refitting with new contact lenses, and switching the patient to rigid gas-permeable lenses may be helpful.

Contact Lens Solutions

THIMEROSAL

Thimerosal (sodium ethylmercuric thiosalicylate) is an organic mercury compound commonly used as a preservative and disinfecting agent. The agent has a static effect against pathogenic microorganisms. Thimerosal alone is insufficiently broad spectrum or fast acting to be an optimal agent for disinfection,[33] and it is often combined with other agents such as chlorhexidine, edetate disodium, benzalkonium chloride, or chlorobutanol. Thimerosal, which does not bind strongly to lens materials, does bind to organic surface deposits. Thimerosal is well tolerated by the cornea.[34] In concentrations as high as 1%, thimerosal does not alter corneal oxygen uptake.[35] In a concentration of 0.004%, it has no effects on corneal epithelial wound healing.[36] Even at a 2% concentration, thimerosal did not cause epithelial defects in the rabbit cornea.[37] However, thimerosal can cause ocular hypersensitivity reactions.[38, 39] The clinician should recognize thimerosal hypersensitivity and should discontinue all solutions containing thimerosal. The use of new soft contact lenses is not recommended because the coating on the soft lens may contain thimerosal.

CHLORHEXIDINE

Chlorhexidine is a biguanide antiseptic with a "cidal" effect against both gram-positive and gram-negative organisms, except *Serratia marcescens*.[40] The agent acts by disrupting the plasma membrane of the bacterial cell. Chlorhexidine is used in a concentration of 0.005% in hydrogel lens chemical disinfection solutions; no cytotoxic effects were observed at this concentration.[41] Chlorhexidine can bind to many polymers; it also can form complexes with tear proteins and mucin to form lens deposits that can cause ocular irritation. However, it does not bind as readily to rigid gas-permeable lenses.[42] Because chlorhexidine has a limited effect against yeast and fungi, it is often combined with ethylenediamine tetraacetate or thimerosal. Chlorhexidine can cause a toxic response. If chlorhexidine is present in a lens soaking solution, a saline rinse should be incorporated into the cleaning schedule.

BENZALKONIUM CHLORIDE

Benzalkonium chloride is a quaternary ammonium compound with a bactericidal effect against a wide spectrum of bacteria. It was introduced in the late 1940s as a preservative for hard contact lens solutions.[43] The preservative is not used with hydrogel lens solutions because the hydrogel lens material binds to the preservative, a process that can cause ocular injury.[44] Benzalkonium chloride can cause toxic ocular symptoms, most notably corneal injection and superficial punctate staining. In addition to toxic reactions, a delayed hypersensitivity reaction can develop to the preservatives thimerosal, chlorhexidine, and benzalkonium chloride. The effectiveness of benzalkonium chloride as a preservative is enhanced when it is combined with ethylenediamine tetraacetate.[43]

ETHYLENEDIAMINE TETRAACETATE

This substance is a chelating agent, not a true preservative. Because it enhances the bacterial action of pure preservatives against *Pseudomonas aeruginosa*,[45] it is commonly used in combination with benzalkonium chloride and other preservatives.

POLYQUAD (POLYQUATERNIUM 1)

Polyquad is effective against many microorganisms, but it is much less effective against *Aspergillus*. Polyquad-preserved saline should not be used with lenses of hydration of more than 50%. Polyquad in a concentration of 0.001% is relatively well tolerated, but higher concentrations can cause toxicity.

Non–Contact Lens–Related Medications

Patients wearing contact lenses and using topical medications may develop an allergic reaction to the drug that should be differentiated from signs and symptoms related to the use of contact lens and contact lens–related solutions. With long-term use of certain medications, toxic follicular conjunctivitis may develop with conjunctival hyperemia and a follicular reaction of the bulbar and palpebral conjunctiva and cul-de-sac. Cycloplegic agents (atropine, homatropine), anti-glaucoma medications (epinephrine, pilocarpine, carbachol, apraclonidine), and antiviral agents have all been implicated in such reactions. Early recognition and discontinuation of the drug are beneficial to the patient. The conjunctival injection and ocular symptoms must be differentiated from those that may be related to contact lens use.

CONDITIONS TO BE CONSIDERED IN THE DIFFERENTIAL DIAGNOSIS

Lens-Related Conditions

LENS SPLITTING

Because soft contact lenses are inherently fragile, they can split as a result of improper handling or lens fatigue. Lens splitting is reported to occur in about 20% of patients using daily-wear lenses.[46] If the patient continues to wear the lens, ocular symptoms such as redness, irritation, foreign body sensation, and tearing can occur. When lens splitting is discovered, the lens should be discarded.

LENS SPOILAGE

Lens spoilage can manifest as either a diffuse surface coating on the lens with fine deposits or localized large deposits. In contrast to daily-wear lenses, this problem is more significant with extended-wear contact lenses.[47] The lens deposits may contain calcium,[48] proteins,[49] and lipoproteins. When lens spoilage is significant, patients experience ocular symptoms including irritation, hyperemia, and even blurred vision when the central region of the lens is involved. If the surface deposits cannot be removed adequately, lens replacement is warranted.

Patient-Related Conditions

Inadequate or improper blinking habits can result in ocular symptoms even if the lens fits properly. Symptoms may include blurred vision, corneal edema resulting in photophobia and decreased vision, corneal staining with fluorescein at the 3 and 9 o'clock positions, and various reading problems.[50] The normal blink rate is approximately 15 to 18 per minute; the rate decreases when the patient reads, is fatigued, and is under the influence of alcohol.[50] Proper blinking exercises may be beneficial.

Eye-Related Conditions

CONJUNCTIVA

VIRAL CONJUNCTIVITIS. Epidemic keratoconjunctivitis, which is highly contagious, is mainly caused by adenovirus serotypes 8 and 19.[51] Symptoms include watery discharge, foreign body sensation, and mild photophobia. Conjunctival follicles, pseudomembrane formation, and preauricular lymph node enlargement may be observed. These symptoms may arise in a contact lens wearer as a result of an adenoviral infection. Contact lens wear should be discontinued, and the viral conjunctivitis should be treated symptomatically. The corneal findings are described later. According to the recommendations of the Centers for Disease Control and Prevention, infected health care providers should avoid direct patient contact for up to 14 days after the onset of epidemic keratoconjunctivitis.[52]

CHLAMYDIAL CONJUNCTIVITIS. Chlamydial conjunctivitis or inclusion conjunctivitis caused by *Chlamydia trachomatis* is a venereal disease most commonly seen in sexually active young adults.[53, 54] Patients complain of foreign body sensation, tearing, photophobia, and redness. A scant mucopurulent discharge may be present. Follicular conjunctivitis is evident in the lower tarsal conjunctiva. The condition is usually unilateral. Epithelial keratitis may present as small, focal epithelial lesions that stain with fluorescein. Subepithelial infiltrates may be present, but they are usually smaller than those observed in epidemic keratoconjunctivitis. Marginal corneal abscesses have been reported, although this finding is not common.[55] If untreated, the condition will persist until a proper diagnosis is made and appropriate treatment is instituted.

EPISCLERA

EPISCLERITIS. Episcleritis is a relatively benign and self-limiting condition with an acute onset. Patients may complain of ocular discomfort and redness; however, the discomfort is usually mild. Photophobia may be present.[56] Most cases of episcleritis are idiopathic, but they may be associated with a number of diseases including rheumatoid arthritis, herpes zoster, and atopy. Visual acuity is unaffected in episcleritis. Bulbar conjunctival injection may be sectorial or diffuse. Conjunctival injection is usually seen in the interpalpebral area.[57] Because episcleritis can occur in a contact lens wearer, this condition needs to be recognized as being unrelated to the contact lens.

CORNEA

SUPERFICIAL PUNCTATE KERATITIS. Contact lens-induced corneal epithelial abnormalities include superficial punctate keratitis (SPK), corneal abrasions, epithelial microcysts, tight lens syndrome, and corneal edema. Contact lens–related SPK may result from flaws in the lens, such as edge damage and surface deposits. Improper lens fit may cause surface SPK. Excessive bearing down of the lens centrally or peripherally leads to SPK from the mechanical effect of the lens, which should be corrected. A steep, tight lens can lead to poor tear flow beneath the lens and may cause accumulation of debris and waste products and compromised flow of nutrients to the corneal surface, resulting in surface SPK.

SPK also can occur secondary to preservatives such as thimerosal and benzalkonium chloride (discussed previously). In such a case, the offending preservative should be eliminated from all solutions including disinfectants, cleaner, lubricants, and wetting and saline solutions. Staining at 3 and 9 o'clock may be associated with desiccation resulting from a rigid lens. Excessive edge lift or an edge that is too thick should be avoided in these cases. Lagophthalmos and incomplete or abnormal blinking patterns can also cause SPK. Central SPK secondary to central corneal desiccation is associated with lenses with a high water content.[58, 59] To correct this, a thicker lens or a hydrogel lens with a lower water content should be prescribed.

CORNEAL ABRASION. Corneal abrasion may be associated with contact lens wear. Patients usually complain of redness, pain, tearing, photophobia, and blurred vision, depending on the severity and location of the corneal abrasion. Contact lens wear should be temporarily discontinued, and the abrasion should be treated with topical antibiotics and cycloplegia. It is best to avoid patching the eye in wearers of contact lenses because of the risk of infection, especially with *Pseudomonas aeruginosa*.

EPITHELIAL MICROCYSTS AND VACUOLES. Epithelial microcysts have been reported in wearers of both daily-wear and extended-wear contact lenses.[60–64] The origin of epithelial microcysts and vacuoles is unknown, but investigators have speculated that the microcysts may be a sign of prolonged hypoxia.[62, 64] If the patient has significant epithelial changes signifying epithelial stress, changing the lens may be necessary, such as from a hydrogel lens to a rigid gas-permeable lens or from an extended-wear to a daily-wear contact lens.

TIGHT LENS SYNDROME. Also known as "toxic lens syndrome" or "acute red eye," this condition usually occurs in patients wearing a soft contact lens on an extended-wear basis. An immobile lens may occur secondary to debris trapped beneath the lens and causing an inflammatory response. Symptoms include acute onset of pain, photophobia, and tearing. Marked limbal injection, peripheral corneal infiltrates, and keratic precipitates may be seen in severe cases.

CORNEAL ULCERATION. This condition is an ocular emergency. The most common organism associated with contact lens–related corneal infection and ulceration is *Pseudomonas aeruginosa*. If not appropriately treated, *Pseudomonas* corneal ulcer can rapidly progress to corneal perforation. Investigators have shown that the risk of ulcerative keratitis is 10 to 15 times greater with extended-wear lenses than with daily-wear soft contact lenses.[65, 66] The risk factors for microbial keratitis include incorrect or no lens disinfection, the absence of hand washing before lens manipulation, lens overwear, contaminated lens care solutions or cases, swimming while wearing contact lenses, and the presence of external diseases, such as blepharitis.[50]

STAPHYLOCOCCAL MARGINAL KERATITIS. Patients usually present with pain, photophobia, foreign body sensation, and conjunctival injection. Staphylococcal marginal keratitis is associated with the presence of localized peripheral stromal infiltrates[67] that are usually separated from the limbus by a thin strip of clear cornea approximately 1 to 2 mm in width. With prolonged inflammation, the overlying epithelium can break down, resulting in ulceration.[67] Usually, staphylococcal marginal keratitis is associated with staphylococcal blepharoconjunctivitis.

VIRAL KERATITIS. The ocular findings associated with adenovirus are described earlier. The corneal epithelial findings initially include small punctate keratitis with photophobia. Subepithelial infiltrates can form later; if located centrally, they can cause decreased visual acuity. The corneal changes may include epithelial keratitis, focal epithelial keratitis, subepithelial opacities, and small gray opacities.

Herpes simplex virus (HSV) of the cornea can be a management problem for the clinician. HSV keratitis may include a variety of manifestations including epithelial keratitis (e.g., dendritic ulcer, geographic ulcer, marginal ulcer), stromal keratitis (e.g., necrotizing stromal keratitis, immune stromal keratitis), neurotrophic keratopathy, and disciform keratitis. When present, classic dendritic keratitis helps to establish the diagnosis of HSV keratitis. The infectious marginal ulcers are more difficult to treat. Patients with HSV marginal ulcers are more symptomatic than those with central dendritic keratitis.

REFERENCES

1. Abelson MB, Udell IJ, Allansmith MR, et al. Allergic and toxic reactions. In: Principles and practice of ophthalmology. Vol. 1. Albert DM, Jakobiec FA, eds. Philadelphia, WB Saunders, 1994, p 77.
2. Meisler DM, Laret CR, Stock EL. Trantas dots and limbal inflammation associated with soft contact lens wear. Am J Ophthalmol 89:66, 1982.
3. Allansmith MR, Korb DR, Greiner JV, et al. Giant papillary conjunctivitis in contact lens wearers. Am J Ophthalmol 83:697, 1977.
4. Refojo MF, Holly FJ. Tear protein absorption on hydrogels: a possible cause of contact lens allergy. Contact Intraoc Lens Med J 3:23, 1977.
5. Friedlaender MH, Ohashi Y, Kelley J. Diagnosis of allergic conjunctivitis. Arch Ophthalmol 102:1198, 1984.
6. Abelson MB, Madiwale N, Weston JH. Conjunctival eosinophils in allergic ocular disease. Arch Ophthalmol 101:555, 1983.
7. Friedlaender MH. Corticosteroid therapy of ocular inflammation. Int Ophthalmol Clin 23: 175, 1983.
8. Spring TF: Reaction to hydrophilic lenses. Med J Aust 1:449, 1974.
9. Fowler SA, Allansmith MR. Evolution of soft contact lens coatings. Arch Ophthalmol 7:1223, 1975.
10. Fowler SA, Allansmith MR. The effect of cleaning soft contact lenses: a scanning electron microscopic study. Arch Ophthalmol 99:1382, 1981.
11. Allansmith MR, Ross RN, Greiner JV. Giant papillary conjunctivitis: diagnosis and treatment. In: Contact lenses: the CLAO guide to basic science and clinical practice. 2nd ed. Dabezies OH Jr, ed. Boston, Little, Brown, 1989, p 43.1.
12. Heidemann DG, Dunn SP. Unusual cases of giant papillary conjunctivitis. Cornea 12:78 1993.
13. Meisler DM, Krachmer JH, Goeken MD. An immunopathologic study of giant papillary conjunctivitis associated with an ocular prosthesis. Am J Ophthalmol 92:368, 1981.
14. Jolson AS, Jolson SC. Suture barb giant papillary conjunctivitis. Ophthalmic Surg 15:139, 1984.
15. Robin JB, Regis-Pacheco LF, May WN, et al. Giant papillary conjunctivitis associated with extruded scleral buckle. Arch Ophthalmol 105:619, 1987.
16. Korb DR, Allansmith MR, Greiner JV, et al. Biomicroscopy of papillae associated with hard contact lens wearing. Ophthalmology 88:1132, 1981.
17. Korb DR, Greiner JV, Allansmith MR, et al. Biomicroscopy of papillae associated with wearing soft contact lenses. Br J Ophthalmol 67:733, 1983.
18. Allansmith MR, Korb DR, Greiner JV. Giant papillary conjunctivitis induced by hard or soft contact lens wear: quantitative histology. Trans Am Acad Ophthalmol Otolaryngol 85:766, 1978.
19. Greiner JV, Covington HI, Allansmith MR. Surface morphology of giant papillary conjunctivitis in contact lens wearers. Am J Ophthalmol 85: 242, 1978
20. Greiner JV, Gladstone L, Covington HI, et al. Branching of microvilli in the human conjunctival epithelium. Arch Ophthalmol 98:1253, 1980.
21. Greiner JV, Weidman TA, Korb DR, et al. Histochemical analysis of secretory vesicles in nongoblet conjunctival epithelial cells. Acta Ophthalmol 63:89, 1985.
22. Butrus SL, Ochsner K, Abelson M, et al. The level of tryptase in human tears. Ophthalmology 97:1678, 1990.
23. Donshik PC, Ballow M. Tear immunoglobulins in giant papillary conjunctivitis induced by contact lenses. Am J Ophthalmol 96:460, 1983.
24. Barishak Y, Zavoro A, Samra Z, et al. An immunological study of papillary conjunctivitis due to contact lenses. Curr Eye Res 3:1161, 1989.
25. Donshik PC, Ballow M, Luistro A, et al. Treatment of contact lens–induced giant papillary conjunctivitis. CLAO J 10:346, 1984.
26. Miller RA, Brightbill FS, Slama SL. Superior limbic keratoconjunctivitis in soft contact lens wearers. Cornea 1:293, 1982.
27. Sendele DD, Kenyon KR, Mobilia EF, et al. Superior limbic keratoconjunctivitis in contact lens wearers. Ophthalmology 90:616, 1983.

28. Stenson S. Superior limbic keratoconjunctivitis associated with soft contact lens wear. Arch Ophthalmol 101:402, 1983.

29. Fuerst DJ, Sugar J, Worobec S. Superior limbic keratoconjunctivitis associated with cosmetic soft contact lens wear. Arch Ophthalmol 101:1214, 1983.

30. Theodore FH. Superior limbic keratoconjunctivitis. Eye Ear Nose Monthly 42:25, 1963.

31. Theodore FH. Further observations on superior limbic keratoconjunctivitis. Trans Am Acad Ophthalmol Otolaryngol 71:341, 1967.

32. Theodore FH, Ferry AP. Superior limbic keratoconjunctivitis: clinical and pathological correlations. Arch Ophthalmol 84:481, 1970.

33. Sibley MJ. Disinfection solutions. Int Ophthalmol Clin 21:237, 1981.

34. Pfister RR, Burnstein N. The effects of ophthalmic drugs, vehicles, and preservatives on corneal epithelium: a scanning electron microscopy study. Invest Ophthalmol Vis Sci 15:246, 1976.

35. Burton GD, Hill RM. Aerobic responses of the cornea to ophthalmic preservatives, measured in vivo. Invest Ophthalmol Vis Sci 21:842, 1981.

36. Collin HB, Grabsch BE. The effect of ophthalmic preservatives on the healing rate of the rabbit corneal epithelium after keratectomy. Am J Optom Physiol Opt 59:215, 1982.

37. Gassett AR, Ishii Y, Kaufman HE, et al. Cytotoxicity of ophthalmic preservatives. Am J Ophthalmol 78:98, 1974.

38. Wilson LA, McNatt J, Reitschel R. Delayed hypersensitivity to thimerosal in soft contact lens wearers. Ophthalmology 88:804, 1981.

39. Molinari JF, Nash R, Badham D. Severe thimerosal hypersensitivity in soft contact lens wearers. Int Contact Lens Clin 9:323, 1982.

40. McLaughlin R, Barr JT, Rosenthal P, et al. The new generation of RGP solutions meets increasing demands. Contact Lens Spectrum 5:45, 1990.

41. Ruben M. Chlorhexidine (CH) and the PHEMA contact lens. Contact Lens J 9:3, 1980.

42. Lieblein JS. Overview of soft contact lens hygiene. Rev Optom 115:29, 1978.

43. Brown MRW, Richards RME. Effect of ethylene diamine tetra-acetate on the resistance of *Pseudomonas aeruginosa* to antibacterial agents. Nature 207:1391, 1965.

44. MacKeen GD, Bulle K. Buffers and preservatives in contact lens solutions. Contacto 21:33, 1977.

45. MacGregor DR, Elliker PR. A comparison of some properties of *Pseudomonas aeruginosa* sensitive and resistant to quaternary ammonium compounds. Can J Microbiol 4:449, 1968.

46. Koetting RA. Frequency of hydrogel lens replacement. Contacto 19:11, 1975.

47. Doughman DJ, Mobilia E, Drago D, et al. The nature of spots on soft lenses. Ann Ophthalmol 7:345, 1975.

48. Klintworth GK, Reed JW, Hawkins HK, et al. Calcification of soft contact lenses in patients with dry eye and elevated calcium concentration in tears. Invest Ophthalmol Vis Sci 16:158, 1977.

49. Ericksen S. Cleaning hydrophilic contact lenses: an overview. Ann Ophthalmol 7:1223, 1975.

50. Stein R, Stein H, Rao G. Contact lens complications. In: Contact lenses: the CLAO guide to basic science and clinical practice. Vol. 3. Kastl PR, ed. Dubuque, IA, Kendall/Hunt Publishing, 1995, p 1.

51. O'Day DM, Guyer B, Hierholzer JC. Clinical and laboratory evaluation of epidemic keratoconjunctivitis due to adenovirus types 8 and 19. Am J Ophthalmol 81:207, 1976.

52. Epidemic keratoconjunctivitis in an ophthalmology clinic: California. MMWR Morb Mortal Wkly Rep 39:598, 1990.

53. Hammerschlag MR. *Chlamydia* infections. J Pediatr 114:727, 1989.

54. Schachter J. *Chlamydia* infections. West J Med 153:523, 1990.

55. Darougar S, Viswalingam ND. Marginal corneal abscess associated with adult *Chlamydia ophthalmia*. Br J Ophthalmol 72:774, 1988.

56. Watson PG, Hayreh SS. Scleritis and episcleritis. Br J Ophthalmol 60:163, 1976.

57. Lyne AJ, Pitkeathley DA. Episcleritis and scleritis. Arch Ophthalmol 80:171, 1968.

58. Zantos SG, Osborn GN, Walter HC, et al. Studies on corneal staining with thin hydrogel contact lenses. J Br Contact Lens Assoc 9:61, 1986.

59. Osborn GN, Zantos SG. Corneal desiccation staining with thin high water content contact lenses. CLAO J 14:81, 1988.

60. Holden BA, Sweeney DF, Vannas A, et al. Effects of long-term extended contact lens wear on the human cornea. Invest Ophthalmol Vis Sci 26:1489, 1985.

61. Ruben M, Brown N, Lobascher D, et al. Clinical manifestations secondary to soft contact lens wear. Br J Ophthalmol 60:529, 1976.

62. Kenyon E, Polse KA, Seger RG. Influence of wearing schedule on extended-wear complications. Ophthalmology 93:231, 1986.

63. Zantos SG, Holden BA. Ocular changes associated with continuous wear of contact lenses. Aust J Optom 61:418, 1978.

64. Zantos SG. Cystic formations in the corneal epithelium during extended wear of contact lenses. Int Contact Lens Clin 10:128, 1983.

65. Schein OD, Glynn RJ, Poggio EC, et al. The relative risk of ulcerative keratitis among users of daily-wear and extended-wear soft contact lenses. N Engl J Med 321:773, 1989.

66. Poggio EC, Glynn RJ, Schein OD, et al. The incidence of ulcerative keratitis among users of daily-wear and extended-wear soft contact lenses. N Engl J Med 321:779, 1989.

67. Mondino BJ. Inflammatory disease of the peripheral cornea. Ophthalmology 95:463, 1988.

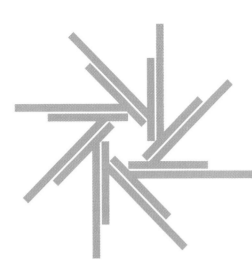

CHAPTER 20

Medicamentosa

MARK B. ABELSON ■ **MICHELLE GEORGE**

In a simple sense, the conjunctiva can be viewed as having limited ways in which to respond to insult. On external examination, the stimulated conjunctiva may appear hyperemic and edematous, and it may secrete mucus. The job of the clinician is to establish the cause of these clinical signs by taking a thorough history, considering differential diagnoses, and obtaining specific laboratory tests when appropriate. Although some causes of toxic keratoconjunctivitis represent a direct reaction to an offending agent, some may be confused with ocular allergies. Appropriate management hinges on establishing a proper diagnosis. The diagnostic term "medicamentosa" is derived from *medicamentosus* or *medicamentous*, meaning "used in or caused by a drug or drugs."[1] Medicamentosa is essentially a toxic response with no underlying immune dysfunction. It is one of the most common disorders seen in the subspecialty of cornea and external disease.

CLINICAL PRESENTATION

The time of onset after contact with the offending agent can vary from within minutes to hours. On slit-lamp examination, the conjunctiva is generally injected and appears "beefy" red. Chemosis may or may not be extensive. If the reaction has been ongoing, diffuse papillae or follicles may have developed.[2] The cornea is often involved, and diffuse pinpoint keratitis typically extends over the entire corneal surface (Fig. 20.1). Heaped-up opaque epithelium or pseudodendrites can occur in severe cases. Dermal involvement of the ocular adnexa includes injection, swelling, and, in some pa-

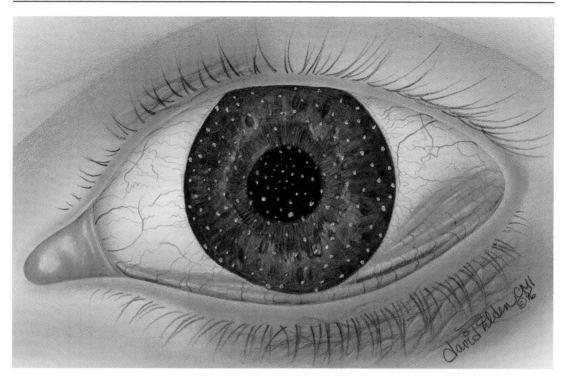

FIGURE 20.1 The conjunctiva is generally injected and can appear "beefy" red. Chemosis may or may not be extensive. If the reaction has been ongoing, diffuse papillae or follicles may have developed. The cornea is often involved, and diffuse pinpoint keratitis typically extends over the entire corneal surface.

tients, excoriation. Involvement of the lid skin is commonly associated with ointment use resulting from extended contact.

The clinician must take a careful history and must review the types and duration of medication used. Skin creams or other over-the-counter agents must not be overlooked. The patient should be instructed to discontinue the use of any suspect products, and a reevaluation should be scheduled for a few weeks later. Readministration of the suspected agents can be performed in the office, thus allowing the clinician to observe the reaction directly. Multiple applications of the offending agent may be required before the toxicity becomes apparent. All too often, additional toxic medications are substituted to treat the initial toxic reaction.

Agents commonly associated with toxic reactions include antibiotics, antivirals, sympathomimetics, miotics, and beta blockers.[3] Topical anesthetics and common ophthalmic preservatives such as benzalkonium chloride and thimerosal have also been identified as causative agents. Prolonged ocular contact time is likely to contribute to the higher incidence of medicamentosa associated with ointments. Eye medications and cosmetics are most frequently found to be the causative factor. Molluscum contagiosum is a nearly identical condition often included in discussions of toxic keratoconjunctivitis, wherein lesions of the lid and palpebral conjunctiva are suspected to result from a toxic viral protein or hypersensitivity to the virus.

PATHOPHYSIOLOGY

Frequently, the development of medicamentosa follows a minor external disease or problem such as dry eye or mild conjunctivitis that is treated for inappropriately long periods with toxic agents. The severity of the reaction is likely to be related to the offending agent's potency and toxicity.[2] Not all patients develop a true reaction to a given agent. The inciting agents may destabilize the tear film,[4] the first barrier to toxicity.

The pathological features of the conjunctival reaction are those of an acute inflammatory response. The reaction does not seem to be characterized by a unique cellular infiltrate profile. When the reaction has been chronic, the conjunctiva can be seen to undergo structural changes supporting the formation of papillae. In more severe cases, particularly seen in response to anti-glaucoma agents, conjunctival scarring may develop, mimicking or inducing ocular cicatricial pemphigoid. Corneal epithelial defects can also develop in severe cases. These defects typically occur inferonasally and are associated with intense superficial keratitis.

TREATMENT

Care must be exercised to avoid confusing the onset of medicamentosa with continuation of the underlying condition for which the irritating agent was being used. For example, the resolution of a bacterial infection may be missed if the prescribed antibiotic is inducing toxic keratoconjunctivitis and is masking recovery. It is easy to see that a self-perpetuating cycle can develop in which the offending antibiotic is continued in an effort to treat the mistakenly diagnosed signs and symptoms.

Removal of the offending agent is imperative. Should the patient be using multiple topical preparations, all should be discontinued. Readministration of medications should be done one at a time only after careful consideration. Improvement may not be immediate. Patients may not be inclined to discontinue the suspected agent when they believe that their signs and symptoms are related to a preceding condition.

Medicamentosa involves the superficial ocular tissues and is amenable to cold compress therapy. This method of treatment is preferable because the addition of topical vasoconstrictors, nonsteroidal anti-inflammatory agents, or mild corticosteroids may merely mask the signs and symptoms in the face of a continuing reaction. Of particular concern is the use of topical anesthetics to treat painful keratitis for which a cause has not been established. In the treatment of suspected medicamentosa, less is better.

REFERENCES

1. Dorland's Illustrated Medical Dictionary, 28th ed. Philadelphia, WB Saunders, 1988.
2. Terry JE. Diseases of the cornea. In: Clinical ocular pharmacology. 2nd ed. Bartlett JD, Jaanus SD, eds. Boston, Butterworths, 1989, p 582.
3. Terry JE. Diseases of the cornea. In: Clinical ocular pharmacology. 2nd ed. Bartlett JD, Jaanus SD, eds. Boston, Butterworths, 1989, p 547.
4. Abelson MB, Udell IJ. Ocular allergy update. Princeton, NJ, Excerpta Medica, 1981, p 20.

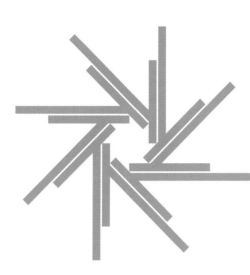

CHAPTER 21

Vernal Keratoconjunctivitis

ANDREA LEONARDI ■ **LISA M. SMITH** ■ **ANTONIO G. SECCHI**

Vernal keratoconjunctivitis (VKC) is a severe inflammatory disease that appears with seasonal recurrence or, less frequently, as a perennially chronic disease.[1, 2] The disease is most commonly seen in children and adolescents. It was first described more than 150 years ago as a *conjunctivitis lymphatica* and subsequently as *spring catarrh, phlyctenula pallida, circumcorneal hypertrophy, recurrent vegetative conjunctivitis, conjunctivitis verrucosa,* and *conjunctivitis aestivale*—all terms illustrating different clinical aspects of the disease, yet none, including VKC, fully describing this disease. VKC is distributed worldwide, but it occurs more frequently in warm climates and subtropical areas. The characteristic features of the two clinical forms of VKC, giant papillae on the upper tarsal conjunctiva and gelatinous limbal infiltrates, leave no doubt as to the diagnosis of vernal disease (Fig. 21.1).

Although VKC has always been considered an allergic disorder, its origin and immunopathogenesis remain unclear. In fact, many patients have no familial or personal history of atopic disease and can have negative results on the standard allergic diagnostic tests. This ambiguity makes the disease a challenge both for researchers, seeking new answers on its immunopathology and treatment, and for ophthalmologists, who have to manage young patients suffering from VKC's grave inflammatory consequences.

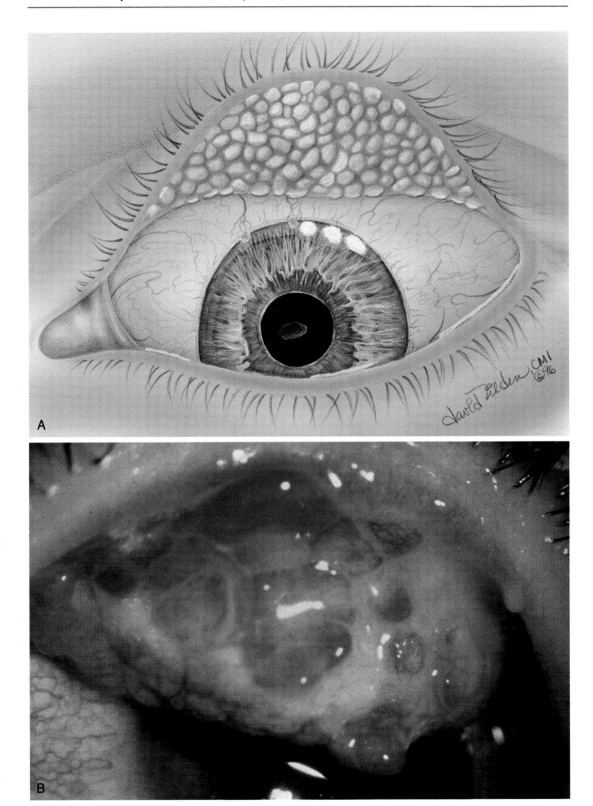

FIGURE 21.1 *A* and *B*, The characteristic features of the two clinical forms of vernal keratoconjunctivitis, giant papillae on the upper tarsal conjunctiva and/or gelatinous limbal infiltrates, leave no doubt as to the diagnosis of vernal disease.

EPIDEMIOLOGY

Clinical manifestations of VKC rarely appear in patients younger than 3 or older than 25 years of age. Males are more commonly affected than females, by a ratio of 2:1.[3, 4] Although the disease usually lasts 4 to 10 years and resolves after puberty, it can still be present, and even worsened, in some adult patients. The notable gender predilection and postpubescent resolution are features that suggest a role of hormonal factors in VKC's development. One report derived from a study of endocrine and immune system intercommunications demonstrated sex hormone receptors on the conjunctival eosinophils of patients with VKC.[5] Continued research should help to elucidate some of the epidemiological aspects of the disease.

VKC occurs over a broad geographical range. It occurs more frequently in the Mediterranean area, central Africa, India, and South America, but it is also reported in North America, Japan, China, and Australia. Considerable contributions to our knowledge of the disease also come from patients studied in cooler climates, such as Great Britain and other northern European countries.[6] The presence of the disease in these northern countries is thought to be a consequence of migratory movements of the susceptible population, a finding suggesting that both genetic and environmental factors contribute to its incidence. Further evidence of a genetic influence is the predominance of the limbal form of VKC in African populations[7] and the appearance of the disease in members of the same family. Until now, however, genetic studies have not been performed that confirm a relationship of VKC with a particular genotype.

In the majority of the cases, the disease is seasonal, lasting from the beginning of spring until fall. Nevertheless, perennial cases have been observed, especially in warm subtropical or desert climates. The predominance of VKC during the high pollen season lends credence to the widely accepted hypothesis that the disease is an immunologically mediated hypersensitivity reaction to environmental antigens. In an Italian population, 40% of young patients presented with associated allergic manifestations such as asthma, eczema, and rhinitis. In the published literature, the association with atopy varies from 15 to 60%.

CLINICAL PRESENTATION

Clinical Forms

VKC is usually bilateral, although monocular forms and asymmetric symptoms do occur. Three clinical forms can be observed: tarsal, limbal and mixed tarsal/limbal. Each is differentiated by the localization of signs and the type of corneal involvement.

Symptoms

All forms of VKC are characterized by intense itching, tearing, mucus secretion, and often severe photophobia that nearly forces children to live in the dark. Continued eyelid rubbing increases mast cell degranulation (and subsequently itching and inflammation) and can also encourage secondary bacterial infections. A foreign body sensation is caused by conjunctival surface irregularity and copious mucosal secretions. The presence of pain is indicative of a compromised cornea (Table 21.1).

Differential Signs

In the *tarsal* form of VKC, abundant mucus secretions are adherent to irregularly sized giant papillae, leading to a cobblestone appearance of the upper tarsal conjunctiva, which is pathognomonic to the disease (Fig. 21.2). The papillae are usually larger than 1 mm, evenly distributed over the entire tarsal area, or limited to one isolated zone. At times, the size of the papillae is not as notable as the diffuse subepithelial fibrosis and increased overall thickness of the conjunctiva. The papillae may be hyperemic and edematous and are surrounded by mucus strands.

An often asymmetric papillary hypertrophy can cause ptosis, which partially resolves in phases of clinical remission. Secretions, easily sampled from the fornix or internal canthus, are yellow, dense, filamentary, and rich in ropy, tenacious mucus and eosinophils.

In the *limbal* form of the disease, single or multiple limbal infiltrates, which are gelatinous and yellow-gray in appearance, are pathognomonic to the disease (Fig. 21.3). The limbus appears thickened and opacified, accompanied by hyperemia of the entire bulbar conjunctiva, especially near the infiltrates (Fig. 21.4). Often at the apices of the infiltrates, punctiform calcified concretions, called Trantas' dots, are observed. Their localization varies in different phases of the disease. In the more severe forms, the infiltrate can form a 360 degree ring around the cornea accompanied by a peripheral, superficial corneal neovascularization. Mucus secretion is present, yet it is less evident than in the tarsal form of the disease. In the *mixed form* of VKC, signs of both tarsal and limbal vernal disease are observed to varying degrees.

Corneal Involvement

Corneal involvement is common in VKC (Fig. 21.5) and can take the form of a superficial punctate keratitis, epithelial macroerosions or ulcers, plaque, subepithelial scarring, or pseudogerontoxon.[8] Punctate epithelial keratitis

---

✳ TABLE 21.1 Symptoms and Signs of Vernal Keratoconjunctivitis

Symptoms	Signs
Itching	Hypertrophic papillae on tarsal conjunctiva
Tearing	Limbal gelatinous infiltrates
Photophobia	Trantas' dots
Foreign body sensation	Mucous discharge
Pain	Punctate corneal epitheliopathy
	Corneal ulcers
	Pseudoptosis
	Tarsal conjunctival subepithelial fibrosis
	Conjunctival redness and edema

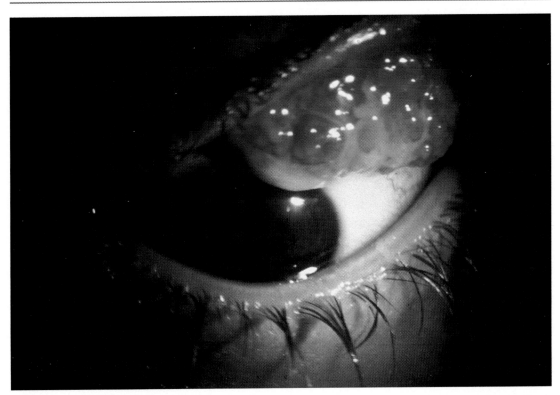

FIGURE 21.2 The cobblestone appearance (each papilla has a diameter greater than 1 mm) of the upper tarsal conjunctiva is pathognomonic to the disease.

can be present in both the tarsal and limbal forms, whereas aseptic corneal ulcers are more often noted in the tarsal form. The formation of "shield ulcers" is preceded by a progressive worsening of the corneal epithelium, which appears rough, irregularly stained, and at times covered with fine filaments. To assist in the treatment of VKC corneal ulcers, a scoring system has been proposed to grade their severity clinically[9]:

Grade 1: Ulcers that extend to the Bowman's membrane yet have a transparent base.
Grade 2: Ulcers with an opaque base that are partially filled with inflammatory debris.
Grade 3: Debris-filled ulcers that remain above the surrounding epithelium, that is, with plaque formation.

The peripheral cornea is almost always involved in limbal VKC, usually as compromised epithelium or superficial pannus (Fig. 21.6). A pseudogerontoxon can appear as a consequence of chronically altered limbal permeability. Transitory modifications in the corneal curvature with variations in astigmatism, which resolve with local therapy, have been demonstrated in association with the limbal infiltration.[10]

Keratoconus is the most common corneal ectasia present in VKC.[11, 12] Pellucid marginal degeneration, keratoglobus, and superior corneal thinning have also been described.[13] Excessive eye rubbing may play a role in the development of keratoconus in VKC.[14]

During the course of the disease, other corneal complications can arise from the stress of chronic inflammation, including bacterial or viral keratoconjunctivitis, delayed corneal healing, strabismus, amblyopia, increased

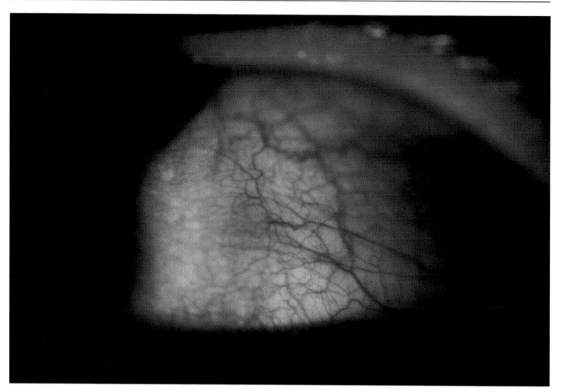

FIGURE 21.3 In the limbal form of vernal keratoconjunctivitis, the limbal vessels are injected. One may also see single or multiple limbal infiltrates that may appear gelatinous and yellow gray.

corneal scarring, and vascularization. Corneal perforation is, fortunately, a rare feature. Corneal complications, as well as glaucoma and cataract formation, may also relate to prolonged steroid treatment.

DIAGNOSTIC APPROACHES

Specific Diagnostic Tests

Given the characteristic history, signs, and symptoms, the diagnosis of VKC is, above all, clinical. However, it is useful to try to identify any specific allergen using skin tests. Specific immunoglobulin E (IgE) may be assayed in serum for systemic hypersensitivity and in tears for local hypersensitivity.[15, 16] The most common offending allergens are airborne, such as pollens, mites, animal epithelium, and molds. Patients with VKC can demonstrate hypersensitivity to food allergens, albeit less frequently. Nevertheless, in many cases the specific offending allergens remain undiscovered. In our study population, systemic tests were negative in approximately 50% of patients with VKC. Results were more often positive for specific tear IgE, a finding reflecting predominantly local production and an exclusively conjunctival hypersensitivity.[17] The measurement of total IgE in serum can be useful for the identification of a generalized atopic state. Blood cell count, in some cases, can also demonstrate modest eosinophilia. The conjunctival provocation test, carried out during the latent phases of the disease, may be

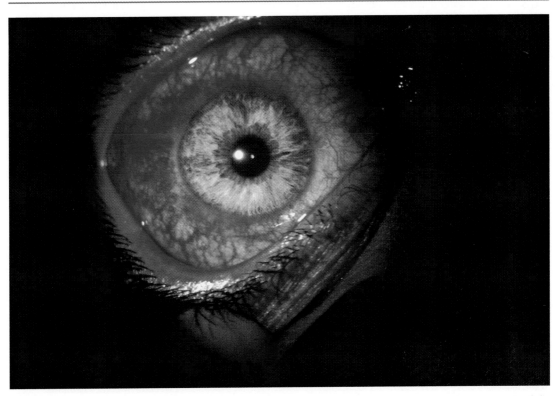

FIGURE 21.4 The limbus may also appear thickened and opacified, accompanied by a more or less intense hyperemia of the entire bulbar conjunctiva, especially near the infiltrates.

useful in the identification of a local specific reactivity to various environmental allergens.

On the basis of skin test results and serum and tear IgE measurement, two VKC populations have been defined: (1) those with negative test results and a negative personal and familial history of atopy; and (2) those with a positive test result who generally also present with some other allergic manifestation such as asthma, rhinitis, or eczema.

Diagnostic Cytology

Conjunctival scrapings and tear cytological examination are easy, useful tools in the diagnosis of allergic diseases. Conjunctival biopsies are not a necessary part of the diagnostic workup and are usually performed solely for research purposes.

Eosinophils, which have a constant and characteristic presence in the conjunctival and lacrimal cytology sampled during the active phase of the disease,[18] constitute as much as 80% of the cytological picture (Fig. 21.7). VKC is also one of the few diseases, ocular or not, in which basophils are frequently observed in the cytological examination. Last, neutrophils are always present in the acute phase, even if their role in allergic disease has not been emphasized.

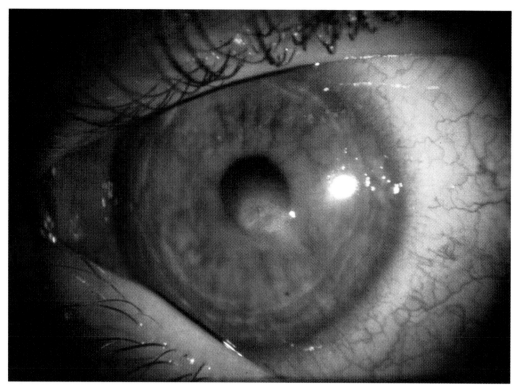

FIGURE 21.5 Corneal involvement is common in vernal keratoconjunctivitis. It can be present in the form of a superficial punctuate keratitis, epithelial macroerosions or ulcers, plaque, subepithelial scarring, or pseudogerontoxon.

Differential Diagnosis

Making the diagnosis of VKC is usually relatively straightforward. However, several conjunctival disorders may be confused with the milder forms of VKC: childhood-onset atopic keratoconjunctivitis in association with atopic eczema, contact lens–associated giant papillary conjunctivitis, trachoma (in endemic areas),[19] ligneous conjunctivitis, phlyctenular keratoconjunctivitis, chronic allergic conjunctivitis, and Theodore's microbio-allergic conjunctivitis. Trachoma and VKC can co-exist.

IMMUNOLOGY

Pathogenesis

Vernal disease is considered an allergic disorder in which an IgE-mediated hypersensitivity is one of the essential pathogenetic mechanisms. The seasonal incidence, the association with other allergic manifestations, the high number of mast cells and eosinophils in tissues, the high levels of specific IgE in serum and in tears, an increased tear level of mast cell–derived and eosinophil-derived mediators, and the therapeutic response to mast cell stabilizers in mild cases are all evidence of an atopic origin. However, the commonly observed absence of one or more of the foregoing characteristics in any individual person suggests that IgG-mediated responses, basophil

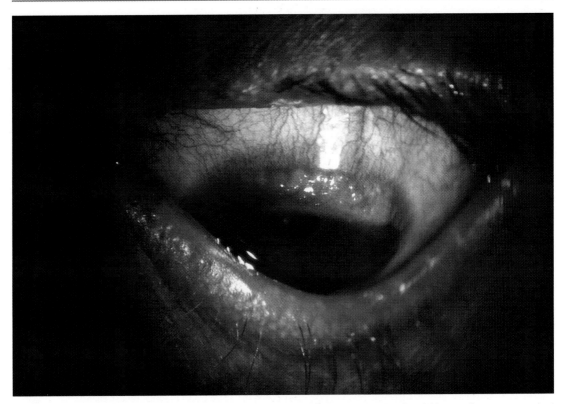

FIGURE 21.6 The peripheral cornea is almost always involved in limbal vernal keratoconjunctivitis, usually as compromised epithelium or a superficial pannus.

hypersensitivity, or cellular delayed-type hypersensitivity may additionally be involved.[20, 21] One or more environmental allergens and, rarely, food allergens are likely to be the initial cause of the hypersensitivity. The finding that a specific sensitivity is not found in many patients could signify only that other allergens, unknown or untested, are responsible. Furthermore, histological or histochemical evidence of differences between patients considered "atopic" or "nonatopic" has not yet been found.[22]

The conjunctival accumulation of T-helper (T_H2) lymphocytes, producing interleukins that mediate many of the histopathological changes seen in VKC, also confirms that it is an allergic disorder.[23] As mentioned previously, allergic persons may, in fact, be genetically predisposed to develop sensitivity to environmental allergens. An imbalance between the activation of the T_H1 and T_H2 subpopulations of lymphocytes, resulting in an overactivation of T_H2 cells, may give origin to hyperreactivity against substances that commonly come in contact with the mucosa. In any case, it is made evident by the severity of the clinical manifestations and the precocity of its onset that exaggerated conjunctival hyperreactivity is necessary for the development of this disease.

Mast cells play a key role in the pathogenesis of VKC both as effector cells in the development of IgE-mediated and non–IgE-mediated reactions and as regulator cells of the extracellular matrix transformed by this disease. In addition to the well-known preformed and newly formed mediators released by mast cells, cytokines and growth factors are liberated, stimulating fibroblast activity that causes the observed epithelial hyperproliferation. We have demonstrated in vitro that histamine also has a stimulating effect

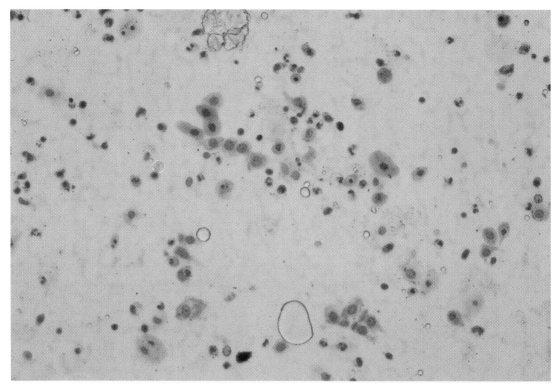

FIGURE 21.7 Eosinophils dominate the histological profile (80%) during the active phase of vernal keratoconjunctivitis.

on conjunctival fibroblasts, thus increasing the production of procollagens I and III. This finding highlights the ever-broadening role of histamine in the pathogenesis of VKC.[24]

Notable evidence indicates that VKC and its acute episodes are triggered or exacerbated by nonspecific stimuli such as heat, wind, and solar radiation. These factors appear to be so critical in the evolution of the disease that photosensitization has been proposed as one pathogenic factor. Nevertheless, its clinical and histopathological characteristics verify that at the root of VKC is an IgE or helper lymphocyte–mediated response stimulating a specific pattern of interleukin production. As in other allergic diseases such as eczema, it has been difficult to identify precisely which factors trigger single acute episodes. The finding that the disease is generally more severe in hot climates also may suggest that, in addition to nonspecific environmental factors, infectious agents may play an adjuvant role in allergic sensitization. Despite the diverse theories proposed for the pathogenetic complexity of this disease (Fig. 21.8), complete understanding of the causes and mechanisms exists that could be pharmacologically manipulated to eliminate or alleviate the symptoms of VKC.

Histopathology and Pharmacology

Histopathological studies reveal the following cellular tissue changes in the conjunctival epithelium and substantia propria of both bulbar and tarsal conjunctivae: (1) proliferative and degenerative changes in the epithelium; (2) prominent cellular infiltration in the substantia propria; and (3) hyperplasia of the connective tissue. Epithelial proliferation occurs early and

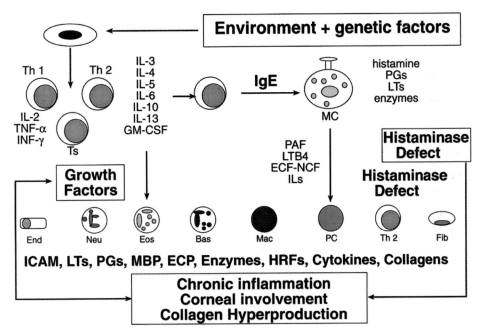

FIGURE 21.8 Despite the diverse theories proposed for the pathogenetic complexity of this disease, no complete understanding exists of the causes and mechanisms, which could be pharmacologically manipulated to eliminate or alleviate the symptoms of vernal keratoconjunctivitis. Bas, basophil; ECF, eosinophil chemotactic factor; ECP, eosinophil cationic protein; Eos, eosinophil; Fib, fibroblast; GM-CSF, granulocyte-macrophage–colony-stimulating factor; HRF, histamine releasing factor; ICAM, adhesion molecules; IgE, immunoglobulin E; IL, interleukin; INF, interferon; LT, leukotriene; LTB, leukotriene B; Mac, macrophage; MBP, major basic protein; MC, mast cell; NCF, neutrophil chemotactic factor; Neu, neutrophil; PAF, platelet-activating factor; PC, plasma cell; PG, prostaglandin; TNF, tumor necrosis factor; Th, T-helper lymphocyte.

concomitantly with degeneration and marked acanthosis.[25] The increased thickening of the epithelium—5 to 10 layers instead of the 2 found normally—results in the transformation of stratified columnar cells to stratified squamous cells, with keratinization sometimes present. Intraepithelial pseudocysts containing cell debris or inflammatory cells are closely associated with the epithelial degenerative changes. Numerous epithelial columnar or triangular down-growths or overgrowths, without penetrating the tarsus, are observed deep in the stroma. In the cul-de-sac formed by the ingrowths, numerous goblet cells are evident, giving a pseudoglandular appearance to these epithelial neoformations (Fig. 21.9).

The inflammatory infiltrate consists of eosinophils, neutrophils, basophils, lymphocytes, and plasma cells. Resident mast cells[26, 27] and fibroblasts are also increased (Fig. 21.10).

The total number of mast cells rises in both the stroma and epithelium—where they are normally absent—with a change in the ratio between their mucosal (tryptase-only–containing mast cells) and connective tissue (tryptase- and chymase-containing mast cells) subpopulations.[28, 29] Although proportionally fewer mucosal mast cells are present, their percentage is increased with respect to connective tissue mast cells. Eighty to ninety percent of mast cells can be completely degranulated and are identifiable only with electron microscopic techniques.[30] Mucosal mast cells have been shown to be less responsive to the mast cell stabilizer, disodium cromoglycate (DSCG).[31]

Histamine, the main inflammatory mediator in allergic diseases, is released by activated mast cells and basophils, both of which have high-

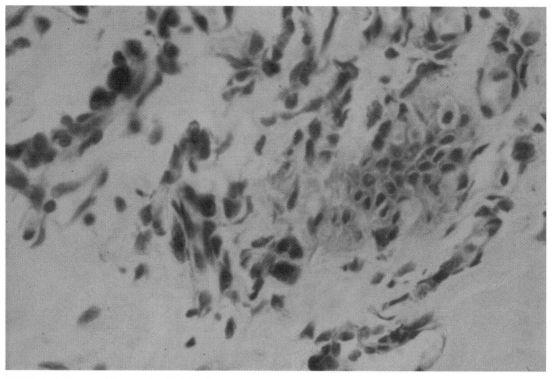

FIGURE 21.9 In the cul-de-sac of epithelial columnar or triangular downgrowths or overgrowths, numerous goblet cells are evident, giving a pseudoglandular appearance to these epithelial neoformations.

affinity receptors for IgE (FcεRI). Tear concentrations of histamine are elevated with respect to healthy persons and those with other inflammatory diseases.[32] Patients affected with VKC respond to a histamine conjunctival challenge at a lower threshold than normal subjects, a finding demonstrating a nonspecific conjunctival hyperreactivity.[33] This conjunctival hyperreactivity was shown to be associated with a deficit in the activity of the histamine-metabolizing enzymes, the histaminases, both at the conjunctival and systemic level.[34] This anomaly, most likely of genetic origin, leads to a greatly reduced inactivation of the histamine released by specific and nonspecific activation of mast cells. This phenomenon would explain the finding of chronically elevated histamine in tears in patients with VKC, even in the absence of stimulation. This phenomenon, together with the greatly increased number of stromal and epithelial mast cells, may also account for the severe exacerbating effect of histamine release stimulated by long-term eyelid rubbing. This finding suggests that VKC may be considered a systemic disease with a predominantly ocular expression.

Eosinophils and neutrophils are characteristic constituents of the cellular infiltrate in all stages of the disease.[35] A massive infiltration of eosinophils is highly characteristic of VKC conjunctival inflammation. The precise stimulus for this infiltration is unknown. Both types of cells can be observed within the microvessel, outside the vessel, in the stroma, and migrating through the epithelium. Increased expression of the adhesion molecule, ICAM-1, was shown in epithelial cells, thus indicating that eosinophils and neutrophils can selectively migrate through endothelial cells, through the epithelium, and into the tear film.[36] For this reason, these cells are easily observed in tear cytological specimens and are considered to be markers for tissue inflammation.

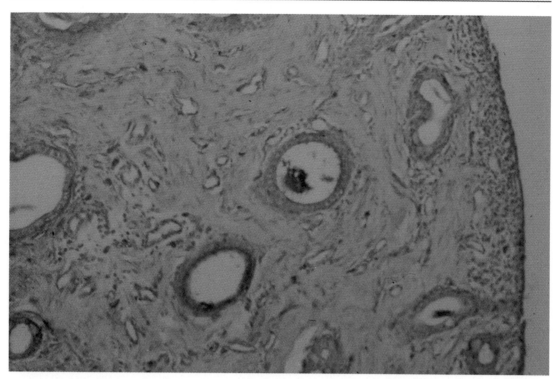

FIGURE 21.10 The presence of mast cells is increased in the stroma and the epithelium. Mast cells enter the stroma through the blood vessels in the limbal area.

Eosinophils can be activated by specific stimuli, because they possess IgE receptors, and by nonspecific stimuli, subsequently releasing proinflammatory mediators (e.g., leukotrienes, prostaglandins, platelet-activating factor), and toxic factors such as major basic protein, eosinophil cationic protein (ECP), eosinophil peroxidase, and eosinophil-derived neurotoxin. Extracellular major basic protein has been identified in the conjunctiva and in inflammatory material covering the de-epithelialized base of vernal ulcers, a finding suggesting a role in the pathogenesis of corneal complications.[37, 38] In vitro studies have shown that both major basic protein and ECP inhibit corneal epithelial migration.[39, 40] Furthermore, in patients with active VKC, high levels of tear ECP were found to correlate significantly with the severity of the disease and were used as a means to monitor local therapies.[41, 42] Abnormally high levels of ECP and eosinophil-derived neurotoxin were also found in the serum of patients with VKC, a finding reflecting the presence of eosinophilic inflammation.[43] Possibly, in situ eosinophils differentiate from stem cells stimulated by the presence of certain growth factors such as interleukin-5 (IL-5) and colony-stimulating factor (CSF).

Lymphocytes T and B and plasma cells are always found in the conjunctival stroma of patients with VKC. In varying amounts, T-helper (CD4+) and T-suppressor/cytotoxic (CD8+) lymphocytes have been identified in lesions; the ratio of CD4+ to CD8+ may depend on the stage of the disease.[44] Some studies have reported CD4+ lymphocytes to be two- to threefold higher in the substantia propria than CD8+, whereas in the epithelium both subsets were found in equal amounts.[45, 46] In tears,[47, 48] in vitro[23, 49] and histochemical studies[50, 51] the major part of tissue T lymphocytes were shown to be the T_H2-like type and are thus capable of producing IL-3, IL-4, IL-5, IL-6, IL-10, IL-13, and granulocyte-monocyte CSF (GM-CSF). This

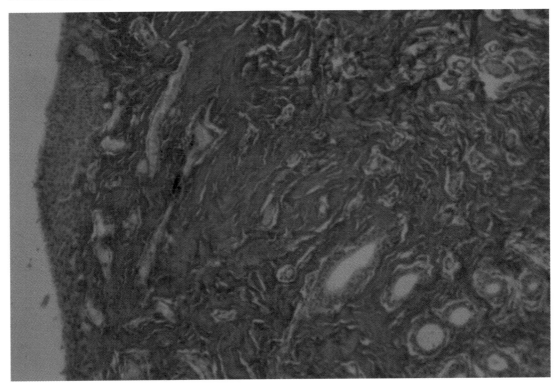

FIGURE 21.11 The conjunctival connective tissue grows to form large, sessile papillae, creating an abundant overflow of collagen fibers.

particular array of cytokines favors local hyperproduction of IgE (IL-4, IL-13),[52, 53] an increased number of eosinophils (IL-5, GM-CSF) and mast cells (IL-3), and the continual activation of both.[54] Plasma cells, staining positive for IgG, IgM, IgA, and IgE, were identified in VKC tissues,[22] explaining the finding of elevated levels of antibodies in tears.[55] As previously mentioned, an exclusively local production of IgE can be shown by measuring tear-specific IgE in 30 to 50% of patients with VKC who are otherwise considered to be nonatopic.[17, 56–60]

Most of the epithelial cells and inflammatory cells present in the tissue stain positively for the major histocompatibility antigens, a finding indicating that these cells are immunologically active.[22, 44, 45, 48] Many are antigen-presenting cells such as Langerhans' cells, which can amplify the local immune response.

Proinflammatory cytokines, such as IL-1α, IL-1β, IL-6, and TNF-α, have been found increased in tears, serum, tissues, and tissue cultures from VKC patients. Significant differences are not demonstrated between the tarsal and limbal forms of the disease or between the atopic and non-atopic VKC cases.[61]

One of the most spectacular events in VKC is the overgrowth of the conjunctival connective tissue forming large, sessile papillae from which overflows an abundance of collagen fibers (Fig. 21.11). In the deep layers of the conjunctiva, the collagen fibers run parallel to the surface, then radiate to form the fibrous structure of the giant papillae. A proliferation of capillaries and vascular neoformations provides vascular support to the papillae. Hyaline degeneration of the conjunctival stroma has been observed in the late stages of the disease.[25] In the limbal form of VKC, the fibrous proliferation is less evident than are the epithelial down-growth and overgrowth extensions, which form epithelial plugs of 30 to 40 cell layers. Studying the extracellular matrix of giant conjunctival papillae, we have demonstrated biochemically a reduction in proteoglycans, an increase in total collagen, and an increase in type III collagen,[62] resulting in an altered ratio between type I and III collagens.[63, 64]

One immunohistochemical study showed, in giant papillae of VKC, an increased deposition of collagen I and VII and an increased expression of the growth factors TGF-β, FGF, PDGF, and TNF-α.[62] In vitro experiments demonstrated that histamine, the metabolism of which is altered in VKC, may also act as a growth factor by increasing fibroblast growth and migration and by stimulating procollagen production.[63]

THERAPY

Preventive measures can be useful, but they are not sufficient for the control of vernal signs and symptoms. A change of climate, especially a move to high mountains during the summer months, can provide much relief to patients. In any case, it is necessary to avoid exposure to nonspecific triggering factors such as sun, wind, and salt water. The last can be avoided with the aid of swimming goggles.

Therapy is always long and involved, requiring frequent examinations, particularly if steroids are used. The first tier of treatment, mast cell stabilizers, should be used continuously throughout the season.[65] Many studies have demonstrated the efficacy of 4% DSCG (cromolyn sodium),[66–68] nedocromil,[69] and lodoxamide.[70, 71] This last mast cell stabilizer was demonstrated to be superior to DSCG in its steroid-sparing effect. It was also shown to be more effective than DSCG in the inhibition of eosinophil activation evaluated by measuring tear ECP before and after therapy.[72] As mentioned previously, mucosal mast cells have been shown to be less responsive to DSCG.

Antihistamines[73] and decongestants are useful adjunctives to mast cell stabilizers only in mild forms of VKC or in adult patients who have demonstrated a notable improvement in symptoms after adolescence. In contrast, even in more severe cases, studies have demonstrated the efficacy of aspirin at doses of 0.5 to 1 g/day, administered either locally or systemically, and of other nonsteroidal anti-inflammatory drugs (NSAIDs), thus proving them to be another valid steroid-sparing option.[74, 75] However, because patients are usually children, the use of aspirin must be evaluated case by case, given that it has its own risks. Gastrointestinal intolerance, Reye's syndrome in adolescents, hypersensitivity reactions, disturbance of renal function, hearing loss, and subconjunctival or retinal hemorrhages have all been reported with the use of aspirin.

Steroids are, undoubtedly, the most efficacious drugs for moderate to severe VKC. When used, they should be administered locally, with an absolute preference for those drugs with low systemic absorption, such as clobetasol, desonide, and fluorometholone. Doses are chosen based on the inflammatory state of the eye, with therapy prescribed in pulses of not more than 10 to 15 days. Prednisolone, dexamethasone, and betamethasone are to be used only when the previously mentioned steroids have proven ineffective. It is not unusual, however, to find steroid-resistant forms of VKC that necessitate alternative therapy.

Cyclosporine 2% ophthalmic emulsion in castor or olive oil is, in our clinic, the first choice for severe VKC.[76, 77] It is used seasonally or perennially, four times daily at first, gradually decreasing to one dose daily during relatively quiet phases of the disease. After long cycles of treatment, cyclosporine has an enormous steroid-sparing effect, and as a consequence, symptoms are successfully controlled solely by mast cell stabilizers. The local route of administration does not allow for systemic drug absorption detectable by clinical laboratory methods. However, the formulation is irritating to the ocular tissue, and many patients complain of burning, which can occasionally lead to mild corneal epithelial alterations.

In the presence of corneal ulcers, attentive monitoring of anti-inflammatory therapy is necessary, in conjunction with debridement of the ulcer, eye patching, and preventive antibiotic coverage for secondary superinfections.[8, 9] In these patients, steroids are preferred over cyclosporine because the former are more effective in inhibiting the inflammatory component of corneal damage, that is, eosinophil and neutrophil-liberated epithelial toxic mediators. Specific immunotherapy is useful only when a clearly defined systemic hypersensitivity to identified allergens exists.[78]

Surgical treatment consisting of giant papillae excision and cryotherapy of the tarsal mucosa is at times indispensable.[79] In our clinic, this procedure is followed by a cycle of local cyclosporine therapy. Oral mucosal grafting and saphenous vein transplantation have also been proposed as surgical treatment of severe tarsal VKC.[78, 80] A corneal transplant is sometimes necessary for adult patients with serious visual deficits and VKC-associated keratoconus. Finally, the iatrogenic consequences of prolonged and sometimes careless use of potent topical steroids can often lead to cataracts and glaucoma that must then be treated.

REFERENCES

1. Allansmith MR. Vernal conjunctivitis. In: The eye and immunology. St. Louis, CV Mosby, 1982, p 118.
2. Duke-Elder S. Diseases of the outer eye. In: System of ophthalmology. Vol. 8. Duke-Elder S, ed. London, Henry Kimpton, 1965, p 475.
3. Beigelman MN. Vernal conjunctivitis. Los Angeles, University of Southern California Press, 1965.
4. Neumann E, Gutmann MJ, Blumenkranz N, et al. A review of four hundred cases of vernal conjunctivitis. Am J Ophthalmol 47:166, 1959.
5. Bonini S, Lambiase A, Schiavone M, et al. Estrogen and progesterone receptors in vernal keratoconjunctivitis. Ophthalmology 102:1374, 1995.
6. Buckley RJ. Vernal keratoconjunctivitis. Int Ophthalmol Clin 28:303, 1988.
7. Dahan E, Appel R. Vernal conjunctivitis in the black child and its response to therapy. Br J Ophthalmol 67:688, 1983.
8. Buckley RJ. Vernal keratopathy and its management. Trans Ophthalmic Soc U K 101:234, 1981.
9. Cameron JA. Shield ulcers and plaques of the cornea in vernal keratoconjunctivitis. Ophthalmology 102:985, 1995.
10. Secchi AG, Leonardi A, Tognon MS, et al. Astigmatism changes in limbal vernal keratoconjunctivitis. Invest Ophthalmol Vis Sci 33 Suppl:994, 1992.
11. Tabbara KF, Butrus SM. Vernal keratoconjunctivitis and keratoconus. Am J Ophthalmol 95:704, 1983.
12. Kahan MD, Kundi N, Saeed N, et al. Incidence of keratoconus in spring catarrh. Br J Ophthalmol 72:41, 1988.
13. Cameron JA, Al-Rajhi AA, Badr IA. Corneal ectasia in vernal keratoconjunctivitis. Ophthalmology 96:1615, 1989.
14. Greiner JV, Peace DG, Baird RS, et al. Effects of eye rubbing on the conjunctiva as a model of ocular inflammation. Am J Ophthalmol 100:45, 1985.
15. Easty DL, Birkenshaw M, Merrett T, et al. Immunological investigations in vernal eye disease. Trans Ophthalmol Soc U K 100:98, 1980.
16. Leonardi A, Fregona IA, Gismondi M, et al. Correlation between conjunctival provocation test (CPT) and systemic allergometric tests in allergic conjunctivitis. Eye 4:760, 1990.
17. Leonardi A, Battista C, Gismondi M, et al. Antigen sensitivity evaluated by tear and serum IgE, skin tests, and conjunctival and nasal provocation tests in patients with ocular allergic disease. Eye 7:461, 1993.
18. Abelson MB, Udell IJ, Weston JH. Conjunctival eosinophils in allergic ocular disease. Arch Ophthalmol 101:555, 1983.
19. Friedlaender MH, Cameron J. Vernal keratoconjunctivitis and trachoma. Int Ophthalmol 12:47, 1988.
20. Khatami M, Donnelly JJ, Johon T, Rockey JH. Vernal conjunctivitis: model studies in guinea pigs immunized topically with fluorescenyl ovalbumin. Arch Ophthalmol; 120:1683–1688, 1984.

21. Allansmith MR, Cornell-Bell AH, Baird RS, et al. Conjunctival basophil hypersensitivity in guinea pigs. J Allergy Clin Immunol 78:919–927, 1986.

22. Montan PG, Biberfeld PJ, Scheynius A. IgE, IgE receptors, and other immunocytochemical markers in atopic and nonatopic patients with vernal keratoconjunctivitis. Ophthalmology 102: 725–732, 1995.

23. Maggi E, Biswas P, Del Prete G, et al. Accumulation of Th2–like helper T cells in the conjunctiva of patients with vernal conjunctivitis. J Immunol 146:1169–1174, 1991.

24. Leonardi A, De Paoli M, Fregona IA, et al. Fibroblast activity and collagen overproduction in VKC. Invest Ophthalmol Vis Sci 36 (Suppl):3866, 1995.

25. Morgan G. The pathology of vernal conjunctivitis. Trans Ophthalmol Soc UK 91:467–478, 1978.

26. Allansmith MR, Baird RS. Percentage of degranulated mast cells in vernal conjunctivitis and giant papillary conjunctivitis associated with contact-lens wear. Am J Ophthalmol 91:71–75, 1981.

27. Lambiase A, Bonini S, Bonini S, Micera A, et al. Increased plasma levels of nerve growth factor in vernal keratoconjunctivitis and relationship to conjunctival mast cells. Invest Ophthalmol Vis Sci 36:2127–2132, 1995.

28. Irani AM, Butrus SI, Tabbara KF, Schwartz LB: Human conjunctival mast cell: distribution of MCT and MCTC in vernal and giant papillary conjunctivitis. J Allergy Clin Immunol 86:34–40, 1990.

29. Morgan SJ, Williams JH, Walls AF, et al. Mast cell number and staining characteristics in the normal and allergic conjunctiva. J. Allergy Clin Immunol 87:111–116, 1991.

30. Henriquez AS, Kenyon KR, Allansmith MR. Mast cell ultrastructure: comparison in contact lens–associated giant papillary conjunctivitis and vernal conjunctivitis. Arch Ophthalmol 99: 1266–1272, 1981.

31. Schwartz LB. Mediators of human mast cells and human mast cell subsets. Ann Allerg 58:226, 1987.

32. Abelson MB, Soter NA, Simon MA, et al. Histamine in human tears. Am J Ophthalmol 85:417–418, 1977.

33. Bonini S, Bonini S, Todini V, et al. Conjunctival hyperresponsiveness to ocular histamine challenge in patients with vernal conjunctivitis. J Allergy Clin Immunol 89:103–107, 1992.

34. Abelson MB, Leonardi A, Smith LM, et al. Histaminase activity in vernal keratoconjunctivitis. Ophthalmology 102:1958–1963, 1995.

35. Trocme SD, Aldave AJ. The eye and the eosinophil. Survey Ophthalmol 39:241–252, 1994.

36. Bacon AS, McGill JI, Anderson D, et al. Adhesion molecules and relationship to leukocyte levels in allergic eye disease. Invest Ophthalmol Vis Sci 39:322, 1998.

37. Trocme SD, Kephart GM, Allansmith MR, et al. Conjunctival deposition of eosinophil granule major basic protein in vernal keratoconjunctivitis and contact lens–associated giant papillary conjunctivitis. Am J Ophthalmol 108:57, 1989.

38. Trocme SD, Kephart GM, Burne WM, et al. Eosinophil granule major basic protein deposition in corneal ulcers associated with vernal keratoconjunctivitis. Am J Ophthalmol 115:640–643, 1993.

39. Trocme SD, Gleich GJ, Kephard GM, Zieske JD. Eosinophil granule major protein inhibition of corneal epithelial wound healing. Invest Ophthalmol Vis Sci 35:3051–3056, 1994.

40. Hallberg CK, Brysk MM, Tyring SK, et al. Toxic effects of eosinophil cationic protein on cultured human corneal epithelium. Invest Ophthalmol Vis Sci 35 Suppl:1943, 1994.

41. Leonardi A, Borghesan F, Smith LM, et al. Eosinophil cationic protein (ECP) in tears as a method to monitor local therapy in vernal keratoconjunctivitis. Invest Ophthalmol Vis Sci 35(Suppl.): 1290, 1944.

42. Leonardi A, Borghesan F, Faggian D, et al. Eosinophil cationic protein in tears of normal subjects and patients affected by vernal keratoconjunctivitis. Allergy 50:610–613, 1995.

43. Tomassini M, Magrini L, Bonini S, et al. Increased serum levels of eosinophil cationic protein and eosinophil-derived neurotoxin (protein X) in vernal keratoconjunctivitis. Ophthalmology 101:1808–1811, 1994.

44. Bahan AK, Fujikawa LS, Foster CS. T-cell subsets and Langerhans cells in normal and diseased conjunctiva. Am J Ophthalmol 94:205–212, 1982.

45. Abu-El-Asrar AM, Van den Oord JJ, Geboes K, et al. Immunopathological study of vernal keratoconjunctivitis. Grafes Arch Clin Exp Ophthalmol 227:374–379, 1989.

46. Abu-El-Asrar AM, Geboes K, Missotten L, et al. Cytological and immunohistochemical study of the limbal form of vernal keratoconjunctivitis by the replica technique. Br J Ophthalmol 71:867, 1987.

47. Leonardi A, DeFranchis G, Zancanaro F, et al. Flow cytometry identification of Th2 and Th0 lymphocytes in tears of vernal keratoconjunctivitis patients. Invest Ophthalmol Vis Sci 39 Suppl:547, 1998.

48. Calder VL, Leonardi A. mRNA expression of INF-γ and IL-4 transcripts in activated T-cells from tears of vernal keratoconjunctivitis patients. Invest Ophthalmol Vis Sci 40 Suppl:683, 1999.

49. Calder VL, Jolly G, Hingorani M, et al. Cytokine production and mRNA expression by conjunctival T cell lines in chronic allergic eye diseases. Clin Exp Allergy (in press).

50. Metz DP, Bacon AS, Holgate S, Lightman SL. Phenotypic characterization of T cells infiltrating the conjunctiva in chronic allergic disease. J Allergy Clin Immunol 98:686, 1996.

51. Metz DP, Hingorani M, Calder VL, et al. T-cell cytokines in chronic allergic eye diseases. J Allergy Clin Immunol 100:817, 1998.

52. Romagnani S. Regulation and deregulation of human IgE synthesis. Immunol Today 11:316, 1990.

53. De Vries JE, Gauchat JF, Aversa GG. Regulation of IgE synthesis by cytokines. Curr Opinion Immunol 3:851, 1991.

54. Ricci M, Rossi O, Bertoni M, Matucci A. The importance of Th2-like cells in the pathogenesis of airway allergic inflammation. Clin Exper Allergy 23:360, 1993.

55. Allansmith MR, Hahn GS, Simon MA. Tissue, tear and serum IgE concentrations in vernal conjunctivitis. Am J. Ophthalmol 81:506–511, 1976.

56. Ballow M, Mendelson L. Specific immunoglobulin E antibodies in tear secretions of patients with vernal conjunctivitis. J Allergy Clin Immunol 66: 112–118, 1980.

57. Sompolinsky D, Samara Z, Zavaro A, Barishak Y. Allergen-specific immunoglobulin E antibodies in tears and serum of vernal conjunctivitis patients. Int Arch Allergy Appl Immunol 75:317–321, 1984.

58. Ballow M, Mendelson L, Donshik P, et al. Pollen specific IgE antibodies in tears of patients with allergic-like conjunctivitis. J Allergy Clin Immunol 73:376–380, 1984.

59. Kari O, Salo OP, Bjoeksten F, Backman A. Allergic conjunctivitis, total and specific IgE in the tear fluid. Acta Ophthalmologica 63:97–99, 1985.

60. Liotet S, Warnet VN, Arrata M. Lacrimal immunoglobulin E and allergic conjunctivitis. Ophthalmologica 186:31–34, 1986.

61. Leonardi A, Borghesan F, DePaoli M, et al. Procollagens and fibrogenic cytokines in vernal keratoconjunctivitis. Exp Eye Res 67:105, 1998.

62. Leonardi A, Albanese C, Abatangelo G, Secchi AG. Collagen type I and III in vernal keratoconjunctivitis. Br J Ophthalmol 79:482–485, 1995.

63. Leonardi A, Brun P, Tavolato M, et al. Growth factors and collagen distribution in giant papillae of vernal keratoconjunctivitis. Invest Ophthalmol Vis Sci 40 Suppl:683, 1999.

64. Leonardi A, Radice M, Fregona IA, et al. Histamine effects on conjunctival fibroblast derived from patients with vernal keratoconjunctivitis. Exp Eye Res (in press).

65. Allansmith MR, Ross RN. Ocular allergy and mast cell stabilizers. Surv Ophthalmol 30:229–244, 1986.

66. Foster CS, Duncan J. Randomized clinical trial of topically administered cromolyn sodium for vernal keratoconjunctivitis. Am J Ophthalmology 90:175–181, 1980.

67. Foster CS. Evaluation of topical cromolyn sodium in the vernal keratoconjunctivitis. Ophthalmology 95:194–201, 1988.

68. Tabbara KF, Arafat NT. Cromolyn effects on vernal keratoconjunctivitis in children. Arch Ophthalmol 95:2184–2186, 1977.

69. Bonini S, Barney NP, Schiavone M, et al. Effectiveness of nedocromil sodium 2% eyedrops on clinical symptoms and tear fluid cytology of patients with vernal conjunctivitis. Eye 6:648–652, 1992.

70. Caldwell DR, Verin P, Hartwich-Young R, et al. Efficacy and safety of lodoxamide 0.1% vs. cromolyn sodium 4% in patients with vernal keratoconjunctivitis. Am J Ophthalmol 113:632, 1992.

71. Santos CI, Huang AJ, Abelson MB, et al. Efficacy of lodoxamide 0.1% ophthalmic solution in resolving corneal epitheliopathy associated with vernal keratoconjunctivitis. Am J Ophthalmol 117:488–497, 1994.

72. Leonardi A, Borghesan F, Avarello A, et al. Effect of lodoxamide and DSCG on tear eosinophil cationic protein in VKC. Br J Ophthalmol 81:23, 1997.

73. Goes F, Blockhuys S, Janssens M. Levocabastine eye drops in the treatment of vernal conjunctivitis. Documenta Ophthalmol 87:271–281, 1994.

74. Abelson MB, Butrus S, Weston JH. Aspirin therapy in vernal conjunctivitis. Am J Ophthalmol 95:502–505, 1983.

75. Meyer E, Kraus E, Zonis S. Efficacy of antiprostaglandin therapy in vernal conjunctivitis. Br J Ophthalmol 71:497–499, 1987.

76. BenEzra D, Pe'er J, Brodsky M, Cohen E. Cyclosporine eyedrops for the treatment of severe vernal keratoconjunctivitis. Am J Ophthalmol 101: 278–282, 1986.

77. Secchi AG, Tognon MS, Leonardi A. Topical use of cyclosporine in the treatment of vernal keratoconjunctivitis. Am J Ophthalmol 110:137–142, 1990.

78. Del Prete A, Chilosi E, Magli A, et al. Surgical treatment and desensitization therapy of giant papillary allergic conjunctivitis. Ophthalmol Surgery 23:776–779, 1992.

79. Sankarkumar T, Panda A, Angra SK. Efficacy of cryotherapy in vernal catarrh. Ann Ophthalmol 24:253–256, 1992.

80. Tse DT, Madelbaum S, Epstein E, et al. Mucous membrane grafting for severe palpebral vernal keratoconjunctivitis. Arch Ophthalmol 101:1879, 1983.

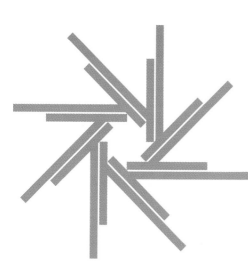

CHAPTER 22

Drug Pharmacokinetics

KRISTINE ERICKSON

In the medical treatment of ocular allergy, it is necessary to deliver a sufficient concentration of drug to the surface of the eye over a sufficient period to obtain optimal results. Pharmacokinetics is the quantitative study of the processes of drug absorption, distribution, metabolism, and excretion. This chapter reviews basic pharmacokinetics concepts, the compartment model for understanding pharmacokinetics of topically applied substances, and considerations required in the treatment of ocular allergy.

ABSORPTION, BIOAVAILABILITY, AND ROUTES OF ADMINISTRATION

Drug Properties that Influence Pharmacokinetics

Many important substances used pharmacologically exist in both an undissociated (lipid-soluble) and dissociated (ionized, lipid-insoluble) form. Such substances are often referred to as bi-phasic. These substances can be transported across membranes by simple diffusion only in undissociated form. The extent to which the drug is in its dissociated and undissociated forms is determined by the dissociation constant (pKa) of the substance and by the pH of its medium.

Solubility is determined in terms of the so-called ether-water partition coefficient or can be calculated using the Henderson-Hasselbalch equation.

Many important alkaloidal salts and synthetic drugs used in ophthalmic diagnosis and treatment are biphasic molecules. For substances with biphasic solubility, fixed percentages of the drug exist in each form at any given instant. Those molecules that are undissociated can penetrate biological membranes by diffusion. Molecules that are dissociated can pass more readily through porous structures provided that the sieve is "coarse enough." Size, shape, and electrical charge are important secondary considerations.

Vehicle Properties

The residence time of a topically applied ophthalmic preparation refers to the duration of its contact with the ocular surface. The residence time can be influenced by the characteristics of the drug vehicle, including osmolarity, pH, viscosity, and ionic strength.[1] The pH and osmolarity of a topical ocular product must be within a relatively limited range to be tolerable to the ocular tissues and to ensure patient comfort. However, the viscosity of the drug vehicle can range from high (e.g., an ointment) to low (e.g., physiological saline). In general, the more viscous the vehicle, the longer is the drug's residence time on the ocular surface. Increased viscosity improves transcorneal penetration and prevents drainage through the nasal lacrimal system. According to Patton and Robinson,[2] the optimal viscosity range of an ocular drug vehicle is 12 to 15 centipoise.

Tissue Barriers

Both dosage form and route of administration can exert significant effects on the clinical results obtained with a given drug. The optimal route of administration is influenced by the way in which the drug crosses various barriers. In the treatment of ocular allergy, the most important route of administration is the topical route, with the systemic route playing a smaller role.

One can think of the eye as a closed compartment that is set off from the external environment by the tear film, cornea, and conjunctiva and from the internal environment by the blood-ocular barrier (i.e., tight junctions among retinal pigment epithelial cells, retinal capillaries, nonpigmented ciliary epithelial cells, and iris capillaries). This model should make it apparent that a drug can gain access to sites inside the eye only after crossing one or more tissue barriers. Such barriers can be thought of (simplistically) as consisting of two principal types: biological (lipid) membranes and sieve-like structures. The only exception to this rule is drug injected directly into the aqueous or vitreous humor.

Cornea as a Tissue Barrier

The cornea presents the most substantial physical barrier to intraocular penetration of a topically applied drug. Although the sclera comprises a larger surface area, its densely packed collagen fibers create an effective diffusion-proof barrier to the inner eye. The cornea contains elements of both a biological barrier and a sieve-like barrier. The most significant barrier to the transfer of nonlipophilic drugs consists of the tight junctions between corneal epithelial cells. For all practical purposes, if these junctions are intact, only compounds of extremely low molecular weight can pass by a paracellular route. Thus, drug transfer across the corneal epithelium favors lipophilic compounds that are able to diffuse across cell membranes. However, once past the corneal epithelium, the corneal stroma consists of hydrated collagenous fibrils that favor the transfer of hydrophilic compounds. Therefore, the maximal ocular absorption is obtained by amphoteric compounds.[3]

Although extremely hydrophobic compounds can easily pass through the epithelium, their rate of absorption is significantly lower through the stroma. Hence, it would be ideal if drugs used to treat ocular allergy had a high octonol/water partition coefficient to help prevent loss of drug to the anterior chamber (and potential side effects), yet would allow penetration into the conjunctival tissue.

Blood-Ocular Barrier

The blood-ocular barrier is a tissue barrier that limits the diffusion of substances from the blood to the eye. Physically, the blood-ocular barrier consists of tight junctions among various cells including capillary endothelial cells in the retina and iris, retinal pigmented epithelial cells, and non-pigmented ciliary body cells. Only extremely small hydrophilic compounds can diffuse passively from the blood into the eye. However, some active transport systems, particularly in the ciliary body, assist the transport of certain organic acids and bases into the eye.[4] The primary tissue barriers encompassing both the cornea and the blood ocular barrier are depicted in Figure 22.1.

Conjunctival vessels are reasonably "leaky." Therefore, systemic administration should be useful in the treatment of allergic conjunctivitis, provided adequate tissue levels can be maintained without significant systemic side effects.

COMPARTMENT THEORY AND DRUG KINETICS OF THE EYE

Topical Administration

The administration of drugs to the ocular surface can be described by a pair of two-compartment models: one describing drug exchange between the precorneal tear film and the cornea and the other describing drug exchange between the cornea and the anterior chamber.[5] Many variables make it difficult to determine the exact fate of a topically applied drug at any given time, including physical factors (e.g., partition coefficient), anatomical factors (e.g., integrity of corneal epithelial tight junctions), physiological factors (e.g., tear flow rate), and pathological conditions (e.g., inflammation).[1] However, the overall concentration of a drug in any given compartment can be approximated using the simplified model depicted in Figure 22.2.

After topical application, significant drug loss from the eye occurs as drug overflows into the nasal-lacrimal system and as it is momentarily diluted by tears. This dilution and draining are the rate-limiting factors in topical drug delivery.[5] The dwell time of the drug on the corneal surface can be maximized by selecting a drop size no larger than 20 μL.[1] Dwell time can be further enhanced by preventing drainage with brief punctal occlusion or tilting the patient's head back.[6] In addition to dilution and drainage, topically applied drug is also lost by adsorption to tear proteins and sur-

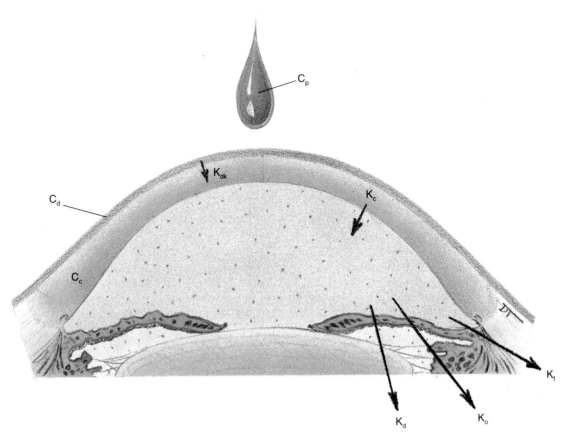

FIGURE 22.1 Drug bioavailability is affected by a number of physiologic factors. Drug penetration is affected by factors such as epithelial and stromal permeability whereas drug residence is determined by factors such as uveoscleral outflow and aqueous dynamics. C_c, tissue concentration; C_d, concentration in the tear film; C_p, drop concentration; K_c, transfer coefficient (aqueous); K_d, coefficient of diffusional exchange; K_{dk}, transfer coefficient (epithelium); K_f, coefficient of outflow; K_o, coefficient of loss. (Adapted from Maurice DM, Mishima S. Ocular pharmacokinetics. In: Pharmacology of the eye: handbook of experimental pharmacology. Vol. 69. Sears ML, ed. Berlin, Springer-Verlag, 1984, p 19.)

Pathways of Potential Drug Loss

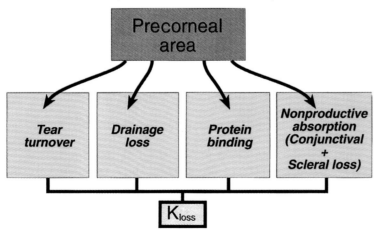

FIGURE 22.2 A significant drug loss occurs initially as drug overflows into the nasal lacrimal system and momentary dilution by tears. In addition to dilution and drainage, topically applied drug is also lost to adsorption by tear proteins and surrounding tissues including the lids, conjunctiva, and sclera.

rounding ocular tissues, including the lids, conjunctiva, and sclera (see Fig. 22.2).

When target tissues are internal (e.g., in the treatment of glaucoma or uveitis), drug absorption is regarded as nonproductive, although recent studies have suggested that noncorneal absorption may be significant with some compounds having poor corneal permeability.[7] In the case of ocular allergy treatment, in which the drug dwell time at the ocular surface should be maximized and intraocular absorption should be minimized, topical administration is advantageous because the surface ocular tissues are the targets for drug treatment.

Drug metabolism by tear and tissue enzymes is another factor influencing the bioavailability of a topically applied drug. Local drug breakdown may be particularly accelerated in cases of ocular inflammation when, in addition to tear enzymes, serum inflammatory enzymes are also present.[1]

REFERENCES

1. Ueno N, Refojo M, Abelson MB. Pharmacokinetics. In: Principles and practice of ophthalmology. Albert DM, Jacobiec FA, eds. Philadelphia, WB Saunders, 1994, p 916.
2. Patton TF, Robinson JR. Ocular evaluation of polyvinyl alcohol vehicle in rabbits. J Pharm Sci 64:1312, 1975.
3. Waltman SR, Hart WM. The cornea. In: Adler's physiology of the eye. 8th ed. Moses RA, Hart WM, eds. St. Louis, CV Mosby, 1987, p 36.
4. Caprioli J. The ciliary epithelia and the aqueous humor. In: Moses RA, Hart WM, eds. Adler's physiology of the eye. 8th ed. St. Louis, CV Mosby, 1987, p 204.
5. Maurice DM, Mishima S. Ocular pharmacokinetics. In: Pharmacology of the eye: handbook of experimental pharmacology. Vol. 69. Sears ML, ed. Berlin, Springer-Verlag, 1984, p 19.
6. Fraunfelder FT. Extraocular fluid dynamics: how best to apply topical ocular medications. Trans Am Ophthalmol Soc 74:457, 1976.
7. Schoenwald RD. Ocular pharmacokinetics/pharmacodynamics. In: Ophthalmic drug delivery systems. Mitra AK, ed. New York, Marcel Dekker, 1993, p 83.

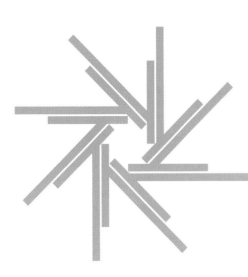

CHAPTER **23**

Antihistamines and Antihistamine/ Vasoconstrictor Combinations

MARK B. ABELSON ■ **KENDYL SCHAEFER** ■ **PAULA J. WUN**

Throughout the 20th century, much information on histamine has been documented, but not until 1977 was histamine detected in the human tear film.[1] Two years later, Abelson et al.[2] demonstrated that topical instillation of histamine produced, in a dose-dependent fashion, the itching and redness associated with allergic conjunctivitis. Subsequently, identification of specific receptors on the ocular surface has made it possible to identify the pathological effects of histamine selectively. Studies have shown that stimulation of H_1 receptors elicits ocular itching,[3] whereas stimulation of H_2 receptors produces vasodilation of conjunctival vessels without itching.[4]

Histamine H_1-receptor antagonists, also known as H_1 antihistamines, compete with histamine at the H_1-receptor site on the effector cell (Fig. 23.1). These agents have been classified by chemical structure into seven major groups: alkylamines, ethanolamines, ethylenediamines, phenothiazines, piperidines, piperazines, and cyclohexylpiperidines.

The H_1 antihistamines are composed of one or two aromatic (heterocyclic) rings connected by a nitrogen, carbon, or oxygen atom to an ethylamine

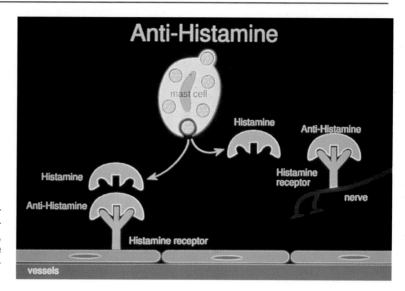

FIGURE 23.1 Antihistamines competitively block histamine from attaching to the histamine receptors, thereby inhibiting the onset of the signs and symptoms of allergic conjunctivitis.

group (Fig. 23.2). The multiple aromatic rings make these compounds extremely lipophilic, a property that contributes to H_1-receptor binding.[5] In addition, both histamine and the H_1 antihistamines have a positively charged amino group believed to be important in receptor recognition.[6]

Histamine H_2-receptor antagonists, also known as H_2 antihistamines, are more similar in structure to histamine than are the H_1 antihistamines. H_2 antihistamines have an imidazole ring and are polar compounds. These compounds are weak bases and are highly water soluble, so they exist uncharged in aqueous solutions at physiological conditions (pH = 7.4).[5]

Antihistamines bind competitively and reversibly to histamine receptors.

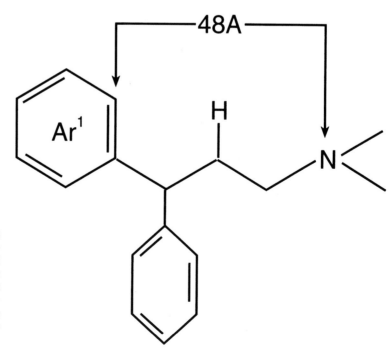

FIGURE 23.2 The H_1 antihistamines are composed of one or two aromatic (heterocyclic) rings connected via a nitrogen, carbon, or oxygen atom to an ethylamine group. The multiple aromatic rings of the H_1 antihistamines make these compounds very lipophilic, a feature that contributes to H_1 receptor binding.

By competing with histamine for receptors on effector cells, both H_1 and H_2 antihistamines effectively prevent the immune response and the manifestation of clinical signs and symptoms of allergic disease.

Histamine affects the vascular system through both H_1 and H_2 receptors.[7, 8] Stimulation of H_1 receptors causes systemic vasodilation and localized erythema and edema resulting from capillary dilation and increased permeability.[9] In the eye, topically applied histamine induces ocular itching and vasodilation. H_1 antihistamines effectively reduce this histamine-induced itching.[10]

OPHTHALMIC ANTIHISTAMINES

Topical ophthalmic preparations of H_1 antihistamines currently include an alkylamine (pheniramine maleate), two ethylenediamines (antazoline phosphate and pyrilamine maleate), two piperidines (levocabastine hydrochloride and ketotifen fumarate), a dibenzoxepin (olopatadine hydrochloride), and a benzimidazole (emedastine fumarate). These drugs provide relief of symptoms associated with seasonal or atopic conjunctivitis (Fig. 23.3). Pheniramine maleate, antazoline phosphate, and pyrilamine maleate have been shown to inhibit ocular itching significantly. However, these agents are only available in combination with alpha-adrenergic agents, which are included to alleviate conjunctival redness. Levocabastine hydrochloride, olopatadine hydrochloride, and emedastine fumarate are available without a vasoconstrictor. Ketotifen fumarate is expected to be on the market presently. Currently, no H_2-receptor antagonists are available for ocular use.

Pheniramine, Pyrilamine, and Antazoline

Pheniramine 0.3%, pyrilamine 0.1%, and antazoline 0.5% are classic antihistamines that have been used since the 1940s. All three agents are specific H_1-receptor antagonists and have been shown to be efficacious in reducing the chemosis and itching associated with allergic conjunctivitis. Antazoline 0.5% has been shown to decrease intraocular pressure.[11] Antazoline 0.5% has also exhibited some anesthetic properties, but it has been shown in rabbit models to be insufficient in preventing ocular irritation.[12] The recommended dose for the relief of ocular allergy symptoms is 1 to 2 drops instilled in the eye up to four times daily.

Levocabastine

Levocabastine hydrochloride 0.05% (Livostin) is a long-acting, highly potent, and selective H_1-receptor antagonist.[12] It is 15,000 times more potent than chlorpheniramine in the rat model of 48/80-induced mortality.[13] Studies using radiolabeled markers have indicated that levocabastine specifically binds to histamine H_1-receptor sites and dissociates from those sites slowly—the dissociation half-life is 116 minutes.[12] In contrast, levocabastine has remarkably low affinity for dopamine, serotonin, alpha-adrenergic, beta-adrenergic, and several other receptor sites. The small amounts of levocabastine that do bind to these sites dissociate rapidly, thereby displaying no pharmacological effect. In clinical trials, a topical preparation of levocabastine 0.05% effectively reduced itching, hyperemia, and chemosis.[13] Levo-

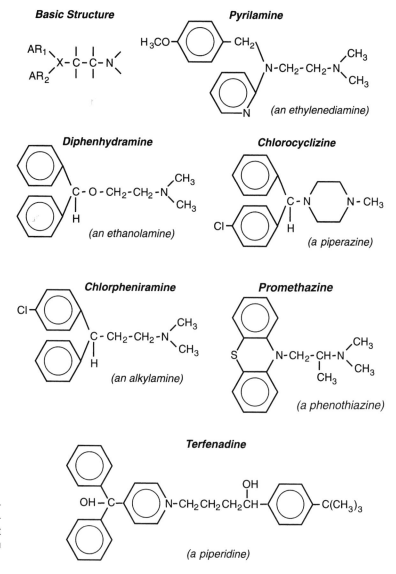

FIGURE 23.3 Numerous antihistamines are available. The basic structure contains two aromatic rings, at least a two-carbon chain, and an amino group.

cabastine 0.05% is used four times daily to relieve signs and symptoms of seasonal allergic conjunctivitis.

Olopatadine

Olopatadine 0.1% (Patanol) is the first dual-action allergy therapy to receive approval as both an antihistamine and a mast cell stabilizer. Olopatadine was shown to be 1,059 times and 4,177 times more selective for H_1 receptors than H_2 and H_3 receptors, respectively.[14] The H_1 selectivity for olopatadine is superior to those of other ocular antihistamines, including ketotifen, levocabastine, antazoline, and pheniramine.[14, 15] Olopatadine has been shown, in a concentration-dependent fashion (IC_{50} = 559 μM), to inhibit histamine, tryptase, and prostaglandin D_2 release from human conjunctival mast cell preparations in vitro.[15, 16] This agent is indicated for the prevention of ocular itching, and the recommended dosing regimen is 1 to 2 drops twice a day, at 6- to 8-hour intervals.

Emedastine

Emedastine difumarate 0.05% (Emadine) is a potent, selective H_1 antagonist possessing a rapid onset and an acceptable duration of action following topical ocular administration. Emedastine's ability to inhibit increases in vascular permeability is agonist specific. Emedastine inhibits the histamine-induced response without significantly affecting increases in vascular permeability induced by either serotonin or platelet-activating factor. Selectivity is further demonstrated by emedastine's lack of interaction with the adrenergic, cholinergic, serotonergic, bradykinin, and prostanoid receptor systems, whereas levocabastine has been shown to possess significant affinity for $dopamine_2$- and $alpha_1$-adrenergic receptors in addition to its interaction at the histamine receptors. This high degree of selectivity may account for emedastine's low side-effect profile.

Both environmental and conjunctival allergen challenge clinical studies have shown that emedastine is both effective in relieving the signs and symptoms of allergic conjunctivitis and superior to levocabastine. In a guinea pig model using a 30-minute interval between topical ocular treatment and histamine challenge, emedastine demonstrated greater antihistaminic potency than brompheniramine, chlorpheniramine, levocabastine, pheniramine, pyrilamine, antazoline, and diphenhydramine and was equipotent to ketotifen.[17] In similar experiments using a 1-minute interval, emedastine was 3, 8, and 17 times more potent than ketotifen, pheniramine, and antazoline, respectively, and was approximately equipotent to pyrilamine. When administered immediately before challenge, emedastine inhibited the histamine-induced response by 92%.[18] Emedastine 0.05% can be used up to four times daily to relieve signs and symptoms of allergic conjunctivitis.

Ketotifen

Ketotifen fumarate is a noncompetitive H_1-receptor antagonist currently marketed as a 0.05% ophthalmic solution in Japan for the treatment of allergic conjunctivitis under the trade name Zaditen. In addition to its antihistaminic properties, ketotifen has been shown to inhibit the release of leukotrienes, to inhibit eosinophil chemotaxis, and to suppress eosinophil activation by cytokines. Ketotifen fumarate 0.025% was filed with the FDA in December of 1998. It was granted primary review and is expected to be available presently.

MARKETED ANTIHISTAMINES

The currently available topical ocular antihistamine preparations are listed in Table 23.1. Topical H_1 antihistamines are not only the most commonly used drugs for the treatment of acute allergic conjunctivitis,[10] but are also frequently used to quiet the manifestations of vernal keratoconjunctivitis and atopic keratoconjunctivitis. For these more severe disorders, the usual

✳ TABLE 23.1 Topical Ocular Antihistamines

Trade Name	Manufacturer	Composition	Concentration (%)
Livostin	CIBA Vision	Levocabastine HCl	0.05
Vasocon-A	CIBA Vision	Antazoline PO_4	0.5
		Naphazoline HCl	0.05
Naphcon-A	Alcon	Pheniramine maleate	0.3
		Naphazoline HCl	0.025
AK-Con-A	Akorn	Pheniramine maleate	0.3
		Naphazoline HCl	0.025
Opcon-A	Bausch & Lomb	Pheniramine maleate	0.315
		Naphazoline HCl	0.027
Patanol	Alcon	Olopatadine HCl	0.1
Emadine	Alcon	Emedastine difumarate	0.05
Ketotifen	CIBA Vision	Ketotifen fumarate	0.025

recommended dose is 1 to 2 drops taken every 3 to 4 hours as needed to relieve symptoms up to four times per day.

CLINICAL TRIALS

The allergen (or antigen) challenge model, developed by Abelson, Chambers, and Smith, has become the standard for demonstrating the efficacy of anti-allergic compounds. It has been used successfully to evaluate the efficacy of Emadine (emedastine difumarate), and Patanol (olopatadine hydrochloride), Livostin (levocabastine hydrochloride), Vasocon-A (naphazoline hydrochloride/antazoline phosphate), and Naphcon-A, AK-Con-A, OcuHist, and Opcon-A (naphazoline hydrochloride/pheniramine maleate) in the treatment of seasonal allergic conjunctivitis.

In this model, allergic conjunctivitis is induced by directly exposing the conjunctiva to a topically applied dilution of antigen. This technique elicits a physiological immune response resulting in a classic picture of allergic conjunctivitis, including the cardinal signs of itching, redness, chemosis, tearing, and, to a lesser extent, lid swelling.[19] Using this model, the previously mentioned antihistamines have been shown to be clinically and statistically significantly better than placebo in the inhibition of the signs and symptoms of allergic conjunctivitis.[20–23]

Despite difficulty with several variables, seasonal environmental studies have also been successfully used to demonstrate the efficacy of these compounds. Seasonal studies rely on patient exposure to allergen through the environment. Environmental allergen concentration may vary from day to day. This variable, intermittent stimulus and the resulting response often do not provide a suitable baseline for evaluating the efficacy of potential antiallergic agents. For example, even inactive controls in environmental studies have been shown to elicit a "drug effect" in approximately 70% of placebo-treated subjects.[19]

PHARMACOKINETICS

Oral Antihistamines

The H_1 antihistamines are rapidly and completely absorbed following oral administration. Drug effects are observed within 30 minutes, with peak efficacy at 1 to 2 hours. Drug action usually lasts 4 to 6 hours, but it may be longer with the piperazines and the piperidines. These antihistamines are lipid soluble and cross the blood-brain, blood-placental, and blood-ocular barriers. All but the newer-generation oral antihistamines are associated with the side effects of sedation and drying of mucosal membranes. Drying of the mucosa presents a special problem in allergic conjunctivitis, in which wetting of the ocular surface provides one of the first barriers to allergen penetration of the conjunctiva. Most of these agents are completely metabolized by the liver, with their metabolites excreted in the urine.[24]

Although oral antihistamines are widely distributed throughout the body, attaining adequate concentrations in ocular tissue is difficult. For therapeutic amounts of drug to be delivered to the ocular tissue, inappropriately high oral doses would be required. For this reason, compounded by the problem of drying of the ocular surface, oral antihistamines are not commonly used in the treatment of ocular allergy. Perhaps the only warranted indication for oral antihistamines is in patients with atopic keratoconjunctivitis, in which antihistamine effect would be beneficial in other involved body systems.

Topical Antihistamines

Pharmacokinetic data following ophthalmic instillation of levocabastine are readily available. Absorption of levocabastine after topical administration is rapid (1–2 hr) and incomplete. The systemic bioavailability of ocular levocabastine ranges from 30 to 60%. Steady-state plasma concentrations of levocabastine were obtained within 7 to 10 days following multiple ocular doses (1 drop bilaterally three times daily). After 2 weeks' administration, mean plasma levels were 1.6 μg/L. However, after multiple doses of topically applied levocabastine, the wheal-and-flare response to intradermal histamine was not significantly inhibited. This finding indicates that minimal systemic absorption occurs with topical administration of the drug.

The elimination half-life of levocabastine is approximately 33 hours. Plasma protein binding is approximately 55%, with most of the drug bound to albumin. Most (65–70%) absorbed drug is excreted in the urine unchanged; 10% is excreted as the acylglucuronide metabolite, and the remaining 20% is excreted unchanged in the feces.[12]

THERAPEUTIC USE

Topical H_1 antihistamines are the most commonly used drugs for the treatment of acute allergic conjunctivitis.[20] In addition, topical H_1 antihistamines, used alone or with vasoconstrictors, may relieve the intense redness and itching associated with vernal keratoconjunctivitis and atopic keratoconjunctivitis.

As with any medication, topical H_1 antihistamines are contraindicated in patients with known allergy to any component of the medication. Combination products containing antihistamines and vasoconstrictors are contraindicated in patients with poorly controlled hypertension, cardiovascular disease with arrhythmias, poorly controlled diabetes mellitus, or in any patient concurrently taking monoamine oxidase inhibitors.

SIDE EFFECTS AND TOXICITY

Oral Antihistamines

The most common adverse effect associated with oral H_1 antihistamines is sedation.[24] Other central nervous system (CNS) side effects include disturbed coordination, dizziness, fatigue, and difficulty in concentration. These effects result from a generalized depression of the CNS. In contrast, some patients may experience euphoria, nervousness, insomnia, or tremors.

Gastrointestinal adverse effects include loss of appetite, nausea, vomiting, epigastric distress, diarrhea, and constipation. These effects occur less frequently than CNS side effects and can sometimes be controlled by administering oral antihistamines with meals.

The anticholinergic properties of the older oral H_1 antihistamines are responsible for dryness of the mucous membranes of the oropharynx and conjunctiva. Conjunctival involvement leads to the appearance of dry eye symptoms, which confound treatment of the underlying allergy.

Topical Antihistamines

Topical ocular antihistamines are associated with an extraordinarily low incidence of systemic side effects. Blood levels are often undetectable following topical ocular application of antihistamines. Local irritation, including burning or stinging, may occur, but it usually resolves within a few seconds after instillation. Medicamentosa and punctate keratitis have been associated with the preservative benzalkonium chloride, which is found in many topical antihistamines.

Because of their anticholinergic effects, some topical antihistamines are contraindicated in patients with narrow-angle glaucoma. The atropine-like effects of the vasoconstrictor component in combination products include mydriasis that could precipitate an attack of acute angle-closure glaucoma in predisposed, untreated persons. Furthermore, antihistamine/vasoconstrictor combination products should be used with caution in patients with poorly controlled hypertension, cardiovascular disease with arrhythmias, and poorly controlled diabetes mellitus.[10] Ciliary muscle paresis with an associated decrease in accommodation may account for visual difficulties experienced by some patients.

REFERENCES

1. Abelson MB, Soter NA, Simon MA, et al. Histamine in human tears. Am J Ophthalmol 83:417, 1977.
2. Abelson MB, Allansmith MR. Histamine and the eye. In: Immunology and immunopathology of the eye. Silverstein A, O'Connor G, eds. New York, Masson, 1979, p 362.
3. Weston JH, Udell IJ, Abelson MB. H_1 receptors in the human ocular surface. Invest Ophthalmol Vis Sci 20 Suppl:32, 1981.
4. Abelson MB, Udell IJ. H_2 receptors in the human ocular surface. Arch Ophthalmol 99:302, 1981.
5. Ganellin CR. Chemistry and structure-activity

relationships of H_2 receptor antagonists. In: Histamine II and anti-histaminics: chemistry, metabolism, and physiological and pharmacological actions. Handbook of experimental pharmacology. Vol. 18. Part 2. Rocha M, Silva M, eds. New York, Springer-Verlag, 1978, p 251.

6. Ariens EJ, Simonis AM. Autonomic drugs and their receptors. Arch Int Pharmacodyn 127:479, 1960.

7. Douglas WW. Histamine and 5-hydroxytryptamine (serotonin) and their antagonists. In: Goodman and Gilman's the pharmacological basis of therapeutics. 6th ed. Gilman A, Goodman L, eds. New York, Macmillan, 1980, p 609.

8. Witiak DT, Lewis NJ. Absorption, distribution, metabolism, and elimination of antihistamines. In: Histamine II and anti-histaminics: chemistry, metabolism, and physiological and pharmacological actions. Handbook of experimental pharmacology. Vol. 18. Part 2. Rocha M, Silva M, eds. New York, Springer-Verlag, 1978, p 513.

9. Harvey RP, Shocket AL. The effect of H_1 and H_2 blockade on cutaneous histamine response in man. J Allergy Clin Immunol 65:136, 1980.

10. Berdy GJ, Abelson MB. Antihistamines and mast cell stabilizers in allergic ocular disease. In: Principles and practice of ophthalmology. Abelson M, Neufeld A, Topping T, eds. Philadelphia, WB Saunders, 1994, p 1028.

11. Krupin T, Silverstein B, Feitl M, et al. The effect of H_1-blocking antihistamines on intraocular pressure in rabbits. Ophthalmology 87:1167, 1980.

12. Dechant KL, Goa KL. Levocabastine: a review of its pharmacological properties and therapeutic potential as a topical antihistamine in allergic rhinitis and conjunctivitis. Drugs 41:202, 1991.

13. Abelson MB, Smith LM. Levocabastine: evaluation in the histamine and compound 48/80 models of ocular allergy in humans. Ophthalmology 95:1494, 1988.

14. Sharif NA, Xu SX, Yanni JM. Olopatadine (AL-4943A): ligand binding and functional studies on a novel, long acting H_1-selective histamine antagonist and anti-allergic agent for use in aller-gic conjunctivitis. J Ocul Pharmacol Ther 12:401, 1996.

15. Sharif NA, Xu SX, Miller ST, et al. Characterization of the ocular antiallergic and antihistaminic effects of olopatadine (AL-4943A), a novel drug for treating ocular allergic diseases. J Pharmacol Exp Ther 278:1252, 1996.

16. Yanni JM, Stephens DJ, Miller ST, et al. The in vitro and in vivo ocular pharmacology of olopatadine (AL-4943A), an effective anti-allergic/anti-histaminic agent. J Ocul Pharmacol Ther 12:389, 1996.

17. Sharif NA, Yanni JM. Emedastine: a potent, high affinity histamine H_1-receptor-selective antagonist for ocular use. Receptor binding and second messenger studies. J Ocul Pharmacol 10:653, 1994.

18. Yanni JM, Stephens DJ, Parnell DW, et al. Preclinical efficacy of emedastine, a potent, selective histamine H_1 antagonist for topical ocular use. J Ocul Pharmacol 10:665, 1994.

19. Abelson MB, Chambers WA, Smith LM. Conjunctival allergen challenge: a clinical approach to studying allergic conjunctivitis. Arch Ophthalmol 108:84, 1990.

20. Berdy GJ, Abelson MB, George MA, et al. Allergic conjunctivitis: a survey of new antihistamines. J Ocul Pharmacol 7:313, 1991.

21. Abelson MB, Paradis A, George MA, et al. The effects of Vasocon-A in the allergen challenge model of acute conjunctivitis. Arch Ophthalmol 108:520, 1990.

22. Smith LM, Abelson MB, George MA, et al. A double-masked study on the effects of ophthalmic levocabastine vs. placebo on the signs and symptoms of allergic conjunctivitis (abstract). Invest Ophthalmic Vis Sci 33 Suppl:1297, 1992.

23. Abelson MB. A double-masked study of the effects of ophthalmic levocabastine vs. placebo on the signs and symptoms of allergic conjunctivitis. Contact Lens Assoc Ophthalmol Presentation, 1993.

24. Hegeman SL. Antihistamines. In: Clinical ocular pharmacology. 2nd ed. Bartlett J, ed. Boston, Butterworths, 1989, p 313.

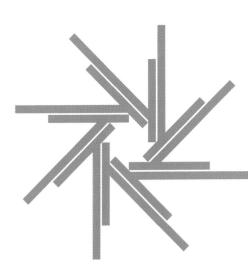

CHAPTER 24

Corticosteroids

MARK B. ABELSON ■ **DONNA WELCH**

In 1949, the clinical results of studies by Hench and co-workers,[1] which focused on arthritis, spurred other scientists to research the possible use of adrenal cortex hormones in other diseases. In 1950, ocular therapy with cortisone was introduced by Gordon and McLean.[2] The development and use of topical compounds reduced the risk of systemic effects; however, the emergence of local, ocular side effects became evident. Since the initiation of corticosteroid treatment in the eye, local treatment has been found to be equal or superior to systemic administration, provided the diseased tissue is supplied with sufficient concentrations of steroid.[3] Topical ocular therapy is generally sufficient for treating inflammatory disorders of the lid, conjunctiva, iris, cornea, and ciliary body. The benefits of topical corticosteroid treatment for anterior segment disease include ease of application, comparatively low cost, and minimal incidence of systemic side effects.

PHARMACOLOGY

Over the decades, corticosteroid research has focused on development of compounds with increased anti-inflammatory activity and reduced side effects. All the anti-inflammatory corticosteroids share a common structural link. A double bond between C-4,5 and the 3-ketone must be present (Fig. 24.1); however, other modifications to the molecular structure can contribute greatly to anti-inflammatory potency. Most of the current corticosteroids have a 17-hydroxyl group; this substitution is associated with optimal anti-inflammatory effects.[4] However, the structure of rimexolone, a novel corticosteroid, differs in that it possesses a 17-methyl group, which may contribute to its altered activity.

211

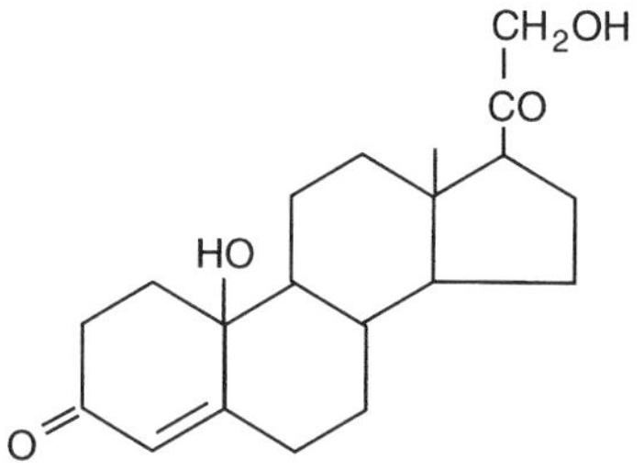

Structural formula common to anti-inflammatory steroids

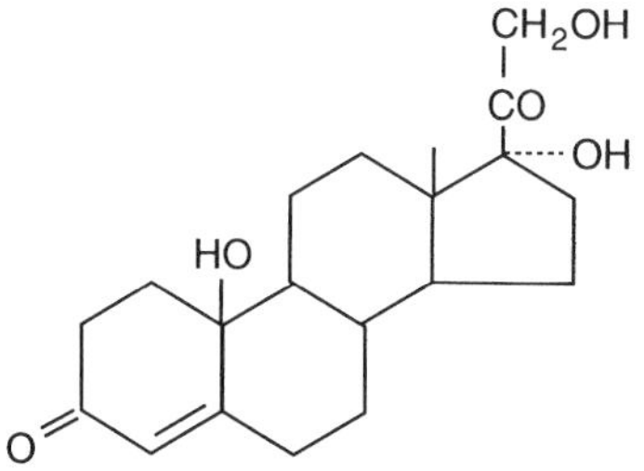

Cortisol
(17-hydroxy-cortisone)

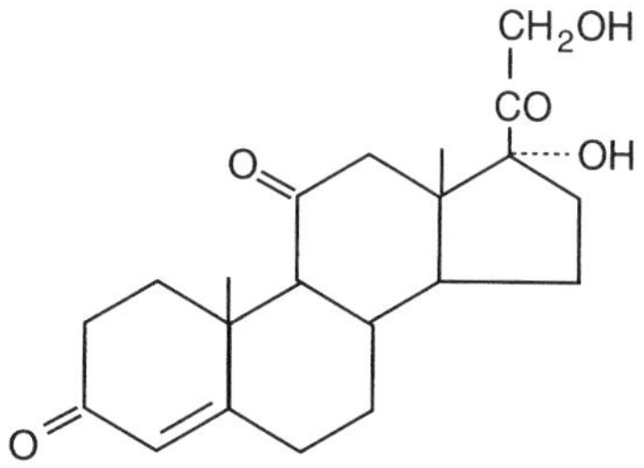

Cortisone
(17-hydroxy-11-dehydrocorticosterone)

FIGURE 24.1 All the anti-inflammatory corticosteroids share a common structural link of double bond between C-4,5 and the 3-ketone. Other modifications to the molecular structure can contribute greatly to the anti-inflammatory potency of a corticosteroid. Most of the current corticosteroids have a 17-hydroxyl group; this substitution is associated with optimal anti-inflammatory effects.[4] (From Haynes RC, Murad F. Adrenocorticotropic hormone: adrenocortical steroids and their synthetic analogs. In: The pharmacological basis of therapeutics. 7th ed. Gilman AG, Goodman LS, Rall TW, et al., eds. New York, Macmillan, 1985, p 1459.)

Corticosteroids pass through target cell membranes and bind to steroid receptor proteins in the cytoplasm. The corticosteroid-receptor complex is then carried into the cell nucleus, where it interacts with specific DNA sequences. This interaction signals the production of messenger RNA, leading to the production of specific proteins that determine the cellular response (Fig. 24.2).[5]

Corticosteroids affect inflammation by producing an involution of inflammatory cells that have invaded the cornea. They slow the migration of additional polymorphonuclear leukocytes to the inflamed site. Clinically, the infiltrate in the cornea disappears with the initiation of corticosteroid therapy.[6]

Corticosteroids available for ophthalmic use are modified derivatives of natural glucocorticoids. The derivative of the steroid base, that is, alcohol, acetate, or phosphate, can affect both the activity and the pharmacokinetics of the product. The derivatives of corticosteroids have different abilities to penetrate the eye.[7] The concentration of drug at the site of inflammation does not seem to equal the anti-inflammatory efficacy. This finding was demonstrated in a comparison of corneal bioavailability and anti-inflammatory effectiveness for three dexamethasones. The lowest concentrations were found in the cornea, where the greatest anti-inflammatory effect was observed.[8]

Another factor that influences absorption and thereby efficacy is the vehicle in which the drug is delivered. In general, the prolonged contact time associated with an ointment results in a higher drug concentration in the ocular tissue.[9] The rate of release of drug particles from a suspension

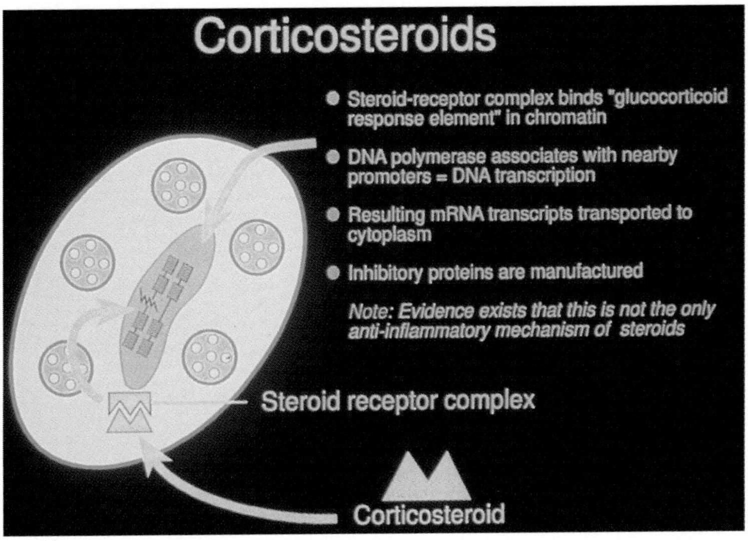

FIGURE 24.2 Corticosteroids pass through target cell membranes and bind to steroid receptor proteins in the cytoplasm. The corticosteroid-receptor complex is then carried into the cell nucleus, where it interacts with specific DNA sequences. This interaction signals the production of messenger RNA, leading to the production of specific proteins that determine the cellular response.

can influence corneal penetration. High-viscosity gels produce higher concentrations of drug in the cornea and aqueous humor; however, dose-related steroid toxicity has limited their use.[9]

TYPES OF OPHTHALMIC CORTICOSTEROIDS

The choice of corticosteroid therapy is often influenced by the physician's clinical experience and preference. Table 24.1 lists the topical ocular preparations that are currently available.

Prednisolone acetate 1% (Fig. 24.3), which is a synthetic analog of hydrocortisone, is considered the most effective anti-inflammatory agent for anterior segment ocular inflammation.[10] Prednisolone is formulated as both acetate and phosphate derivatives. Results from experiments using inflamed rabbit corneas indicate that the mean decrease in corneal inflammation is greater for the acetate derivative than for the phosphate.[11] Prednisolone acetate is available as a 0.125% and a 1% suspension. Raising the concentration from 1% to either 1.5% or 3% has not been shown to enhance the anti-inflammatory effects.[12, 12a]

Dexamethasone (see Fig. 24.3), which is also structurally related to hydrocortisone, is available as the alcohol derivative in a 0.1% suspension or the phosphate derivative in a 0.1% ophthalmic solution. Dexamethasone sodium phosphate ointment 0.05% is also available. Studies show that dexamethasone alcohol is a more effective anti-inflammatory agent than dexamethasone sodium phosphate.

Fluorometholone (see Fig. 24.3) is a fluorinated structural analog of progesterone. Initially formulated as an alcohol, fluorometholone 0.1% (FML) has proved to be effective in reducing external ocular inflammation with low potential for elevating intraocular pressure (IOP). Increasing the concentration of fluorometholone in an ocular preparation does not always increase the anti-inflammatory effects, but it does increase the tendency to raise IOP. In comparative studies, fluorometholone alcohol is less effective in reducing inflammation than are dexamethasone alcohol and prednisolone acetate.[13, 14] Fluorometholone is available as the alcohol derivative in a 0.1% suspension and ointment (FML) and in a 0.25% suspension (FML Forte).

TABLE 24.1 Types of Ophthalmic Corticosteroids

Preparation	Trade Name	Concentration (%)
Prednisolone sodium phosphate solution	AK-Pred	0.125
	Inflamase	0.125
	AK-Pred	1.0
	Inflamase Forte	1.0
Prednisolone acetate solution	Pred Mild	0.12
	Econopred	0.125
	AK-Tate	1.0
	Econopred Plus	1.0
	Pred Forte	1.0
Dexamethasone suspension	Maxidex	0.1
Dexamethasone sodium phosphate solution	AK-Dex	0.1
	Decadron	0.1
Dexamethasone sodium phosphate solution ointment	AK-Dex	0.05
	Decadron	0.05
	Maxidex	0.05
Fluorometholone acetate suspension	Flarex	0.01
Fluorometholone suspension	Fluor-Op	0.1
	FML	0.1
	FML Forte	0.25
Fluorometholone ointment	FML S.O.P.	0.1
Medrysone suspension	HMS	1.0
Rimexolone	Vexol	1.0

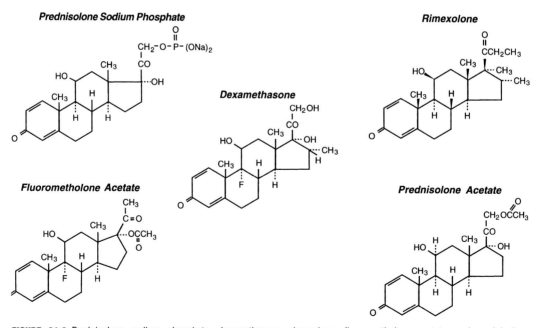

FIGURE 24.3 Prednisolone sodium phosphate, dexamethasone, rimexolone, fluorometholone acetate, and prednisolone acetate are five corticosteroids used in ocular allergic disease.

Fluorometholone is also available as the acetate in a 0.1% suspension (Flarex). Fluorometholone acetate has demonstrated greater anti-inflammatory activity than has fluorometholone alcohol in clinical evaluations of patients with conjunctivitis, episcleritis, and scleritis. In a comparison study, fluorometholone acetate 0.1% demonstrated anti-inflammatory effects equal to those of prednisolone acetate 1.0% in patients with moderate inflammation.[15]

Medrysone, another synthetic derivative of progesterone, is commercially available as a 1% ophthalmic suspension (HMS). In clinical use, medrysone is the least potent anti-inflammatory of the available ophthalmic steroids. Medrysone is useful for mild cases of allergic and atopic conjunctivitis. Clinical experience has indicated that medrysone is not likely to cause a significant rise in IOP.

Loteprednol etabonate, which is available commercially in the United States as a 0.2% ophthalmic solution, was designed according to the "soft drug" concept proposed by Bodor.[15] Soft drugs are designed to maximize therapeutic effect while minimizing side effects. Although loteprednol is rapidly transformed to an inactive metabolite in the anterior chamber, it does exhibit significant anti-inflammatory activity in the rabbit cornea.[16] In studies by Bartlett and associates,[17] use of 0.5%, 0.3%, and 0.2% loteprednol in patients with seasonal allergic conjunctivitis resulted in an improvement in symptoms and a reduction of the redness and chemosis of the eyes associated with allergic conjunctivitis, in comparison with its vehicle alone.

Rimexolone (see Fig. 24.3) is a novel synthetic topical corticosteroid that alleviates the signs and symptoms of allergic conjunctivitis including itching and tearing with limited systemic absorption.[19] Rimexolone is commercially available as a 1.0% ophthalmic suspension (Vexol) preserved with 0.01% benzalkonium chloride. Rimexolone is indicated for the treatment of postoperative inflammation following ocular surgery and in the treatment of anterior uveitis.

Rimexolone is chemically and pharmacologically related to prednisolone acetate, but multiple modifications to the pentane D ring and its side chain have been made. Rimexolone is non-fluorinated and possesses methyl groups at C16, C17, and C21. The methyl groups increase the lipophilicity of rimexolone in comparison with other steroids, appear to contribute to rimexolone's high affinity for human glucocorticoid receptor, and may contribute to rimexolone's ability to penetrate ocular tissue. The binding affinity of rimexolone to the human glucocorticoid receptor is twice that of dexamethasone and about 10 times higher than prednisolone. Notably, the increased lipophilicity and poor aqueous solubility limit rimexolone's systemic absorption from the site of application and may contribute to the clinical safety of the product.[20] The advantage of rimexolone is that it possesses the anti-inflammatory efficacy of 1.0% prednisolone, but it has no greater associated increase in the risk of elevating IOP than fluorometholone.[21]

PRINCIPLES OF THERAPEUTIC USE

Clinical experience with corticosteroids has led to some common therapeutic principles for their use[22]:

- Route of administration may be determined by the type and location of the inflammation. Topical, systemic, periocular, or multiple routes may be most appropriate. For most allergic disease, topical administration is the logical choice.

- Treatment should be instituted as early as possible with a dosage high enough to suppress the inflammatory response.
- The treatment regimen should be reevaluated at frequent intervals, and dosages should be readjusted as needed.
- Therapy should be tapered, rather than abruptly discontinued.
- Topical ocular therapy of short duration with low doses usually does not result in significant side effects.

When determining treatment, the most appropriate approach should be the minimal effective dose for the shortest amount of time to achieve the desired response. In managing any ocular condition, the therapeutic effects of the steroid on the disease, as well as the potential side effects, must be monitored.

The choice of steroid and dosage depends on the amount of inflammation present. Side effects are also a factor to be considered in choosing a treatment. Drugs such as fluorometholone and medrysone appear to be less likely to result in IOP elevations.[23] This safety advantage may be due to rapid metabolism that limits corneal penetration.

Topical therapy should be tapered slowly over several days to weeks after the symptoms of inflammation have disappeared. Abrupt discontinuation of therapy may be hazardous. A reduction of leukocytic elements in the blood occurs as a result of the use of corticosteroids. The proliferation of immature white blood cells that occurs after discontinuation of corticosteroids can lead to the production of great quantities of antibodies to residual antigen in the tissue. This reaction is followed by a massive polymorphonuclear leukocytic reaction, which, if not interrupted, can lead to a serious necrotizing inflammatory reaction.[24]

CORTICOSTEROID THERAPY IN OCULAR ALLERGIC DISORDERS

Corticosteroids are used most often in the treatment of vernal keratoconjunctivitis, and on rare occasions they may be used as supplemental therapy in atopic keratoconjunctivitis. They are not often used for treating giant papillary keratoconjunctivitis or acute allergic conjunctivitis. Corticosteroids are generally chosen when medications such as antihistamines, vasoconstricting agents, or mast cell stabilizers are ineffective.[23]

The less potent steroids such as fluorometholone alcohol are rarely required in severe seasonal allergic conjunctivitis, and then they should be used only under strict supervision. Topical steroids should be used only for short-term management of allergic conjunctivitis when alternative measures have not been effective. In clinical trials, topical prednisolone 0.12% two or three times per day resulted in few complications.[24]

Pulsed doses used over short periods are indicated for recalcitrant acute allergic conjunctivitis. Allansmith[25] investigated pulse therapy with dexamethasone 1% every 2 hours eight times daily, which was then tapered over several days to weeks. In vernal keratoconjunctivitis, a more typical regimen four times daily can be employed during periods of exacerbation. Prednisolone 1% every 2 hours can be used in treatment of severe cases. Corticosteroids such as medrysone and fluorometholone produce a moderate decrease in corneal inflammation compared with prednisolone. Fluorometholone is generally used for conditions that require more extensive periods of therapy, whereas medrysone is used for minor conditions.[21]

When using steroids for vernal keratoconjunctivitis, care must be taken to watch closely for concomitant shield ulcers. Steroids should be used with great caution in atopic keratoconjunctivitis because these patients are already at risk for corneal melting. As previously mentioned, corticosteroids are not used in treating giant papillary conjunctivitis. Following removal of contact lenses, giant papillary conjunctivitis usually resolves without further treatment.

SIDE EFFECTS

Systemic absorption of topical corticosteroids is evident by the observation of side effects associated with their use. Toxic effects have been reported[25] with all routes of administration and with all compounds currently available. As steroid dosages increase, evidence shows increased side effects. Prolonged treatment with steroids results in more side effects than short-term treatment with higher dosages. A wide range of ocular complications from actual damage to the ocular tissue to interference with healing and the immune response can occur with topical steroid use.

Following the introduction of systemic use of steroids for rheumatoid arthritis, a high incidence of lens opacities in patients receiving long-term therapy was reported by Black and associates.[26] Later studies showed an increased incidence of post-steroid subcapsular cataracts in children receiving systemic steroid therapy for rheumatoid arthritis, systemic lupus erythematosus, and nephrotic syndrome. Children manifested lens changes at lower doses and within shorter periods of time compared with adults, who generally did not manifest cataracts during the first year of therapy, regardless of steroid dose.[27, 28]

The development of cataracts has also been associated with topical ocular steroid administration.[29] In many cases, lens changes accompanying steroid therapy do not significantly impair visual acuity. In one study, fewer than 10% of the patients receiving long-term therapy had vision reduced to less than 20/60.[30] Photophobia and glare, rather than visual problems, were most often reported. Once vision was affected, a decrease or discontinuation of steroid therapy rarely resolved the opacity.[31]

The mechanism for the development of lens opacities is not completely understood. Perhaps cataract formation may be caused by glucocorticoids entering the lens fiber cells. A reaction with amino groups of lens crystallins causes a conformational change within the cells exposing sulfhydryl groups. Disulfide bonds are then formed, which lead to protein aggregation and deposition of complexes that refract light.[23] Studies to determine risk factors indicate that the most important factor may be variability in individual susceptibility to side effects of corticosteroids.

Topical steroid use can also induce elevation of IOP.[32] Goldman reported in 1962 that these agents could produce clinical signs of open-angle glaucoma.[33] Later controlled studies confirmed the observation that patients developed reversible elevations of IOP with repeated use of topical steroids.[34] In both healthy and glaucomatous eyes, the hypertensive response usually develops 2 to 8 weeks following the start of therapy with dexamethasone, prednisolone, hydrocortisone, topical betamethasone, or topical triamcinolone. The reduction of outflow facility and the effects on pressure are generally reversible. Pressures return to baseline levels within 1 to 3 weeks after steroids are discontinued. Cases have been reported in which pressures did not return to baseline levels and vision loss occurred. Other findings demonstrated the elevated pressures to be higher in glaucomatous eyes and were higher than normal in children of patients with glaucoma.[35] Patients with primary open-angle glaucoma and their relatives show a high prevalence of increased IOP with topical steroids.[9] These findings bring to mind the importance of ascertaining family history when considering the use of corticosteroids. In addition to genetic predisposition, other factors can influence pressure elevation associated with topical steroid use. These include myopia of 5 diopters or more, patient age, Krukenberg's spindles, and diabetes.[36]

The specific corticosteroid used may also influence the risk of corticosteroid-induced ocular hypertension. Dexamethasone 0.1% and betamethasone 0.1% seem to be more likely to induce pressure elevations than does prednisolone, fluorometholone, or medrysone.[37, 38] Ocular pressure elevations were compared in male volunteers who were treated with 0.1% dexamethasone phosphate, 0.1% fluorometholone, or 1% medrysone administered four times daily for 6 weeks. At the conclusion of the 6 weeks, mean pressure increases for dexamethasone, fluorometholone, and medrysone were 63.1%, 33.8%, and 8.3%, respectively.[39]

The cause of steroid-induced pressure elevations may be related to the steroid's ability to penetrate the anterior chamber. Plasma dilution and reduced ocular drug levels may contribute to the lower incidence of pressure elevation observed with systemic therapy. Corticosteroid receptors have been identified in human trabecular cells.[40–42] This finding makes it a possibility that alterations in outflow facility could be mediated by a direct corticosteroid action on the meshwork cells. Extracellular materials including glycosaminoglycans have been found in steroid-treated trabecular specimens.[43] Possibly, these glycosaminoglycans could obstruct the meshwork, which would cause resistance to aqueous outflow[44] and fluid retention.

Resistance to infection is lowered while using corticosteroids as a result of their ability to reduce immunological defense mechanisms. Steroid administration increases the risk of developing viral, bacterial, and fungal infections.[45]

Systemic and ocular steroid use can inhibit corneal healing. Investigators have proposed that steroid effects on collagenase activity are the mechanism by which steroids affect corneal epithelial regeneration.[38]

The development of anterior uveitis has been reported with topical use of corticosteroids. The incidence is higher in blacks (5.4%) than in whites (0.5%). No single particular steroid preparation seems most likely to cause this side effect.[9]

Dilation of the pupil and ptosis can occur with topical steroid administration. Dexamethasone 0.1% has produced mydriasis as early as 1 week following initiation of therapy. The average increase in pupil diameter was about 1 mm. The effect disappears following cessation of the drug therapy.[46] Steroids were also tested without their vehicles, and the effects on IOP, pupil size, and upper lid were not observed. The responses to the vehicle alone were identical to the responses to steroid-containing drops. However, corticosteroid in saline did not produce the observed changes. Investigators have suggested that the combined vehicle mixture may cause the effects.[47, 48]

Systemic effects of topically administered steroids are infrequent.[49] In studies by Krupin and associates,[50] subjects showed decreased plasma levels of cortisol after using topical dexamethasone sodium phosphate four times daily for 6 weeks. However, administration of the oral metyrapone tartrate test demonstrated the pituitary-adrenal axis to be intact. Intraocular steroid injection has been known to lead to adrenal suppression, particularly in infants and small children. Adrenal suppression can result in weight loss and growth retardation and may last up to 5 months.[51]

Other side effects such as temporary ocular discomfort may also occur following topical ocular administration. Causative factors such as the mechanical effects of the steroid in suspension, the vehicle itself, and the severity of the ocular inflammation could contribute to the discomfort. Additionally, occasional refractive changes, blurred vision, and increases in corneal thickness have been reported. Dry eye syndrome in the post-infection period was reported when topical steroids were used to treat epidemic keratoconjunctivitis.[9] Calcium deposits in the cornea have been reported as a result of topical steroid use, particularly in patients with epithelial defects such as postoperative inflammation, penetrating keratoplasty, history of herpetic keratitis, and dry eye.[52]

CONTRAINDICATIONS

Corticosteroids should always be used with caution because of their potential side effects. Caution should be used particularly with patients who have diabetes mellitus, infectious disease, congestive heart failure, chronic renal failure, or systemic hypertension. Topical steroids must be used only when necessary, and with caution, in patients with glaucoma.[9]

The concurrent use of other medications may interfere with steroid metabolism and may alter the effects of corticosteroids. Rifampin has been known to interfere with the pharmacological effects of corticosteroids by causing an increase in the metabolism of the corticosteroid.[53] Barbiturates may also enhance metabolism, decreasing the anti-inflammatory and immunosuppressive effects of systemic corticosteroids.

When treating a patient with topical ocular steroids, one must observe the patient for potential side effects. The patient should be examined for development of corneal, lens, and IOP changes. The slit-lamp examination must include observation for microbial or herpetic keratitis.

REFERENCES

1. Hench PS, Kendall EC, Slocumb CH, et al. The effect of a hormone of the adrenal cortex and of pituitary adrenocorticotropic hormone on rheumatoid arthritis. Mayo Clin Proc 24:181, 1949.
2. Gordon DM, McLean JM. Effects of pituitary adrenocorticotropic hormone (ACTH) therapy in ophthalmologic conditions. JAMA 142:1271, 1950.
3. Basu PK, Avaria M, Jankie R. Effect of hydrocortisone on mobilization of leukocytes in corneal wounds. Br J Ophthalmol 65:694, 1981.
4. Haynes RC, Murad F. Adrenocorticotropic hormone: adrenocortical steroids and their synthetic analogs. In: The pharmacological basis of therapeutics. 7th ed. Gilman AG, Goodman LS, Rall TW, et al., eds. New York, Macmillan, 1985, p 1459.
5. Schwartz B. Physiological effects of corticosteroids on the eye. Int Ophthalmol Clin 6:753, 1966.
6. Leopold IH, Sawyer JL, Green H. Intraocular penetration of locally applied steroids. Arch Ophthalmol 54:916, 1955.
7. Leibowitz HM, Stewart RH, Kupferman A. Evaluation of dexamethasone acetate as a topical ophthalmic formulation. Am J Ophthalmol 86:419, 1978.
8. Cope CL. Adrenal steroids and disease. Philadelphia, JB Lippincott, 1964.
9. Jaanus SD. Anti-inflammatory drugs: clinical ocular pharmacology. Boston, Butterworths, 1989, p 163.
10. Leibowitz HM, Kupferman A. Bioavailability and therapeutic effectiveness of topically administered corticosteroids. Trans Am Acad Ophthalmol Otolaryngol 79:78, 1975.
11. Leibowitz HM, Kupferman A. Antiinflammatory effectiveness in cornea of topically administered prednisolone. Invest Ophthalmol 13:757, 1974.
12. Leibowitz HM, Kupferman A. Kinetics of topically administered prednisolone acetate: optimal concentrations for treatment of inflammatory keratitis. Arch Ophthalmol 95:311, 1977.
12a. Whitcup SM, Ferris FL. New corticosteroids for the treatment of ocular inflammation. Am J Ophthalmol 127:597, 1999.
13. Leibowitz HM, Ryan WJ, Kupferman A. Comparative antiinflammatory efficacy of topical corticosteroids with low glaucoma-inducing potential. Arch Ophthalmol 110:118, 1992.
14. Kass M, Cheetham J, Duzman E, et al. The ocular hypertensive effects of 0.25% fluorometholone in corticosteroid responders. Am J Ophthalmol 102:159, 1986.
15. Bodor N. The application of soft drug approaches to the design of safer corticosteroids. In: Topical corticosteroid therapy: a novel approach to safer drugs. Christophers E, ed. New York, Raven Press, 1988, p 13.
16. Leibowitz A, Kupferman A, Ryan WS, et al. Corneal anti-inflammatory efficacy of loteprednol etabonate: a new steroidal soft drug. Invest Ophthalmol Vis Sci 32 Suppl:735, 1991.

17. Bartlett JD, Howes JF, Chormley NR, et al. Safety and efficacy of loteprednol etabonate for treatment of papillae in contact lens associated giant papillary conjunctivitis. Curr Eye Res 12: 313, 1993.

18. Abelson M, Howes J, George M. The conjunctival provocation test model of ocular allergy: utility for assessment of an ocular corticosteroid, loteprednol etabonate. J Ocul Pharmacol 14:533, 1998.

19. Gordon DM. Diseases of the uveal tract. In: Medical management of ocular disease. Gordon DM, ed. New York, Harper & Row, 1964, p 245.

20. Becker B, Kolker AE. Intraocular pressure response to topical corticosteroids. In: Ocular therapy: complications and management. Leopold IH, ed. St. Louis, CV Mosby, 1967, p 79.

21. Leibowitz HM, Kupferman A. Anti-inflammatory medications. Int Ophthalmol Clin 20:117, 1980.

22. Leopold IH. The steroid shield in ophthalmology. Trans Am Acad Ophthalmol Otolaryngol 71:273, 1967.

23. Trocme SD, Raizman MB, Bartley GB. Medical therapy for ocular allergy. Mayo Clin Proc 647: 557, 1992.

24. Abelson MB, Schaefer K. Conjunctivitis of allergic origin: immunologic mechanisms and current approaches to therapy. Surv Ophthalmol 38:115, 1993.

25. Haynes RC, Murad F. Adrenocorticotropic hormone: adrenocortical steroids and their synthetic analogs. In: The pharmacological basis of therapeutics. 7th ed. Gilman AG, Goodman LS, Rall TW, et al., eds. New York, Macmillan, 1985, p 1459.

26. Black RL, Oglesby RB, Von Sallmann L, et al. Posteriod subcapsular cataracts induced by corticosteroids in patients with rheumatoid arthritis. JAMA 174:166, 1960.

27. Havre DC. Cataracts in children on long-term corticosteroid therapy. Arch Ophthalmol 73:818, 1965.

28. Loredo A, Rodriguez RS, Murillo L. Cataracts after short-term corticosteroid treatment. N Engl J Med 286:160, 1972.

29. Becker B. Cataracts and topical corticosteroids. Am J Ophthalmol 58:872, 1964.

30. Becker B. The side effects of corticosteroids. Invest Ophthalmol 3:492, 1964.

31. Urban RC, Cotlier E. Corticosteroid-induced cataracts. Surv Ophthalmol 31:102, 1986.

32. Francois J. Cortisone et tension oculaire. Ann Ocul 187:805, 1954.

33. Goldman H. Cortisone glaucoma. Arch Ophthalmol 68:621, 1962.

34. Armaly MF. Effect of corticosteroids on intraocular pressure and fluid dynamics. I. The effect of dexamethasone in the normal eye. Arch Ophthalmol 70:482–491.

35. Becker B, Mills DW. Corticosteroids and intraocular pressure. Arch Ophthalmol 70:500, 1963.

36. Akingbekin T. Corticosteroid-induced ocular hypertension. J Cut Ocul Toxicol 5:45, 1986.

37. Armaly MF. Genetic factors related to glaucoma. Ann N Y Acad Sci 151:861, 1968.

38. Becker B. The genetic problem of chronic simple glaucoma. Ann Ophthalmol 3:351, 1971.

39. Mindel JS, Tovitian HO, Smith H, et al. Comparative ocular pressure elevations by medrysone, fluorometholone, and dexamethasone phosphate. Arch Ophthalmol 98:1577, 1980.

40. Schwartz B. The response of ocular pressure to corticosteroids. Int Ophthalmol Clin 6(4):929, 1966.

41. Weinreb RN, Bloom E, Baxter JD, et al. Detection of glucocorticoid receptors in cultured human trabecular cells. Invest Ophthalmol Vis Sci 21:403, 1981.

42. Hernandez MR, Wenk EJ, Weinstein BI, et al. Glucocorticoid target cells in human trabeculectomy specimens. Invest Ophthalmol Vis Sci 20 Suppl:23, 1981.

43. Francois J. Corticosteroid glaucoma. Ophthalmologica 188:76, 1984.

44. Godel V, Rogenbogen L, Stein R. On the mechanism of corticosteroid-induced ocular hypertension. Ann Ophthalmol 10:191, 1978.

45. Leopold IH. The steroid shield in ophthalmology. Trans Am Acad Ophthalmol Otolaryngol 71:273, 1967.

46. Spaeth GL. Effects of topical dexamethasone on intraocular pressure and the water drinking test. Arch Ophthalmol 76:772, 1966.

47. Kern R, Marci FJ. Steroid eye drops and their components. Arch Ophthalmol 8:794, 1967.

48. Newsome DA, Wong VG, Cameron TP, et al. Steroid-induced mydriasis and ptosis. Invest Ophthalmol 10:424, 1971.

49. Charap AD. Corticosteroids. In: Duane's foundations of clinical ophthalmology. Tasman W, Jaeger EA, eds. Philadelphia, JB Lippincott, 1992.

50. Krupin T, Mandell AI, Podos SM, Becker B. Topical corticosteroid therapy and pituitary-adrenal function. Arch Ophthalmol 94:919, 1976.

51. Weiss AH. Adrenal suppression after corticosteroid injection of periocular hemangiomas. Am J Ophthalmol 107:518, 1989.

52. Travella MJ, Stulting RD, Mader TH, et al. Cacific band keratopathy associated with the use of topical steroid-phosphate preparations. Arch Ophthalmol 112:608, 1994.

53. Buffington GA, Dominguez JH, Piering WF, et al. Interaction of rifampin and glucocorticoids. JAMA 236:1958, 1976.

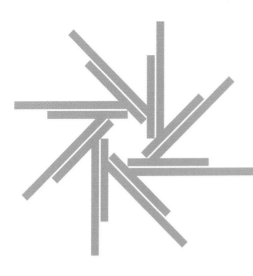

CHAPTER 25

Nonsteroidal Anti-inflammatory Drugs

MARK B. ABELSON ■ **ANNE GIOVANONI**

The therapeutic effects of willow bark were first described in the mid-18th century by Reverend Edmund Stone, who described "an account of the success of the bark of willow in the cure of agues" (fever). The active ingredient in the willow bark, a bitter glycoside called salicin, was isolated in 1829 by Leroux. When hydrolyzed, salicin yields glucose and salicylic alcohol, which can be converted to salicylic acid. Sodium salicylate was first used as an antipyretic in 1875, and the discovery of its usefulness in the treatment of gout soon followed. The success of this drug prompted Hoffmann, a chemist at Bayer, to prepare acetylsalicylic acid. After the anti-inflammatory effects of this compound were demonstrated, it was introduced into medicine at the end of the 19th century by Dreser under the name of aspirin.[1]

The chief therapeutic actions of aspirin were elucidated by the beginning of the 19th century. Synthetic analogs eventually replaced the more expensive natural derivatives. Toward the end of the 19th century, compounds were discovered that shared some or all of the therapeutic actions of aspirin. Of these, only the derivatives of *para*-aminophenol (e.g., acetaminophen) are still in use today. Beginning with indomethacin, many new agents have been introduced into medicine in various countries during the past 30 years.

The nonsteroidal anti-inflammatory drugs (NSAIDs) can be divided into several chemical groups: salicylates, fenamates, propionic acid derivatives, alkanones, indole and indene acetic acids, oxicams, heteroaryl acetic acids, pyrazolidinedione derivatives, and *p*-aminohypnol derivatives. The NSAIDs all have to some degree anti-inflammatory, antipyretic, and analgesic properties. Systemic NSAIDs at therapeutic doses can produce changes in the gastrointestinal, respiratory, hepatic, endocrine, coagulation, and renal systems. This broad spectrum of pharmacological effects is directly related to the diverse range of actions of prostaglandins, whose production is inhibited by the NSAIDs.[2]

MECHANISM OF ACTION

The primary precursor of prostaglandins, leukotrienes, and related compounds is arachidonic acid, which is bound to phospholipids in the plasma membrane and is released by phospholipases. The currently marketed NSAIDs block prostaglandin biosynthesis by inhibiting the activity of cyclooxygenase. This enzyme is responsible for the conversion of arachidonic acid to endoperoxides (prostaglandin D_2 [PGD_2], PGE_2) in ocular and nonocular tissues (Fig. 25.1).[3]

Correlation between the inhibitory activity of NSAIDs on cyclooxygenase and its anti-inflammatory activity has been demonstrated. Experimental studies demonstrating that certain prostaglandins are potent mediators of ocular inflammation have confirmed this view.[4, 5] Topical application of arachidonic acid or certain prostaglandins produces dilation of conjunctival vessels with chemosis, changes in intraocular pressure, and miosis.[6] Elevated levels of prostaglandins are present in aqueous humor following argon iridectomy,[7] cataract surgery,[8] and trauma.[4] By inhibiting cyclooxygenase, NSAIDs have been shown to reduce the de novo synthesis of prostaglandins.[4, 9]

Most NSAIDs do not inhibit the formation of eicosanoids such as the leukotrienes, which also contribute to inflammation, because these inflammatory mediators are formed through the lipoxygenase arm of the arachidonic acid pathway. However, certain NSAIDs (ketoprofen, diclofenac) may have an inhibitory effect on the lipoxygenase pathway.

Leukotrienes have been detected in tear fluids by high-performance liq-

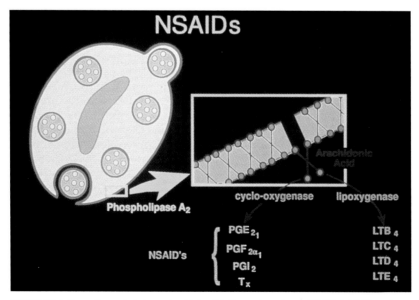

FIGURE 25.1 Currently marketed nonsteroidal anti-inflammatory drugs (NSAIDs) inhibit cyclooxygenase activity, thereby reducing prostaglandin formation. LT, leukotriene; PGF, prostaglandin F; PGI, prostaglandin I; Tx, thromboxane.

uid chromatography following allergen challenge.[10] Topical application of leukotriene B_4 (LTB_4) to hamster conjunctiva did not cause a change in the conjunctival vascular permeability,[11] although it did lead to primary eosinophil and secondary neutrophil chemotaxis in the guinea pig[12] and rat.[13] In rabbits, LTB_4 elicited chemosis, vasodilation, and a leukocytic infiltrate in the conjunctiva, peaking at 3 hours. Conjunctival smears from patients with chronic vernal keratoconjunctivitis have shown that LTB_4 and other leukotrienes are present. Application of LTB_4 topically to the human conjunctiva did not produce vasodilation, but biopsy revealed polymorphonuclear leukocyte infiltrates (our unpublished observations). Although they have yet to be developed sufficiently in the eye, various leukotriene receptor antagonists and 5-lipoxygenase inhibitors are being evaluated in asthmatic patients with promising results.

THERAPEUTIC USE

When employed as analgesics, the NSAIDs are usually effective against pain of low to moderate intensity. Pain arising from integumental structures is well controlled, whereas pain originating from the hollow viscera is not relieved. As antipyretics, NSAIDs reduce the body temperature in febrile states. Fever enhances the formation of cytokines, which induce the synthesis of PGE_2 in circumventricular organs in and near to the preoptic hypothalamic area. The prostaglandin triggers the hypothalamus to promote increases in heat generation and decreases in heat loss, producing an elevation of body temperature. The NSAIDs suppress this response by inhibiting the synthesis of PGE_2.[1]

Orally ingested NSAIDs are rapidly and completely absorbed from the gastrointestinal tract. Peak plasma concentrations are observed within 0.5 to 4 hours. All NSAIDs are highly protein bound. Most NSAIDs require hepatic metabolism; however, others (including ketorolac) are excreted unchanged in the urine. Therefore, patients with underlying hepatic or renal dysfunction may face a greater risk of developing toxic effects even with therapeutic doses of NSAIDs. Because of the reduced potential for systemic toxicity, topical NSAID therapy appears to be safer than oral therapy for ocular diseases.

Several NSAIDs are currently available for the treatment of ocular disease states. Choice of NSAID therapy is generally based on the degree of therapeutic effect and the patient's tolerance to treatment. Table 25.1 lists the most commonly used NSAIDs in clinical practice today.

NSAIDs have shown promise in the management of allergic disorders of the eye. However, the only NSAID currently approved by the United States Food and Drug Administration for the relief of itch due to seasonal allergic conjunctivitis is ketorolac tromethamine 0.5% (Acular). The recommended dose is 1 drop (0.25 mg) four times a day.[14] Evaluation of ketorolac tromethamine in two separate seasonal environmental studies revealed the 0.5% ophthalmic solution to be an effective and well-tolerated treatment for alleviating the signs and symptoms associated with seasonal allergic conjunctivitis. Other studies have found the ophthalmic solution superior to placebo in reducing conjunctival inflammation, itching, swollen eyes, burning or stinging, discharge or tearing, foreign body sensation, and photophobia.[15]

The efficacy of diclofenac sodium 0.1% (Voltaren) in relieving ocular signs and symptoms of acute seasonal allergic conjunctivitis has been evaluated. In one study, diclofenac sodium 0.1% proved to be statistically superior to placebo in the physicians' global evaluation and the primary compos-

TABLE 25.1 Nonsteroidal Anti-inflammatory Drugs Approved for Use as Topical Ophthalmic Preparations

Name and Preparation	Trade Name	Concentration (%)	Indication
Diclofenac solution	Voltaren	0.1	Inhibition of postsurgical inflammation Treatment of photophobia
Flurbiprofen solution	Ocufen	0.03	Inhibition of intraoperative miosis
Ketorolac solution	Acular	0.5	Relief of itch due to seasonal allergic conjunctivitis Inhibition of postsurgical inflammation
Suprofen solution	Profenal	1.0	Inhibition of intraoperative miosis

ite score (itching and bulbar or palpebral conjunctival injection) following 2 weeks of dosing four times daily.[16] In a comparative trial, Voltaren demonstrated similar efficacy to ketorolac tromethamine 0.5% in reducing the ocular signs and symptoms associated with acute seasonal allergic conjunctivitis.[17, 18]

Flurbiprofen 0.03% topical ophthalmic solution was found to be superior to vehicle control in reducing conjunctival, ciliary, and episcleral hyperemia and ocular itching following topical antigen challenge.[19] Aspirin, piroxicam, and indomethacin administered topically have all shown promise as well. All three NSAIDs have blocked lid closure and chemosis induced by topical challenge with 0.25% and 0.5% arachidonic acid in humans and animals.[5]

Oral aspirin therapy has proven successful in the relief of conjunctival and episcleral hyperemia and in the resolution of keratitis and limbal infiltrates associated with vernal conjunctivitis.[21] Patients with vernal keratoconjunctivitis who remained symptomatic following treatment with topical steroids or sodium cromoglycate showed a dramatic improvement of signs and symptoms following treatment with up to 1.0 g aspirin daily for 6 weeks.[22] Oral aspirin appears to be useful as both primary and adjunctive therapy for recalcitrant cases of vernal keratoconjunctivitis. Because of the high doses required, the potential side effects of aspirin should be given careful consideration before initiating treatment.

Suprofen 1.0% has provided symptomatic relief in vernal conjunctivitis and has suppressed the primary ocular signs (papillae and discharge) when compared with vehicle. Suprofen 1.0% has also proven effective in the management of contact lens–associated giant papillary conjunctivitis. Following 4 weeks of therapy four times daily, eyes treated with suprofen 1.0% showed greater than twofold reduction in papillary and ocular discharge and mucous strand scores.[25]

The second generation of NSAIDs, cyclooxygenase-2 inhibitors, selectively inhibit COX-2 while sparing COX-1.[26] COX-1 is constitutively expressed in most tissues and is involved in the de novo synthesis of the small amount of prostaglandins required for the mediation and modulation of normal physiological functions. COX-2 is rapidly induced by cytokines, growth factors, and bacterial endotoxins. High levels of de novo synthesized prostaglandins are produced during inflammation due to COX-2 activity. Currently available NSAIDs are nonselective inhibitors of both cyclooxygenase isoforms. COX-1 inhibition has been associated with the more serious side effects of the NSAIDs. Celecoxib (Celebrex) was the first selective COX-2 inhibitor approved.[27] Clinical trials have shown that it is as effective as nonselective NSAIDs in relieving pain and inflammation of arthritis, but causes less systemic side effects. The current effort to develop highly selective COX-2 inhibitors is expected to yield a new approach to the treatment of ocular inflammation.

Indomethacin 1% showed highly significant improvement in itching, lacrimation, conjunctival injection, and papillae.[28] Moreover, three of four patients with corneal involvement obtained complete relief.

Pranoprofen has proven to be an effective anti-inflammatory agent given either systemically or topically in animal models. Clinical trials have demonstrated that pranoprofen is an effective analgesic agent when administered systemically. When given topically after cataract surgery, pranoprofen exhibited anti-inflammatory effects similar to those of diclofenac and was effective in treating uveitis. In a clinical study comparing pranoprofen 0.1% with fluorometholone 0.1%, the two treatments were equally effective in attenuating the signs and symptoms of inflammation. Whereas fluorometholone had a tendency to increase intraocular pressure, the pranoprofen treatment group exhibited a slight decrease in mean intraocular pressure.[29]

COMPLICATIONS

The therapeutic use of oral NSAIDs can result in a variety of complications. The most common side effect is gastrointestinal irritation, which can lead to nausea, vomiting, cramps, and gastric or intestinal ulceration with potentially significant blood loss and anemia.[30, 31] Prostaglandins normally play a protective role against erosion of the gastrointestinal mucosa; oral administration of NSAIDs may inhibit certain key gastric prostaglandins contributing to local irritative effects.

NSAIDs may increase the bleeding time by inhibiting platelet production of thromboxane A_2, a potent aggregating agent.[32] A single dose of 0.65 g of aspirin approximately doubles the mean bleeding time of persons with normal blood clotting times for a period of 4 to 7 days.[1] The extent and duration of antiplatelet effects with non-aspirin NSAIDs vary.

The NSAIDs can produce acute renal failure in patients with chronic renal disease, congestive heart failure, cirrhosis with ascites, volume depletion secondary to diuretics, or hypotension secondary to hemorrhage. Prostaglandins protect the kidneys in disease states in which renal perfusion is compromised by stimulating vasodilation and maintaining renal perfusion. The use of NSAIDs blocks this prostaglandin-mediated compensatory response.

Because of the low concentrations applied, the aforementioned adverse effects are not likely to be an issue with topical use of NSAIDs for ocular allergy. However, when NSAIDs are used to maintain pupillary mydriasis during surgery, some concern of increased bleeding complications exists. The most common adverse effect associated with topical ocular use of NSAIDs is a stinging sensation following application. The benefits of greater comfort cannot be overemphasized, because comfort is clearly an important factor in the adherence of the patient to a therapeutic regimen.

No adequate, well-controlled studies have been conducted in pregnant women or nursing mothers to evaluate possible adverse effects of NSAIDs. Reproductive studies performed in rabbits and rats for a number of NSAIDs at various systemic doses have resulted in an increased incidence of fetal resorption associated with maternal toxicity, increased stillbirths, and decreased postnatal survival. The NSAIDs should be used by pregnant women only if the potential benefit justifies the potential risk to the fetus. Systemic use of NSAID drugs should be discontinued during late pregnancy to avoid complications such as prolongation of labor, increased risk of postpartum hemorrhage, and intrauterine closure of the ductus arteriosus. Similar precautions are used with topical preparations in the absence of data to support NSAID use in these situations.

Orally administered NSAIDs have been detected in human milk. Owing to the potential for systemic absorption of topically applied NSAIDs, mothers should consider the discontinuation of either nursing or NSAID therapy because the safety of these drugs in human neonates has not been established.

Knowledge of the safety of NSAIDs in neonates, children, and the elderly at this time is incomplete. The association of Reye's syndrome in children with the administration of aspirin for the treatment of febrile viral illnesses precludes its use in this setting. Investigators have suggested that NSAIDs may produce renal compromise in the elderly. However, no such consequences have been reported secondary to topical ophthalmic NSAID use.

The NSAIDs bind firmly to plasma proteins, competing with certain other drugs for binding sites and often displacing them. Such competitive interactions can occur in patients given NSAIDs together with warfarin, sulfonylurea hypoglycemic agents, methotrexate, or some antibiotics. The dosage of such agents may require adjustment, or concurrent administration should be avoided.

REFERENCES

1. Insel PA. Analgesic-antipyretics and antiinflammatory agents: drugs employed in the treatment of rheumatoid arthritis and gout. In: Goodman and Gilman's the pharmacological basis of therapeutics. 8th ed. Gilman AG, Rall TW, Nies AS, et al., eds. New York, Pergamon Press, 1990, p 638.
2. Rainsford KO. Anti-inflammatory and anti-rheumatic drugs. In: Inflammation mechanisms and actions of traditional drugs. Vol. 1. Boca Raton, FL, CRC Press, 1985.
3. Bhattacherjee P. The role of arachidonate metabolites in ocular inflammation. Prog Clin Biol Res 312:211, 1989.
4. Eakins KE. Prostaglandin and inflammatory reactions in the eye. Methods Find Exp Clin Pharmacol 2:17, 1980.
5. Abelson MB, Butrus SI, Kliman GH, et al. Topical arachidonic acid: a model for screening antiinflammatory agents. J Ocul Pharmacol 3:63, 1987.
6. Unger WG, Bass MS. Prostaglandin and nerve-mediated response of the rabbit eye to argon laser irradiation of the iris. Ophthalmologica 175:153, 1977.
7. Miyake K, Sugiyama S, Norimatsu I, et al. Prevention of cystoid macular edema after lens extraction by topical indomethacin: radioimmunoassay measurement of prostaglandins in the aqueous during and after lens extraction procedures. Graefes Arch Klin Exp Ophthalmol 68:581, 1984.
8. Conquet P, Plazonnet B, LeDouarec J. Arachidonic acid-induced elevation of intraocular pressure and anti-inflammatory agents. Invest Ophthalmol Vis Sci 14:772, 1975.
9. Podos SM. Prostaglandin, nonsteroidal anti-inflammatory agents and eye disease. Trans Am Ophthalmol Soc 74:637, 1976.
10. Bisgaard H, Ford-Hutchinson AW, Charleson S, et al. Production of leukotrienes in human skin and conjunctival mucosa after specific allergen challenge. Allergy 40:417, 1985.
11. Woodward DF, Ledgard SE. Comparison of leukotrienes as conjunctival microvascular permeability factors. Ophthalmic Res 17:318, 1985.
12. Spada CS, Woodward DF, Hawley SB, et al. Leukotrienes cause eosinophil emigration into conjunctival tissue. Prostaglandins 31:795, 1986.
13. Trocme SD, Gilber CM, Allansmith MR, et al. Characteristics of the cellular response of the rat conjunctiva to topically applied leukotriene B$_4$. Ophthalmic Res 21:297, 1989.
14. Rooks WH, Maloney PJ, Shott LD, et al. Clinical evaluation of ketorolac tromethamine 0.5% ophthalmic solution for treatment of seasonal allergic conjunctivitis. Surv Ophthalmol 38 Suppl:141, 1993.
15. Tinkelman D, Rupp G, Kaufman H, et al. Ketorolac tromethamine 0.5% ophthalmic solution in the treatment of seasonal allergic conjunctivitis: a placebo-controlled clinical trial. Surv Ophthalmol 38 Suppl:133, 1993.
16. Laibovitz RA, Zimmermann KE, Friley CK. A placebo-controlled trial of 0.1% diclofenac ophthalmic solution in acute seasonal allergic conjunctivitis. Invest Ophthalmol Vis Sci 35 Suppl:179, 1994.
17. Tauber J, Abelson M, Ostrov C, et al. A multicenter comparison of diclofenac sodium 0.1% (DS) to ketorolac tromethamine 0.5% (KT) in patients with acute seasonal allergic conjunctivitis

(SAC). Invest Ophthalmol Vis Sci 35 Suppl:180, 1994.

18. Tauber J, Raizman MB, Ostrov C, et al. A multicenter comparison of the ocular efficacy and safety of diclofenac 0.1% solution with that of ketorolac 0.5% solution in patients with acute seasonal allergic conjunctivitis. J Ocul Pharmacol Ther 14:137, 1998.

19. Bishop K, Abelson MB, Cheetham J, et al. Evaluation of flurbiprofen in the treatment of antigen-induced allergic conjunctivitis. Invest Ophthalmol Vis Sci 31 Suppl:487, 1990.

20. Appiotti A, Gualdi L, et al. Comparative study of the analgesic efficacy of flurbiprofen and diclofenac in patients following excimer laser photorefractive keratectomy. Clin Ther 20:913, 1998.

21. Abelson MB, Butrus SI, Weston JH. Aspirin therapy in vernal conjunctivitis. Am J Ophthalmol 95:502, 1983.

22. Meyer E, Kraus E, Zonis S: Efficacy of antiprostaglandin therapy in vernal conjunctivitis. Br J Ophthalmol 71:497, 1987.

23. Wood TS, Stewart RH, Bowman RW, et al. Suprofen treatment of contact lens associated giant papillary conjunctivitis. Ophthalmology 95:822, 1988.

24. Gupta S, Khurana AK, Ahluwalia BK, et al. Topical indomethacin for vernal keratoconjunctivitis. Acta Ophthalmol 69:95, 1991.

25. Notivol R, Martinez M, Bergamini MVW. Treatment of chronic bacterial conjunctivitis with a cyclooxygenase inhibitor or a corticosteroid. Am J Ophthalmol 117:651, 1994.

26. Masferrer JL, Kulkarni PS. Cyclooxygenase-2 inhibitors: a new approach to the therapy of ocular inflammation. Surv Ophthalmol 41 Suppl: S35, 1997.

27. Mandell BF. COX 2-selective NSAIDs: biology, promises, and concerns. Cleve Clin J Med 66: 285, 1999.

28. Langman MJS. Peptic ulcer complications and the use of non-aspirin non-steroidal anti-inflammatory drugs. Adverse Drug React Bull 120:448, 1986.

29. Paulus HE. Arthritis Advisory Committee Meeting: risks of agranulocytosis aplastic anemia, flank pain and adverse gastrointestinal effects with the use of nonsteroidal antiinflammatory drugs. Arthritis Rheum 30:593, 1987.

30. Hamberg M, Svensson J, Samuelsson B. Thromboxane: a new group of biologically active compounds derived from prostaglandin endoperoxides. Proc Natl Acad Sci U S A 72:2994, 1975.

31. Clive DM, Stoff JS. Renal syndromes associated with nonsteroidal antiinflammatory drugs. N Engl J Med 310:563, 1984.

32. Gurwitz JH, Avorn J, Ross-Degnan D, et al. Nonsteroidal anti-inflammatory drug-associated azotemia in the very old. JAMA 264:471, 1990.

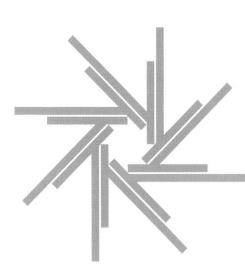

CHAPTER **26**

Mast Cell Stabilizers

MARK B. ABELSON ■ **PAULA J. WUN** ■ **JACQUELINE M. NEVIUS**

The first mast cell stabilizing compound was developed in the 1960s from khellin, an extract derived from the seed of *Ammi visnaga,* an eastern Mediterranean plant[1] that had been used by the ancient Egyptians as an antispasmodic.[2] Successive modifications in structure yielded disodium cromoglycate (cromolyn sodium, or cromolyn)[2] first reported to have antiasthmatic properties when Altounyan demonstrated on himself that cromolyn protected against a provoked asthmatic attack.[3] In the effort to determine cromolyn's mechanism of action as an antiasthmatic, investigators discovered that cromolyn inhibited the release of histamine and other granule contents from sensitized mast cells.[2] The development of cromolyn as an ophthalmic preparation for the treatment of ocular allergic disease was a natural evolution from the asthma research.

Cromolyn sodium (Opticrom) became the first widely used mast cell stabilizer for the treatment for allergic conjunctivitis, atopic keratoconjunctivitis, and vernal keratoconjunctivitis. Lodoxamide tromethamine (lodoxamide trometamol) is a mast cell stabilizer that is 2,500 times more powerful than cromolyn sodium in inhibiting the signs and symptoms associated with allergic disease.[4, 5, 6] Nedocromil sodium (nedocromil) is a compound that has demonstrated mast cell stabilizing effects in clinical asthma models. Further clinical trials may demonstrate its safety and efficacy in the treatment of ocular allergic disease. Nedocromil is not currently available as an ophthalmic preparation in the United States. Olopatadine hydrochloride (Patanol) is a unique antiallergic agent that possesses both mast cell stabilizing and antihistaminic properties.

Cromolyn Sodium

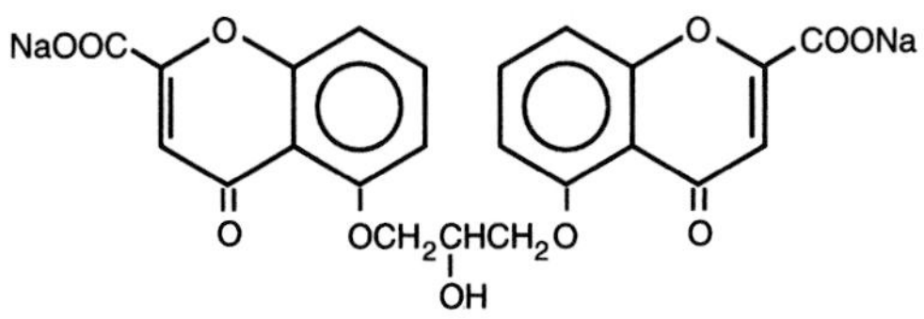

Nedocromil Sodium

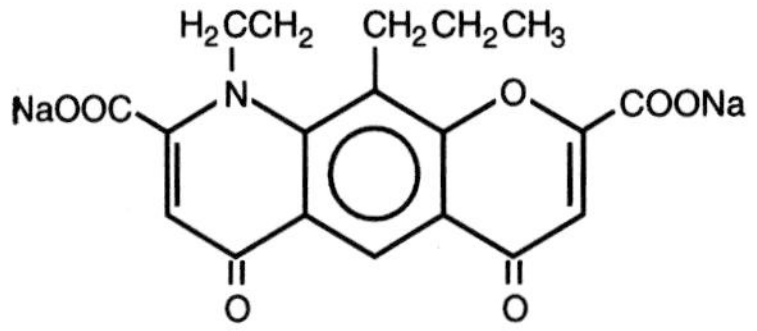

Lodoxamide

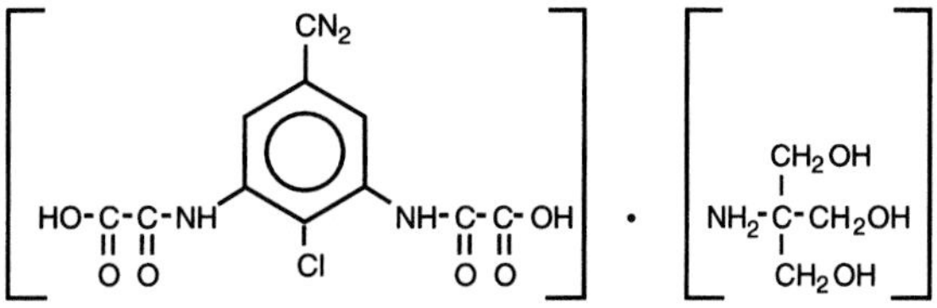

Olopatadine Hydrochloride

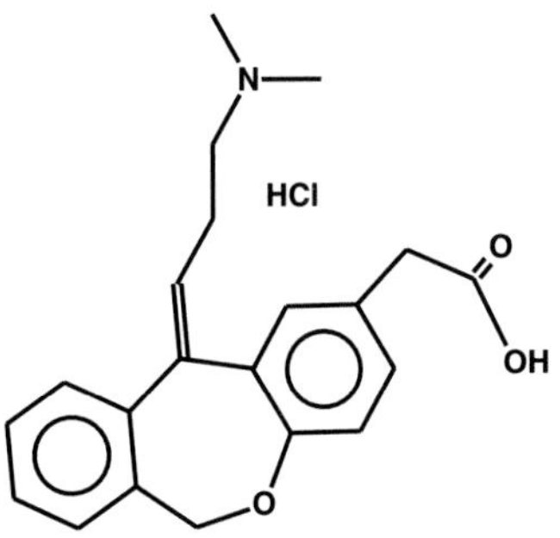

FIGURE 26.1 Variations in the chemical structures of four of the most common mast cell stabilizers: olopatadine hydrochloride, cromolyn sodium, nedocromil sodium, and lodoxamide, are illustrated.

OFFICIAL DRUG NAME AND CHEMISTRY

Figure 26.1 shows the chemical structures of the four most common mast cell stabilizers: olopatadine hydrochloride, cromolyn sodium, nedocromil sodium, and lodoxamide.

MECHANISM OF ACTION

Mast cell stabilizers repress type I hypersensitivity reactions by inhibiting the degranulation of mast cells and by preventing the release of histamine and other mediators of hypersensitivity reactions. Although the specific mechanisms of action remain unknown, studies have shown that lodoxamide, for example, prevents the release of histamine and leukotrienes as well as eosinophil chemotaxis. These actions are reportedly achieved through the prevention of calcium (Ca^{2+}) influx into mast cells following antigen stimulation (Fig. 26.2). Investigators have also suggested that lo-

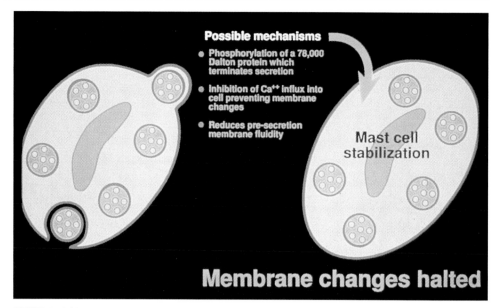

FIGURE 26.2 Mast cell stabilizers repress type 1 hypersensitivity reactions by inhibiting the degranulation of mast cells, and preventing the release of histamine and other mediators of hypersensitivity reactions. Although the specific mechanisms of action remain unknown, membrane changes may be halted through the phosphorylation of a protein, inhibition of calcium influx into the mast cell, or reduction of pre-secretion membrane fluidity.

doxamide blocks the action of eosinophil major basic protein, thereby preventing the release of eosinophils.[7]

Notably, lodoxamide, cromolyn, and nedocromil act to prevent the degranulation of the mast cell. They have no direct vasoconstrictor, antihistaminic, or anti-inflammatory actions. As such, once the mediators of inflammation are released, these compounds are unable to reverse the reaction, but they can prevent further mediator release. Olopatadine hydrochloride, available as Patanol (Alcon), has both mast cell stabilizing ability and antihistaminic properties.

CROMOLYN SODIUM

Clinical and Therapeutic Use

Sodium cromoglycate (cromolyn sodium) has been proven beneficial in the treatment of ocular allergies, including seasonal and perennial allergic conjunctivitis, vernal keratoconjunctivitis, giant papillary conjunctivitis, and atopic keratoconjunctivitis.[4, 6, 8, 9] Cromolyn acts by inhibiting the release of histamine, which is coupled to Ca^{2+} influx. Disodium cromoglycate may prevent mast cell histamine release by altering the plasma membrane, which, in turn, inhibits an increase in membrane permeability to Ca^{2+}.[10-12] Stabilizing the mast cell inhibits further degranulation, thereby suppressing the barrage of inflammatory events following the release of histamine mediators.

Other data indicate that cromolyn may also be effective in inhibiting chemotaxis, activation, degranulation, and cytotoxicity of neutrophils, eosinophils, and monocytes.[4, 6, 8] Additionally, cromolyn sodium may be effective in prolonging the tear break-up time in patients with chronic conjunctivitis.[4]

In a clinical trial comparing cromolyn sodium 4% solution with placebo for the treatment of vernal keratoconjunctivitis, investigators noted a statistically significant improvement in favor of cromolyn sodium for several assessments, including conjunctival injection, limbal injection, edema, nodules, and tearing.[8] Systemic absorption of cromolyn appears to be minimal following topical application to the eye. Less than 0.07% of administered doses was found to be systemically absorbed following multiple doses instilled in rabbit eyes. Analysis of human patients indicated that approximately 0.03% of the administered dose of cromolyn sodium was absorbed by the eye.[4]

Side Effects

Cromolyn sodium solutions are well tolerated. The most common adverse reaction to cromolyn is transient ocular burning or stinging on instillation.[4, 6, 8] The risks of long-term cromolyn sodium use appear to be minimal. A long-standing safety record, including documentation from 1 to 10 years of use, makes this a safe and effective maintenance and preventive agent for controlling allergic symptoms.[8]

Investigators have reported that cromolyn sodium is the only topical medication acceptable for long-term treatment of allergic eye conditions because of its lack of side effects.[9] However, the recommended dosing regimen requiring instillation of drops four to six times per day may be problematic for some patients. It may take up to 7 days of treatment to obtain relief, and a 10- to 14-day period is recommended to evaluate the efficacy of the therapy.[4] Although Opticrom was recalled from the market in 1990,[13] cromolyn sodium has been re-released as Crolom (Cromolyn Sodium Ophthalmic Solution USP, 4%) by Bausch & Lomb Pharmaceuticals.

LODOXAMIDE

Clinical and Therapeutic Use

Lodoxamide has been available for use in the United States since 1993 for the treatment of vernal keratoconjunctivitis, vernal conjunctivitis, and vernal keratitis. In addition, clinical trials have suggested that lodoxamide is effective in the treatment of other types of allergic conjunctivitis, including acute allergic conjunctivitis and superior limbic keratitis.[14, 15] The mechanism of action of lodoxamide as a mast cell stabilizing agent is believed to be similar to that of cromolyn sodium.[13]

Lodoxamide and cromolyn are both indicated for the treatment of vernal keratoconjunctivitis (or vernal conjunctivitis or vernal keratitis). In particular, lodoxamide showed particularly powerful effects in preventing keratitis and shield ulcers in vernal keratoconjunctivitis. This finding is of particular importance because these changes are typically resistant to treatment. In a double-masked, parallel-group 120-patient clinical study, lodoxamide 0.1% was statistically superior to cromolyn sodium 4% in alleviating the symptoms (itching, tearing, foreign body sensation, and discomfort) and signs (Trantas' dots, palpebral conjunctival changes, bulbar conjunctival hyperemia, erythema or swelling of the eyelids and periorbital tissues, and epithelial disease) of vernal conjunctivitis.[16] Lodoxamide 0.1% was also shown to be clinically more effective than N-acetyl aspartylglutamic acid 6% ophthalmic drops in alleviating the signs and symptoms of vernal conjunctivitis in another 120-patient study.[17] In another clinical study, lodoxamide 0.1%

ophthalmic solution was significantly more effective than placebo in lowering severity scores for epithelial disease and corneal staining, complications commonly associated with moderate to severe vernal keratoconjunctivitis.[18] Lodoxamide 0.1% has also been shown to be significantly superior to placebo in alleviating the signs and symptoms associated with pollen-induced allergic conjunctivitis.[19]

In comparison with cromolyn sodium, lodoxamide has been found to be equally or more effective in relieving symptoms of conjunctivitis. The onset of action is earlier, the clinical improvement is significantly greater, and the incidence of the adverse effects of stinging and burning is reportedly lower.[4, 6, 13]

Side Effects

Lodoxamide is available as Alomide Ophthalmic Solution 0.1% (Alcon), and the recommended dose is 1 to 2 drops per affected eye four times per day for up to 3 months. Systemic absorption of lodoxamide appears to be negligible. Transient burning, stinging, and ocular discomfort after instillation were experienced by approximately 15% of patients participating in clinical trials with this drug.[13]

NEDOCROMIL

Clinical and Therapeutic Use

Nedocromil sodium, like cromolyn sodium, was developed as a result of research into compounds to control asthma. Nedocromil appears to be more potent than cromolyn, and it has a wider spectrum of potential as an antiallergic and anti-inflammatory medication.[4, 9] This mast cell stabilizing agent prevents not only the release of preformed mediators, but also the release of newly generated mast cells. Additionally, nedocromil sodium has the ability to stabilize both mucosal and connective tissues, whereas cromolyn acts only on the connective tissue mast cells. The variety of activity of nedocromil sodium suggests that it may be acting on a pathway common to mast cells, eosinophils, epithelial cells, and sensory nerves, thereby qualifying it as first-rate maintenance therapy in the treatment of ocular allergy.[9]

In clinical trials, 2% nedocromil was shown to be superior to placebo in both the relief of allergic symptoms and in patient satisfaction in both seasonal allergic conjunctivitis and perennial allergic conjunctivitis. Further investigation is required in the use of nedocromil for other ocular allergic diseases.[6] In comparison trials with 2% cromolyn, nedocromil was found to be statistically superior in the treatment of seasonal and perennial allergic conjunctivitis, by relieving symptoms such as itching, burning, grittiness, and tearing that persisted during the use of cromolyn.[4, 6]

The significant benefit of nedocromil sodium over both cromolyn and lodoxamide is its dosing requirements. Nedocromil is administered twice daily, rather than four to eight times daily as with the other mast cell stabilizers discussed. The onset of action is rapid, and the dosage regimen is easily adhered to by patients.

Side Effects

Topical administration of nedocromil has caused transient burning and stinging. Additionally, a side effect of an unusual taste sensation has been reported following drop instillation.[20] Nedocromil sodium is formulated as a 2% preserved ophthalmic solution, under the trade name of Tilavist (Fisons Corporation), but it is not currently available in the United States.

OLOPATADINE HYDROCHLORIDE

Clinical and Therapeutic Use

The only topical ocular dual-action antiallergic medication available in the United States, olopatadine hydrochloride 0.1% ophthalmic solution (Patanol) has been proven safe and effective through extensive clinical research. This formulation contains both antihistaminic and mast cell stabilizing properties, potentially reducing the need for multiagent therapy for ocular allergies. As with nedocromil sodium, olopatadine 0.1% is administered only twice daily.

In preclinical studies, 0.1% olopatadine inhibited allergic inflammation in a passive conjunctival anaphylaxis model in guinea pigs. In a study of in vitro human conjunctival mast cells, olopatadine was found to be superior to cromolyn and nedocromil in stabilizing activity. Additionally, 0.1% olopatadine was found to inhibit histamine-induced vascular permeability.[21]

In more than 10 clinical trials, more than 492 patients have received olopatadine 0.1% in comfort, safety, and efficacy models. In a conjunctival antigen challenge study, mean itching and total redness in the treatment group were statistically and clinically lower than in the placebo group at all time points. The treatment was effective at 27 minutes, and after 8 hours.[21]

Side Effects

Systemic absorption of olopatadine at doses 1.5 times higher than the marketed solution was negligible, and, similarly, no accumulation was detected over a 2-week trial period. In a 6-week safety trial, 0.1% olopatadine solution was found to be well tolerated, especially in children 3 to 16 years of age. Safety and efficacy have not been determined in children younger than 3 years of age. No treatment-related adverse events were reported in this age group, and in patients older than 17 years, the rate of adverse events of the treatment group was not statistically significant from the placebo group. The most frequently reported treatment-related side effects were dry eye, pruritus, stickiness, taste perversion, and abnormal dreams.[21] Olopatadine hydrochloride ophthalmic solution 0.1% is available as Patanol (Alcon) and is indicated for the temporary prevention of ocular itching resulting from allergic conjunctivitis.[22]

KETOTIFEN AND PEMIROLAST

Among the more recently approved antiallergic drugs are ketotifen and pemirolast. Ketotifen is a combination of a mast cell stabilizer and an antihistamine. It has antihistamine and antiplatelet activating–factor properties as well as mast cell–stabilizing features. Ketotifen may down-regulate mast cell degranulation to below baseline measurements[23] by preserving the NO pathway, which may be involved in degranulation.[24] Pemirolast is thought to be a mast cell stabilizer that inhibits the release of the phospholipid byproducts histamine and leukotriene. It may also prevent the migration of eosinophils from the bloodstream to the site of infection and the subsequent release of mediators.[25]

REFERENCES

1. Cox JSG, Beach JE, Blair AMJN, et al. Disodium cromoglycate (Intal). Adv Drug Res 5:115, 1970.
2. Rall TW. Drugs used in the treatment of asthma: the methylxanthines, cromolyn sodium, and other agents. In: Goodman and Gilman's the pharmacological basis of therapeutics. 8th ed. Gilman A, Rall T, Nies A, et al., eds. New York, Pergamon Press, 1990, p 619.
3. Berdy GJ, Abelson MB. Antihistamines and mast cell stabilizers in allergic ocular disease. In: Principles and practice of ophthalmology. Abelson M, Neufeld A, Topping T, eds. Philadelphia, WB Saunders, 1994, p 1028.
4. Jaanus SD, Hegeman SL, Swanson MW. Antiallergy drugs and decongestants. In: Clinical ocular pharmacology. 3rd ed. Bartlett JD, Jaanus SD, eds. Boston, Butterworth-Heinemann, 1995, p 347.
5. Abelson MB, Schaefer K. Conjunctivitis of allergic origin: immunologic mechanisms and current approaches to therapy. Surv Ophthalmol 38 Suppl:115, 1993.
6. Hingorani M, Lightman S. Therapeutic options in ocular allergic disease. Drugs 50:208, 1995.
7. Grutzmacher RD, Foster RS, Feiler LS. Lodoxamide tromethamine treatment for superior limbic keratoconjunctivitis. Am J Ophthalmol 120: 400, 1995.
8. Foster CS. Evaluation of topical cromolyn sodium in the treatment of vernal keratoconjunctivitis. Ophthalmology 95:194, 1988.
9. Calonge M, Montero JA, Herreras JM, et al. Efficacy of nedocromil sodium and cromolyn sodium in an experimental model of ocular allergy. Ann Allergy Asthma Immunol 77:124, 1996.
10. Spataro AC, Bosmann HB. Mechanism of action of disodium cromoglycate-mast cell calcium ion influx after a histamine-releasing stimulus. Biochem Pharm 25:505, 1976.
11. Alvarez RG, Arruzazabala ML. Current views of the mechanism of action of prophylactic antiallergic drugs. Allergol Immunopathol 9:501, 1981.
12. Garland LG, Green EF, Hodson HF. Inhibitors of the release of anaphylactic mediators. In: Anti-inflammatory drugs: handbook of experimental pharmacology. Vol 50. Part 2. Vane JR, Ferreira SH, eds. Berlin, Springer-Verlag, 1979, p 467.
13. Lee S, Allard T. Lodoxamide in vernal keratoconjunctivitis. Ann Pharmacother 30:535, 1996.
14. Johnson HG, VanHout CA, Wright JB. Inhibition of allergic reactions by cromoglycate and by a new antiallergy drug U-42,585E. II. Activity in primates against aerosolized *Ascaris suum* antigen. Int Arch Allergy Appl Immunol 56:481, 1978.
15. Cerqueti PM, Ricca V, Tosca MA, et al. Lodoxamide treatment of allergic conjunctivitis. Int Arch Allergy Immunol 105:185, 1994.
16. Caldwell DR, Verin P, Hartwich-Young R, et al. Efficacy and safety of lodoxamide 0.1% vs cromolyn sodium 4% in patients with vernal keratoconjunctivitis. Am J Ophthalmol 113:632, 1992.
17. Gunduz K, Ucakhan O, Budak K, et al. Efficacy of lodoxamide 0.1% versus *N*-acetyl aspartyl glutamic acid 6% ophthalmic solutions in patients with vernal keratoconjunctivitis. Ophthalmic Res 28:80, 1996.
18. Santos CI, Huang AJ, Abelson MB, et al. Efficacy of lodoxamide 0.1% ophthalmic solution in resolving corneal epitheliopathy associated with vernal keratoconjunctivitis. Am J Ophthalmol 117:488, 1994.
19. Cerqueti PM, Ricca V, Tosca MA, et al. Lodoxamide treatment of allergic conjunctivitis. Int Arch Allergy Immunol 105:185, 1994.
20. Blumenthal M, Casale T, Dockhorn R, et al. Efficacy and safety of nedocromil sodium ophthalmic solution in the treatment of seasonal allergic conjunctivitis. Am J Ophthalmol 113:56, 1992.
21. Abelson MB, Casey R, Discepola MJ. Ocular allergy and its management: a state-of-the-art approach. Alcon, Slide Presentation Kit, Fort Worth, TX, February, 1997.
22. 1999 Physicians' Desk Reference for Ophthalmology. Montvale, NJ, Medical Economics, 1998, p 219.
23. Costa JJ, Harris AG, Delano FA, et al. Mast cell degranulation and parenchymal cell injury in the rat mesentery. Microcirculation 6:257, 1999.
24. Kimura M, Mitani H, Bandoh T, et al. Mast cell degranulation in rat mesenteric venule: effects of L-NAME, methylene blue, and ketotifen. Pharmacol Res 39:397, 1999.
25. Unpublished manuscript.

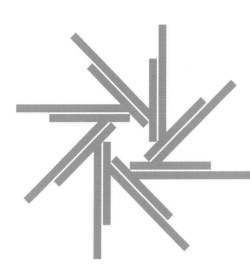

CHAPTER **27**

Vasoconstrictors

MARK B. ABELSON ■ **BETSEY ZBYSZYNSKI**

The most prevalent sign associated with ocular allergic diseases is hyperemia. Whether the condition is mild seasonal allergic conjunctivitis or a severe form of vernal conjunctivitis, patients consider injection to be a significant sign warranting treatment. Once the physician has determined the cause of the condition, vasoconstrictors become a therapeutic option. More than a million bottles of vasoconstrictors are purchased in the United States each month (Table 27.1).

Vasoconstrictors provide symptomatic relief by decreasing conjunctival edema and hyperemia. These drugs activate the postjunctional alpha-adrenergic receptors found on the precapillary and postcapillary blood vessels. Activation of these receptors causes the conjunctival vessels to constrict, thus decreasing blood flow and resulting in shrinkage of the tissue.[1] Following topical instillation, constriction of conjunctival blood vessels occurs at drug concentration levels that generally do not cause pupillary dilation (Fig. 27.1). These agents are chemically compatible with a variety of compounds and can be combined with other agents, including antihistamines.

VASOCONSTRICTORS

Naphazoline

Naphazoline, like tetrahydrozoline and oxymetazoline (discussed later), is classified chemically as an imidazole derivative. These agents differ structurally from other adrenergic agonists by replacement of the benzene ring with an unsaturated ring. Naphazoline is currently available in concentrations ranging from less than 0.012% to 0.1%. Abelson, Yamamota, and

TABLE 27.1 Topical Ocular Adrenergic Medications

Generic Name	Trade Name	Manufacturer	Concentration (%)
Naphazoline HCl	AK-Con	Akorn	0.1
	AK-Con A	Akorn	0.025
	Albalon	Allergan	0.1
	Allergy Drops*	Bausch & Lomb	0.012
	Clear Eyes*	Ross	0.012
	Degest 2*	Barnes-Hind	0.012
	Naphcon	Alcon	0.1
	Naphcon A*	Alcon	0.02675
	OcuHist*	Pfizer	0.025
	Opcon	Bausch & Lomb	0.1
	Opcon A*	Bausch & Lomb	0.05
	Vasoclear*	CIBA Vision	0.02
	Vasocon	CIBA Vision	0.1
	Vasocon A*	CIBA Vision	0.05
Phenylephrine HCl	AK-Nefrin	Akorn	0.12
	Isopto Frin	Alcon	0.12
	Prefrin Liquifilm	Allergan	0.12
	Relief	Allergan	0.12
Oxymetazoline HCl	Ocuclear*	Schering-Plough	0.25
	Visine LR*	Pfizer	0.025
Tetrahydrozoline HCl	Murine Plus*	Ross	0.05
	Visine Original*	Pfizer	0.05
	Visine Moisturizing*	Pfizer	0.05
	Visine Maximum Strength	Pfizer	0.05

*Over-the-counter preparations.

Allansmith[2] found naphazoline 0.02% to be significantly better than other nonprescription decongestant preparations in relieving histamine-induced erythema. Smith and Lanier et al.[3] evaluated the therapeutic efficacy of three ocular decongestant products containing varying concentrations of naphazoline in combinations with the antihistamines antazoline phosphate or pheniramine maleate in relieving signs and symptoms in patients with allergic conjunctivitis. All three products significantly reduced conjunctival inflammation as well as itching and discomfort in patients suffering from allergic conjunctivitis.

Rebound vasodilation has been associated with the use of vasoconstrictors. Although the specific mechanism is still unclear, rebound vasodilation may result from receptor desensitization. In a study of 0.02% naphazoline in healthy subjects, no rebound vasodilation was observed 6 and 24 hours following treatment.[4] Although a rebound effect possibly may have occurred between the 6- and 24-hour time points, most rebound vasodilation would be manifested within 6 hours of treatment and would most likely persist at 24 hours.

Tetrahydrozoline is currently marketed for ophthalmic use in a 0.05% solution. This vasoconstrictor has been shown to produce "good" results in 67% and "fair" results in 30% of patients suffering from allergic conjunctivi-

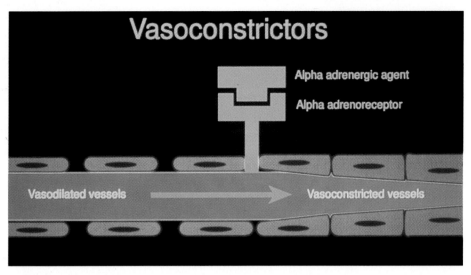

FIGURE 27.1 Alpha-adrenergic drugs activate the postjunctional alpha-adrenergic receptors found on the precapillary and postcapillary blood vessels. Activation of these receptors causes the vessels to constrict. The vasoconstriction decreases the blood flow and results in shrinkage of the tissue.

tis.[5, 6] Most eyes whiten within 1 minute of instillation of the medication, and the effect of a single application has been shown to last up to 4 hours. As with naphazoline, rebound effects were not evident after discontinuation of tetrahydrozoline treatment.[4]

Tetrahydrozoline 0.05% did not alter pupil size or raise intraocular pressure,[5] two other possible side effects that can occur with extended use of a vasoconstrictor. Butler, Thompson, and Yolton[6] demonstrated that tetrahydrozoline 0.05% significantly lowered intraocular pressure at 30 minutes when compared with phenylephrine 0.12% and naphazoline 0.012%.

Phenylephrine

Phenylephrine is the oldest of the currently available vasoconstrictor agents and is present in many ophthalmic combination products. Phenylephrine differs chemically from epinephrine by the absence of the hydroxyl group on position 4 of the benzene ring. Although phenylephrine in low concentration is indicated as a vasoconstrictor, higher concentrations (2.5%, 5%, and 10%) of phenylephrine are used as a mydriatic. Phenylephrine is used for pupillary dilation in uveitis (to prevent or disrupt posterior synechia formation), for ophthalmic surgical procedures, and for refraction without cycloplegia. Phenylephrine may also be used for funduscopy and other diagnostic procedures.[8] At the higher concentrations (10%), phenylephrine may cause hypertension and possible reflex atropine-sensitive bradycardia. There have been rare cases in elderly patients of phenylephrine leading to ventricular arrhythmia and myocardial infarctions. Also more prevalent in elderly patients is an increased incidence of rebound miosis one day after instillation, and transient pigment floaters found 30–45 minutes after instillation.

Caution should be exercised when administering phenylephrine to children with low body weight, the elderly, insulin-dependent diabetics, patients with cardiovascular disease, and patients with hypertension and hyperthyroidism, because a significant increase in blood pressure may occur. Phenylephrine use should also be carefully monitored in patients with narrow angle glaucoma, as it may increase the patient's intraocular pressure.

Oxymetazoline

Oxymetazoline is available without a prescription in a 0.025% solution. A double-masked, multicenter study compared 0.025% oxymetazoline with placebo in relieving signs and symptoms of allergic conjunctivitis.[9] Of the 158 patients who instilled 2 drops of oxymetazoline or placebo in each eye 4 times daily for 1 week, 84% of patients using oxymetazoline showed improvement, compared with 58% in the placebo group.

DOSING REGIMEN AND SIDE EFFECTS

Clinicians generally recommend that ocular vasoconstrictors be applied two to four times daily. There have been reports that usage of nonprescription decongestant eyedrops can produce acute and chronic forms of conjunctivitis by pharmacological, toxic, and allergic mechanisms.[10, 11] However, to minimize side effects, the solutions should be used as infrequently as possible. Fortunately, because of the relatively low concentrations required for ocular decongestion, side effects infrequently occur with the recommended dosage. Transient stinging can occur with use of all ophthalmic vasoconstrictors. Smith and Lanier et al.[3] compared the comfort of three ocular decongestant products containing a vasoconstrictor and an antihistamine. The results significantly favored the decongestant with the lowest concentration of vasoconstrictor and antihistamine.

USE OF VASOCONSTRICTORS

The release of histamine and other vasoactive amines is largely responsible for the hyperemia, tearing, and itching that occur with allergic conjunctivitis. Vasodilation occurring during allergic conjunctivitis results in endothelial cell gaping. This facilitates fluid transudation, leading to chemosis, a swelling of the conjunctiva, and lid edema. It has been noted that agents countering vasodilation—vasoconstrictors and antihistamines—play a role in reducing tissue congestion. By constricting the conjunctival blood vessels, vasoconstrictors are able to alleviate the conjunctival hyperemia and edema associated with allergic conjunctivitis. The signs and symptoms of vernal keratoconjunctivitis are often more severe and difficult to control than those of allergic conjunctivitis. However, the use of vasoconstrictors is effective for mild symptomatic control.

REFERENCES

1. Johnson DA, Hricik JG. The pharmacology of alpha-adrenergic decongestants. Pharmacotherapy 13:110s, 1993.

2. Abelson MB, Yamamota GK, Allansmith MR. Effects of ocular decongestants. Arch Ophthalmol 98:856, 1980.

3. Smith JP, Lanier BQ, Tremblay N, et al. Treatment of allergic conjunctivitis with ocular decongestants. Curr Eye Res 2:141, 1982.

4. Abelson MB, Butrus SI, Weston JH, et al. Tolerance and absence of rebound vasodilation following topical ocular decongestant use. Ophthalmology 91:1364, 1984.

5. Menger HC. New ophthalmic decongestant tetrahydrozoline hydrochloride. JAMA 170:178, 1958.

6. Butler K, Thompson JP, Yolton DP. Effects of nonprescription ocular decongestants. Rev Optom 115:49, 1978.

7. Ciprandi G, Buscaglia S, Cerqueti PM. Drug treatment of allergic conjunctivitis. Drugs 43: 154, 1992.

8. Grossman EE, Lehman RH. Ophthalmic use of Tyzine. Am J Ophthalmol 42:121, 1956.

9. Samson CR, Danzig MR, Sasovetz D, et al. Safety and toleration of oxymetazoline ophthalmic solution. Pharmatherapeutica 2:347, 1980.

10. Soparkar CN, Wilhelmus KR, et al. Acute and chronic conjunctivitis due to over-the-counter ophthalmic decongestants. Arch Ophthalmol 115: 34, 1997.

11. Resano A, Esteve C, Fernandez Benitez M. Allergic contact blepharoconjunctivitis due to phenylephrine eye drops. J Investig Allergol Clin Immunol 9:55, 1999.

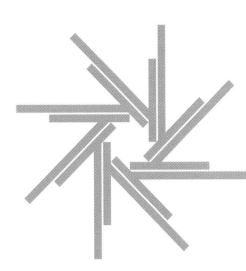

CHAPTER 28

Novel Treatments and Targets

MARK B. ABELSON ▪ **JENNIFER SLOAN** ▪ **PAULO J. GOMES**

Exploring the advances in ocular allergy necessitates a proper understanding of basic allergy mechanisms. The mast cell acts as the foundation of allergic disease by mediating type I hypersensitivity reactions. These cells are found in the substantia propria of the normal human conjunctiva, and they contain hundreds of vesicles. Antigen-antibody complexes may adhere to the mast cell membrane leading to mast cell degranulation and the subsequent release of chemical mediators, such as histamine and arachidonic acid metabolites. This release attracts neutrophils and eosinophils to the inflammatory site, where they release secondary mediators to either perpetuate inflammation or restore homeostasis. Many topical ocular medications are currently approved for treatment of seasonal allergic conjunctivitis for which they provide relief of redness, swelling, and itching.

MAST CELL STABILIZERS

Mechanism of Action

Mast cell stabilizing agents inhibit degranulation of all mast cell mediators[1] including histamine, eosinophil chemotactic factors, eosinophil granule major basic protein, platelet-activating factor, and prostaglandin D_2.[2]

Conventional thought has been that mast cell stabilizers (e.g., lodoxamide, cromolyn, and nedocromil) act by preventing calcium influx across the cell membrane; however, more recent evidence shows they may exert their effects by other mechanisms. For instance, cromolyn has been shown in vitro to inhibit activation of human neutrophils, eosinophils, and monocytes. Thus, investigators have proposed that this drug may inhibit leukocyte activation directly, thereby preventing tissue damage caused by inflammatory cells.[3]

Lodoxamide

Lodoxamide 0.1%, a relatively new mast cell stabilizer, inhibits the immediate (type I) hypersensitivity reaction and is marketed for treatment of vernal keratoconjunctivitis. Like cromolyn, lodoxamide blocks degranulation of mast cells; however, once a hypersensitivity reaction is under way and symptoms are present, this drug is ineffective except to prevent a reaction to the next exposure.

Lodoxamide was judged to be more effective than cromolyn 2.0% and 4.0% in relieving the signs and symptoms (discomfort, itching, and tearing) of vernal conjunctivitis.[4, 5] Lodoxamide 0.1% has also been effective in treating superior limbic keratoconjunctivitis.[6]

Although the efficacy of lodoxamide in the treatment of other allergic diseases is still under investigation, the drug may be superior to cromolyn in treatment of atopic and giant papillary conjunctivitis. The efficacy of lodoxamide on mast cells and eosinophils after allergen challenge was studied. Lodoxamide 1% significantly reduced tryptase levels, neutrophils, and eosinophils in the tear fluid and significantly inhibited ocular itching when compared with placebo.[7] Neither lodoxamide nor cromolyn is approved for treatment of seasonal or hay fever–type conjunctivitis. The efficacy of lodoxamide in the treatment of seasonal allergic conjunctivitis is questionable, because it does not have any intrinsic vasoconstrictor, antihistaminic, or anti-inflammatory activity.

Olopatadine

Olopatadine hydrochloride 0.1% ophthalmic solution (Patanol) is the only ocular dual-action antiallergic medication available in the United States that has been proven safe and effective through extensive clinical research. This formulation contains both antihistaminic and mast cell stabilizing properties, potentially reducing the need for multiagent therapy for ocular allergies. Olopatadine was found to be superior to ketotifen, cromolyn, and nedocromil in stabilizing activity of in vitro human conjunctival mast cells. In a clinical conjunctival allergen challenge study, mean itching and total redness in the treatment group were statistically and clinically lower than in the placebo group at all time points. Another study performed a comparative evaluation of olopatadine 0.1% versus ketorolac 0.5% using the allergen challenge model. Olopatadine significantly reduced both ocular itching and hyperemia in all three vascular beds compared with placebo. Olopatadine was significantly more effective than ketorolac in reducing hyperemia and ocular itching at all time points and was more comfortable in use than ketorolac as reported by subjects immediately following drug instillation.[8] Finally, because of its long duration of action of at least 8 hours, olopatadine is effective when used only twice per day.

ANTIHISTAMINE

Emedastine

A novel addition to the antihistamines available in the United States is emedastine difumarate (Emadine). Emedastine is a potent, selective H_1 antagonist possessing a rapid onset and an acceptable duration of action following topical ocular administration. The ability of emedastine to inhibit increases in vascular permeability is agonist specific. Emedastine's high degree of selectivity may account for its low side-effect profile.

Both environmental and conjunctival allergen challenge clinical studies have shown that emedastine is effective in relieving the signs and symptoms of allergic conjunctivitis and is superior to levocabastine. Emedastine has demonstrated greater antihistaminic potency than brompheniramine, chlorpheniramine, levocabastine, pheniramine, pyrilamine, antazoline, and diphenhydramine, and it was equipotent to ketotifen in studies conducted in guinea pigs. Emedastine 0.05% can be used up to four times daily to relieve symptoms of allergic conjunctivitis.

Ketotifen

Ketotifen fumarate is a selective, noncompetitive antagonist of histamine (H_1-receptor) that also inhibits the release of inflammatory mediators from mast cells.[9, 10] Ketotifen fumarate has also been shown to inhibit the release of inflammatory mediators from basophils and neutrophils. It is known to inhibit the production and release of leukotriene C4 and the production of leukotriene B4.[11] Ketotifen fumarate inhibits platelet activating factor (PAF) production by normal human neutrophils and significantly inhibits PAF-induced eosinophil chemotaxis.[12–14] In vitro studies have shown that ketotifen fumarate inhibits eosinophil viability and eosinophil chemotactic functions.[15, 16] Clinical studies have begun to test whether ketotifen is effective in preventing the development of ocular itching associated with allergic conjunctivitis prior to allergen challenge.

NON–IMMUNOGLOBULIN E MAST CELL ACTIVATION

In addition to allergen–immunoglobulin E (IgE) bridging, several non-IgE mechanisms of mast cell activation are possible. Hypothetically, the tears of some patients may be primed with histamine-releasing factors that are released by lymphocytes and macrophages on activation by known allergens or other stimuli.[17]

Nonspecific Conjunctival Hyperreactivity

A nonspecific conjunctival hyperreactivity has been associated with vernal conjunctivitis and may account for the variability of symptoms observed in this disease. Accordingly, nonspecific natural stimuli such as wind, dust, or sunlight may induce an abnormal nonspecific reaction of the conjunctiva regardless of environmental or seasonal changes.

Fourteen asymptomatic patients with vernal conjunctivitis and 10 healthy volunteers were challenged unilaterally, in a dose-dependent fashion, with histamine diphosphate. Post-challenge ocular redness was significantly more intense in patients with vernal conjunctivitis than in control subjects. In addition, the mean concentration of histamine required to cause a significant reaction was substantially lower in patients than controls.[7] These results demonstrate that non–IgE-mediated mechanisms also play a role in ocular allergy.

OTHER CONSIDERATIONS

Inhibitors of kinin pathways, lipoxygenase blockers, combination lipoxygenase-cyclooxygenase blockers, methylxanthines, and anti-IgE compounds are currently under investigation.

Lipoxygenase Blockers

Development of leukotriene receptor antagonists and biosynthesis inhibitors has been focused on treatment of asthma. Various approaches are available for inhibiting leukotriene synthesis, including antagonism of 5-lipoxygenase activating protein (FLAP) and inhibition of lipoxygenase (5-LO). Inhibitors of FLAP (MK-886 and MK-591) prevent the translocation of the enzyme to the cell membrane.[18]

Inhibitors of 5-LO–mediated reactions can act through a number of mechanisms, including trapping radical intermediates, chelation or reduction of iron, and reversible binding at either an active or a regulatory site. Combinations of these mechanisms also may be used.[19] The benzofurans (L-670,630 and L650,224), hydroxamates (BWA4C), N-hydroxyurea derivatives (A-64077 or zileuton), and indazolinones (ICI 207,968) directly inhibit 5-LO with good selectivity and potency by an iron-catalyzed redox mechanism.[20] The methoxyalkylthiazoles (ICI D2138), a new series of non-redox 5-LO inhibitors, are the most potent and selective inhibitors of 5-LO.[21]

The two classes of receptors for leukotrienes are those for the dihydroxyleukotriene leukotriene B_4 (LTB_4), termed LTB receptors, and those for cysteinyl leukotrienes (LTC_y, LTD_4, LTE_4), termed CysLT receptors. Early antagonists lacked sufficient potency to be effective. However, the newer-generation antagonists (ICI 204,219, MK-571, RG-12,525, ONO-1078, and SK&F 104,353) provide greater promise.[19]

Although these compounds have yet to be evaluated in the eye, they represent an important breakthrough in the treatment of allergy. In addition, although these therapies have demonstrated efficacy in asthmatic patients, the origin of ocular allergies may differ considerably. Therefore, little can be said about the role of these therapeutic agents for ocular allergy until they are evaluated in the eye.

Immunoglobulin E Pentapeptide

Human IgE pentapeptide (HEPP), a synthetic antiallergic agent (peptide sequence: Asp-Ser-Asp-Pro-Arg), is thought to prevent the immediate wheal-and-flare response in humans by competitively blocking binding of intact IgE to specific cell receptors. However, limited evidence has supported this hypothesis, and its true mechanism of action remains unknown. In a study of 50 patients diagnosed with allergic conjunctivitis, a 0.5% ophthalmic solution of HEPP was found safe and effective at relieving the signs and symptoms of allergic conjunctivitis.[22]

Another strategy based on the IgE receptor is the use of nonanaphylactogenic antibodies specific for IgE. The rationale is that antibodies directed against IgE would stop the degranulation of the mast cell by preventing allergen-IgE interaction. Clinical studies are currently underway.

Cyclosporine

Cyclosporine, a cyclic peptide, is a potent immunomodulator that inhibits the actions of interleukin-2 on T lymphocytes. Cyclosporine 2% in castor oil has decreased the signs and symptoms of vernal keratoconjunctivitis; however, its use in the treatment of other allergic disease remains unknown.[23]

FK506, another potent immunodulator, has the potential to be effective therapy in allergic disease. FK506 has been shown along with cyclosporine to inhibit mast cell proliferation and survival.[24] FK506 eyedrops in animal models suppress signs of allergic conjunctivitis by inhibiting the release of histamine and other chemical mediators from mast cells and by reducing the cytokine production from T lymphocytes. Clinical studies have begun to investigate the efficacy of FK506 using the allergen challenge model in allergic conjunctivitis.

The inhibition of cytokine production, namely that of IL-5, is also a new area of interest. IL-5 is an important growth and chemotactic factor for eosinophils. The rationale behind this strategy is to prevent the late-phase inflammation associated with allergic disease through the inhibition of eosinophil recruitment. A novel antiallergic drug, betotastine besilate, potently inhibits IL-5 production at concentrations as low as 10 microM.[27] Antibodies directed against IL-5 have also been shown to prevent eosinophil recruitment and infiltration in mice asthma models.

Eosinophil Regulation of Allergic Inflammation

Eosinophils play a prominent role in both chronic and acute allergic disease. Eosinophil-derived leukotrienes and eosinophil granule proteins such as eosinophil major basic protein have been associated with pathological inflammatory changes associated with corneal damage. In addition, eosinophil-generated cytokines are thought to regulate or to amplify the responses of inflammatory cells.

The biological mechanism responsible for eosinophil production and release of cytokines is not well elucidated; however, once released, cytokines are capable of regulating inflammation. Possibly, the same chemotactic agonists responsible for activating eosinophils may also trigger them to generate cytokines. Thus, eosinophils may provide a novel perspective for regulation of allergic inflammation by an autocrine or paracrine mechanism.[25]

The question of the role of adhesion molecules in allergic disease has generated much research. Adhesion molecules located on vascular endothelial cells are vital to the recruitment process of eosinophils in late-phase inflammation. Adhesion molecules (e.g., ICAM-1, P-selectin) bind to eosinophils initiating a cascade of rolling and diapedesis. New strategies of preventing adhesion molecules from binding to eosinophils have shown promising results. A study using a soluble P-selectin glycoprotein ligand showed the inhibition of eosinophil recruitment, tissue infiltration, and late-phase inflammation in the conjunctiva of challenged mice.[26]

As basic science further elucidates the intricacies of the pathways of allergic inflammation, so, too, does clinical science test new methods of mediating these pathways. New treatments with greater potency and efficacy and fewer side effects are constantly evolving. Advances in cytokine blocking and up-regulating suppressor systems will provide novel means of treatment. An ideal approach will influence the inflammatory systems at the first point of breakdown, that is, the recognition of normal environmental proteins as foreign invaders.

REFERENCES

1. Foster CS. Immunologic disorders of the conjunctiva, cornea, and sclera. In: Principles and practice of ophthalmology: clinical practice. Vol. 1. Albert DM, Jakobiec FA, eds. Philadelphia, WB Saunders, 1994, p 191.
2. Abelson MB, Udell IJ, Allansmith MF, et al. Allergic and toxic reactions. In: Principles and practice of ophthalmology: clinical practice. Vol. 1. Albert DM, Jakobiec FA, eds. Philadelphia, WB Saunders, 1994, pp 79, 93.
3. Rodriguez RD, Smith LM, George M, et al. Recent advances in the therapy of ocular allergy. Ophthalmol Clin North Am 3:563, 1990.
4. Fahy GT, Easty DL, Collum LM, et al. Randomized double-masked trial of lodoxamide and sodium cromoglycate in allergic eye disease: a multicentre study. Eur J Ophthalmol 2:144, 1992.
5. Caldwell DR, Verin P, Hartwich-Young R, et al. Efficacy and safety of lodoxamide 0.1% vs. cromolyn sodium 4% in patients with vernal keratoconjunctivitis. Am J Ophthalmol 113:632, 1992.
6. Grutzmacher RD, Foster RS, Feiler LS. Lodoxamide tromethamine treatment for superior limbic keratoconjunctivitis. Am J Ophthalmol 120:400, 1995.
7. Bonini S, Schiavone M, Bonini S, et al. Efficacy of lodoxamide eye drops on mast cells and eosinophils after allergen challenge in allergic conjunctivitis. Ophthalmology. 104:849, 1997.
8. Deschenes J, Discepola M, Abelson M. Comparative evaluation of olopatadine ophthalmic solution (0.1%) versus ketorolac ophthalmic solution (0.5%) using the provocative antigen challenge model. Acta Ophthalmol Scand 228 Suppl: 47, 1999.
9. Martin U, Romer D. The pharmacological properties of a new, orally active antianaphylactic compound: ketotifen, a benzocycloheptathiophene. Arzneimittelforschung. 28:770, 1978.
10. Kimura M, Mitani H, Bandoh T, et al. Mast cell degranulation in rat mesenteric venule: effects of 1-NAME, methylene blue and ketotifen. Pharmacol Res 39:397, 1999.
11. Fink A, Bibi H, Eliraz A, et al. Ketotifen, disodium cromoglycate, and verapamil inhibit leukotriene activity: determination by tube leukocyte adherence inhibition assay. Ann Allergy 57:103, 1986.
12. Devillier P, Arnoux B, Lalau KC, et al. Inhibition of human and rabbit platelet activation by ketotifen. Fundam Clin Pharmacol 4:1, 1990.
13. Wang XD, Bian RL. Effects of ketotifen on rabbit platelet aggregation and platelet activating formation from rat neutrophils. Chung Kuo Yao Li Hsueh Pao 11:524, 1990.
14. Arnoux B, Denjean A, Page CP, et al. Accumulation of platelets and eosinophils in baboon lung after paf-acether challenge. Inhibition by ketotifen. Am Rev Respir Dis 137:855, 1988.
15. Soto J, Tchernitchin AN, Poloni P, et al. Effect of ketotifen on the distribution and degranulation of uterine eosinophils in estrogen-treated rats. Agents Actions 28:198, 1989.
16. Hossain M, Okubo Y, Sekiguchi M, et al. Effects of various drugs (staurosporine, herbimycin A, ketotifen, theophylline, FK 506, and cyclosporin A) on eosinophil viability. Arerugi 43:711, 1994.
17. Bonini S, Bonini S. IgE and non-IgE mechanisms in ocular allergy. Ann Allergy 71:296, 1993.
18. Brideau C, Chan C, Charleson S, et al. Pharmacology of MK-0591 (3[1-(4-chlorobenzyl)-3-(t-butyl thio)-5-(quinolin-2-yl-methoxy)-indol-2-yl]-2,2-dimethylpropanoic acid), a potent, orally active leukotriene biosynthesis inhibitor. Can J Physiol Pharmacol 70:799, 1992.
19. Chung KF. Leukotriene receptor antagonists and biosynthesis inhibitors: potential breakthrough in asthma therapy. Eur Respir J 8:1203, 1995.
20. McMillan RM, Girodeau JM, Foster SJ. Selective chiral inhibitors of 5-lipoxygenase with anti-inflammatory activity. Br J Pharmacol 101:501, 1990.
21. McMillan RM, Spruce KE, Crawley GC, et al. Preclinical pharmacology of ICI D2138, a potent orally-active non-redox inhibitor of 5-lipoxygenase. Br J Pharmacol 107:1042, 1992.
22. Floyd R, Kalpaxis J, Thayer T, et al. Double-blind comparison of HEPP™ (IgE pentapeptide) 0.5% ophthalmic solution (H) and sodium cromolyn ophthalmic solution, USP 4% (O) in patients having allergic conjunctivitis (abstract). Invest Ophthalmol Vis Sci 29 Suppl:24, 1988.
23. Trocme SD, Raizman MB, Bartley GB. Medical therapy for ocular allergy. Mayo Clin Proc 67:557, 1992.
24. Ito F, Toyota N, Sakai H, et al. FK506 and cyclosporin A inhibit stem cell factor–dependent cell proliferation/survival, while inducing upregu-

lation of c-kit expression in cells of the mast cell line MC/9. Arch Dermatol Res 291:275, 1999.

25. Miyamasu M, Hirai K, Takahashi Y, et al. Chemotactic agonists induce cytokine generation in eosinophils. J Immunol 154:1339, 1995.

26. Strauss EC, Larson KA, Brenneise I, et al. Soluble P-selectin glycoprotein ligand 1 inhibits ocu-

lar inflammation in a murine model of allergy. Invest Ophthalmol Vis Sci. 40:1336, 1999.

27. Kaminumka O, Ogawa K, Kikkawa H, et al. A novel antiallergic drug, betotastine besilate, suppresses interleukin-5 production by human peripheral blood mononuclear cell. Biol Pharm Bull 21:411, 1998.

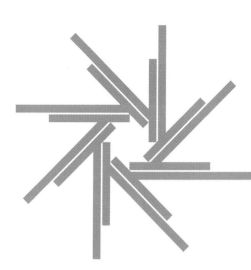

CHAPTER **29**

Nonpharmacological Management of Ocular Allergic Disease

ANDREA LEONARDI ■ **LISA M. SMITH**

ENVIRONMENTAL CONTROLS

The primary approach to the management of ocular allergic disease should be education of the patient and family on the nature of the causative allergens and their environmental control.[1] Avoidance and control of allergen exposure, both indoor and out, can substantially decrease the patients' signs and symptoms and the need for pharmacological therapy (Table 29.1).

During high pollen seasons, patients need to limit their time outdoors in high-exposure activities such as country trips, bicycling, and games in grassy fields. Windows should be closed and air conditioning or filtering should be used when driving or riding in the car. Wearing sunglasses or protective eyewear when outdoors can sometimes be useful. When entry into the house is not limited, grass pollen and fungal spores can quickly invade the house and may become the primary indoor allergens as well. Doors and windows should be kept closed and an air filtering system should be used, when possible. When planning vacations, patients, especially those with vernal conjunctivitis, should avoid high pollen seasons in other regions and should opt for cooler climates and higher altitudes.

TABLE 29.1 Preventive Environmental Measures That Can Significantly Reduce Allergic Symptoms

Avoidance measures for pollens
  Limit outdoor activities
  Use air conditioning or air filtering system
  Drive or ride in car with windows closed and with air conditioning or filtering
  Wear protective eyewear when outdoors
Avoidance measures for mites
  Use effective barrier cover for mattress and pillows
  Wash bedding regularly at 60°C (130°F)
  Remove carpets, upholstered furniture, curtains, books, stuffed animals, and any other reservoirs of dust
  Reduce humidity
  Vacuum and damp dust entire house weekly
Avoidance measure for animal allergens
  Eliminate animals from house
  Reduce exposure to all reservoirs for allergen (carpets, upholstered furniture, curtains, etc.)

Mite allergens[2] and molds are the most frequent causes of chronic or recurrent allergic conjunctivitis. Foremost in the bedroom, dust mites must be controlled by using impermeable covers on mattresses and pillows, by switching from feather and down to polyester fillers, and by changing bedding weekly and washing it in 60°C (130°F) hot water cycles. Ideally, bedroom upholstered furniture, curtains, carpets and rugs, books, and stuffed animals should be eliminated. In the remainder of the house, upholstered furniture should be kept to a minimum and periodically cleaned with commercially available acaricides. The entire house should be vacuumed and damp dusted at least weekly. Houseplants should be eliminated.

Mechanical devices can help to modify the indoor environment. Air conditioners and air cleaners have been proven to reduce airborne particles. Humidifiers and dehumidifiers can be used to maintain optimal conditions to avoid mold and mite growth. By producing negative ions that combine with air particles, negative ion generators may help to remove air impurities.

Maintaining humidity at 35 to 50% is essential for the control of mite and mold growth. If the region is dry, increasing ventilation can be helpful; in humid weather and in subtropical areas, reducing ventilation and using dehumidifiers and air conditioning is recommended. In the case of mold sensitivity, basements should be avoided, and fungicides and dehumidifiers should be used regularly. For domestic pet or rodent sensitivity, eliminating the source is the only effective measure because carpets, upholstery, and clothing are all reservoirs for animal allergens. Finally, because hypersensitivity to nonspecific environmental stimuli is an important aspect of allergic eye disease, all patients should avoid not only allergen exposure but also nonspecific irritants such as smoking and smoke-filled rooms, air pollution, and strong odors or perfumes.

SPECIFIC IMMUNOTHERAPY

Allergic desensitization or hyposensitization, also called specific immunotherapy, involves the long-term administration of low but progressively increasing doses of the offending allergen until the evoked clinical reaction is reduced or eliminated.[3] Subcutaneous administration is the usual route; however, specific immunotherapy has also been attempted sublingually, nasally, bronchially, and ocularly. Immunotherapy is indicated most often in the treatment of patients with seasonal or perennial allergic rhinoconjunctivitis, asthma or Hymenoptera venom allergy. The most common allergens used with success in specific immunotherapy are dust mites, long-term environmental pollens such as Graminacae, Parietariae, and Compositae, and, less frequently, mold spores. The decision to commence immunotherapy must be made with the following considerations:

1. The type of allergen and thus the chance of success.
2. The severity of the disease.
3. The possibility of significantly increasing the quality of the patient's life.
4. The quantity and type of pharmacological agents taken by the patient to control signs and symptoms.

Immunotherapy is contraindicated in the presence of other immunological or neoplastic diseases, severe asthma, and atopic dermatitis, in patients in whom the use of epinephrine is contraindicated, and in children younger than 5 years of age. Therapy should not be initiated but can be continued during pregnancy.

Once initiated, immunotherapy must be continued for at least 3 to 5 years before conclusive evidence on its long-term efficacy can be assessed. The maintenance dose is that maximally tolerated by the patient and cannot be predicted by laboratory or skin tests. Clinical evaluation is still the only method of monitoring the therapeutic and collateral effects of specific immunotherapy.

Local and systemic adverse reactions must be closely monitored. Redness and swelling can occur at the site of administration, requiring a subsequent adjustment in dose. Systemic reactions include generalized erythema, pruritus, urticaria, angioedema, bronchospasm, laryngeal edema, shock, and cardiac arrest. An emergency anti-anaphylactic kit must always be available.[4]

Among the many hypotheses for its mechanism of action, immunotherapy is thought to modify the allergic response by inducing a shift from the lymphocyte helper T_H2 cell type, predominant in allergic disorders, to the lymphocyte helper T_H1 cell type.[5] This shifts the production of cytokines interleukin-3 (IL-3), IL-4, IL-5, and IL-13 to the production of IL-2 and interferon-gamma. Of the former interleukins, IL-4 and IL-13 are known to stimulate immunoglobulin E production, IL-3 stimulates the growth and activation of mast cells, and IL-5 stimulates eosinophil activation.

LOCAL IMMUNOTHERAPY

Following the tendency to administer the vaccine directly to the shock organ,[6] topical local ocular immunotherapy is being attempted in a limited group of patients with allergic conjunctivitis resulting from Graminacae or the Dermatophagoides.[7] The therapeutic protocol involves identifying for each patient the topical ocular dose of lyophilized allergen extract dissolved in an aqueous solution that initiates ocular allergic signs and symptoms. Subsequently, subclinical doses are instilled daily, progressively increasing until the maintenance dose, as in systemic immunotherapy, for 6 months to 3 years. The provocation test evoking a clinical allergic response is periodically identified for the monitoring of upward shifts in threshold sensitivity. Results of up to 5 years of experience demonstrate a beneficial clinical effect during subsequent pollen seasons, a reduction in the use of antiallergic agents, and an increase in the threshold of local reactivity to the offending allergen. Tolerability is excellent, although the patient may have local collateral effects such as mild itching. Positive results have also been obtained in a similar study using a different method of local allergen application.[8]

REFERENCES

1. Middleton E Jr, Reed C, Ellis E, eds. Allergy: principles and practice. St. Louis, CV Mosby, 1998.
2. Platts-Mills TAE, Chapman MD. Dust mites: immunology, allergic disease, and environmental control. J Allergy Clin Immunol 80:755, 1987.
3. European Academy of Allergy and Clinical Immunology. Position Paper: immunotherapy. Malling HJ, Weeke B, eds. Allergy 48 9, Suppl:9, 1992.
4. Norman PS, Van Metre TE Jr. The safety of allergenic immunotherapy. J Allergy Clin Immunol 85:522, 1990.
5. Durham SR, Varney V, Gaga M, et al. Immunotherapy and allergic inflammation. Clin Exp Allergy 21:206, 1991.
6. Georgitis JW, Nickelsen JA, Wypych JI, et al. Local intranasal immunotherapy with high dose polymerized ragweed extract. Int Archs Allergy Appl Immunol 81:170, 1986.
7. Leonardi A, Fregona I, Miorin S, et al. Local immunotherapy in allergic conjunctivitis. Invest Ophthalmol Vis Sci 33 Suppl:851, 1992.
8. Del Prete A, Loffredo C, Carderopoli A, et al. Local specific immunotherapy in allergic conjunctivitis. Acta Ophthalmol 72:631, 1994.

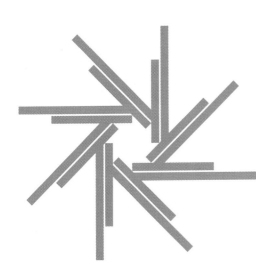

CHAPTER 30

Comparison of the Conjunctival Allergen Challenge Model with the Environmental Model of Allergic Conjunctivitis

MARK B. ABELSON ■ **MICHELLE GEORGE** ■ **KELLY K. GRANT**

DESCRIPTION OF ALLERGIC CONJUNCTIVITIS

Four types of allergic conjunctivitis are generally recognized: vernal, atopic, panseasonal, and seasonal conjunctivitis. These conditions differ in their clinical and histological appearance, although the basic pathophysiological mechanism is similar (Table 30.1). The most prevalent by far is seasonal allergic conjunctivitis (SAC), which accounts for more than 90% of ocular allergies. This disease is exogenously triggered by an allergen coming into contact with the mast cell–bound immunoglobulin E (IgE) antibody. The binding of the allergen results in degranulation and release of chemical mediators. These mediators directly cause vasodilation and increased per-

TABLE 30.1 Four Types of Allergic Conjunctivitis

Vernal

Clinical	Hyperemia of conjunctiva; keratitis and corneal ulcers possible; large cobble-like papillae on the tarsal conjunctiva and/or papillae at the limbus; thick, tenacious mucus and severe itching always present
Epidemiology	Can occur year round with seasonal exacerbation; a chronic severe ocular disease during prepuberty and puberty, mostly in males; less than 1% of allergic conjunctivitis cases
Histology	Mast cells and eosinophils present in epithelium; eosinophils and basophils present in substantia propria

Atopic

Clinical	Hyperemia of the conjunctiva; moderate to severe itching; indurated and lichenified lid margins; tearing with a watery or mucopurulent discharge; keratoconus; corneal ulcers and anterior polar cataract also can develop
Epidemiology	Often accompanied by atopic dermatitis and eczema; males in thirties predominantly; perennial; less than 1% of allergic conjunctivitis cases
Histology	Lymphocyte infiltration and eosinophils

Panseasonal

Clinical	Hyperemia, chemosis, itching, and lid edema
Epidemiology	Perennial; approximately 5% of allergic conjunctivitis cases
Histology	Cellular infiltrates including eosinophils in conjunctiva

Seasonal

Clinical	Hyperemia, chemosis, itching, mucous discharge, and lid edema; papillary reaction rare and never large
Epidemiology	Seasonal; accounts for more than 90% of allergic conjunctivitis cases; males and females of all ages
Histology	No cellular changes to superficial tissues

meability of the conjunctiva, leading to redness and swelling of the conjunctiva and, in extreme cases, the lid. Itching is always associated with SAC. SAC lasts less than a few hours and has no associated cellular response. The clinical course of SAC can be best described as a series of episodes in which exposure to pollen leads to transient ocular allergic reactions.

DISEASE PATHOLOGY

Histology

Scrapings of the conjunctiva in more than a hundred cases of SAC were conducted, and no cellular infiltration was observed. Only in chronic panseasonal and vernal conjunctivitis could eosinophils be identified.[1] Mast cells, the critical cells in allergic conjunctivitis, are neither increased in number nor more superficially located in SAC, unlike in the more chronic allergic diseases.

Cellular Biology

Quiescent mucosal mast cells have been identified in the normal conjunctiva of rats[2] and humans.[3] Although these cells are located primarily in the substantia propria of normal patients, mast cells have been identified in other structures of the eye during disease states.[3, 4, 34] Approximately 50 million mast cells have been found in the ocular and adnexal tissues of the human eye, each containing several hundred vesicles filled with immune mediators.[5]

Immunoglobulin E Receptors

The allergic reaction is elicited via a classic type I hypersensitivity reaction in which allergen dissolves in the tear film and traverses the conjunctiva to crosslink two IgE antibodies on the surface of mast cells.[6] IgE antibodies are attached to the mast cell by FcεRI receptors unique to mast cells and basophils.[7] The allergen IgE–mast cell union results in the activation of a serine esterase that in turn initiates a change in the Fc portion of the IgE molecule attached to the mast cell membrane. Once activated, an intracellular biochemical cascade results in mast cell degranulation and the release of chemical mediators.[5]

Histamine

All signs and symptoms of SAC are associated with the release of preformed mediators from the mast cell. Analyses of the effects of histamine when exogenously applied have shown that histamine is the cardinal mediator of allergic reactions.[8] Twenty patients were topically administered 100 μL of increasing concentrations of histamine (5, 10, 50, and 100 ng/mL). At a dose of 5 ng/mL, histamine induced itching in 10% of the patients and redness in 10% of the patients. The incidence of the manifestations was directly proportional to the dose of histamine. At a dose of 100 ng/mL, histamine elicited an 80% response with respect to itching and a 100% response with respect to redness. This reaction can be blocked with the administration of an H_1 antihistamine, which is confirmation of its causative role.

In addition to producing itching, histamine induces vasodilation and increases vascular permeability when it binds to H_1 receptors.[8, 9] A second histamine receptor, H_2, has been found to induce hypotension,[10] as well as vasodilation.[11] The differentiation of these responses between the two receptors is not absolute. A third class of histamine receptors, known as H_3 receptors, has been identified in the nerve tissue in animals.[12] These receptors have yet to be identified in the ocular tissues.

Other Mediators

Other mediators released by mast cells include arachidonic acid, eosinophilic chemotactic factor,[13] platelet-activating factor,[14] tryptase,[15] and chymase.[16] The metabolism of arachidonic acid results in the production of prostaglandins and leukotrienes. Prostaglandin D_2 is the primary prostaglandin produced by the mast cell in type I hypersensitivity reactions.[17] When applied topically to the guinea pig or human eyes, prostaglandin D_2 causes redness, conjunctival chemosis, mucous discharge, and eosinophilic infiltrates. Eosinophilic chemotactic factor also elicits an influx of eosinophils. Eosinophils release a number of enzymes including histaminase, phospholipase, and aryl sulfatase, which modulate the response through the negative feedback mechanism.[5] As an eosinophilic chemotactic factor, platelet-activating factor is approximately 100 times more effective than eosinophilic chemotactic factor.[18] When applied topically to the eye, platelet-activating factor elicited clinically significant hyperemia and chemosis in a dose-dependent fashion.[19] Tryptase is a tetrameric serine endoprotease that is stored in its active form in mast cells. Although its physiologic role is not yet understood, its regional specificity for mast cells makes it an excellent marker.[15] Chymase, another serine endoprotease, is also stored in its active form in mast cells.[16]

STUDYING THE DISEASE CLINICALLY

Environmental Model

Environmental or seasonal studies are currently used in Europe and have been used in the United States to evaluate the efficacy of a variety of agents.[20–24] An environmental study consists of a fixed dosing regimen with the investigational drug lasting from several days to several weeks during the allergy season. The patient maintains a diary listing the frequency or severity of allergic episodes during the time allotted. At predetermined intervals, the patient receives an examination by the investigator to determine the effect of the agent on the study parameters. The environmental studies provide important safety and comfort information on a drug's behavior in the seasonal allergic population.

Shortcomings of the Environmental Model

VARIED EXPOSURE TO POLLEN

Not all patients in a study group are exposed to comparable degrees of pollen; varied exposure can arise from reasons such as work habits (outdoors versus indoors), use of air conditioning, lifestyle, and natural variation in pollen count. This variance can be exacerbated by the intentional avoidance behavior practiced by some patients to the allergen, a particular concern in parallel-controlled studies.

RELIANCE ON DIARIES

Examinations performed by the investigators may fail to reveal the drug's activity if the patient is asymptomatic at the time of the visit or if the patient's symptoms have resolved by the time the patient is actually seen. Even when exceptional provisions are made for an ophthalmologist to be on call to examine patients, the reaction can be dramatically diminished or completed by the time the patients have arrived at the examination site. This, in turn, eliminates the only objective evaluation of the drug's activity. Researchers therefore are often forced to rely on the patients' diaries to determine the efficacy of the investigational agent, a blunt instrument at best. However, even the patients' diaries are not always reliable because of the variations in subjective interpretation of allergic reactions, and they may be insufficient to provide an accurate measure of the drug's activity. The patients are also not skilled in grading, and they cannot grade clinical signs as precisely as trained investigators. Although large numbers of patients may sometimes show statistical significance, a clinically significant difference between drug and placebo is rarely possible or reproducible.

PLACEBO EFFECT

The identification of truly effective agents is further complicated by the high rate of placebo effect observed in environmental studies. Studies have reported placebo effects as high as 50 and 60%.[21, 25] The vehicle controls used as placebos can be soothing and essentially "rinse" the eye of the allergen.

COMPLIANCE

Compliance is always an issue in environmental studies. Environmental studies involve weeks of regular dosing and daily recording in the diaries. Noncompliance with test articles and excluded medication produce a dramatic amount of background interference. These factors may overwhelm the response either to an effective drug or to a comparison of an effective agent versus an ineffective agent.

Conjunctival Allergen Challenge Model

The conjunctival antigen challenge model (CAC) was developed to create a controlled setting in which to evaluate antiallergic agents.[26] The study design includes two baseline visits, during which skin test–positive subjects are administered a bilateral ocular challenge with standardized extracts of allergen. Hyperemia, itching, chemosis, and mucous discharge are graded on a well-established scale (Table 30.2) ranging from 0 (none) to 4 (severe). Threshold reactivity is defined as 2+ itching and hyperemia, a level that closely reflects the severity of allergic conjunctivitis and from which improvement may be measured. At the first visit, the threshold dose of reactivity is determined by increasing allergen doses at 10-minute intervals. At the second baseline visit 7 days later, the responsive subjects are challenged with the final, highest dose determined on visit 1 to ensure the reproducibility of the allergic reaction. Subjects who demonstrate a sufficient repeatable response to the dose of allergen return for the third visit 14 days later. After a slit-lamp examination, subjects are pretreated with the test drug in one eye and the placebo in the fellow eye in a randomized, double-masked fashion. After 10 minutes, the study subjects are challenged bilaterally with the allergen dose identified on the previous visits as being sufficient to induce 2+ itching and redness. Hyperemia, itching, chemosis, eyelid swelling, and tearing are evaluated at specific time points postchallenge. A fourth visit is used to assess duration of action by challenging the subject at a selected time point after pretreatment with the test drug.

TABLE 30.2 Grading Scale

Itching
0.0 None
0.5 Intermittent tickling sensation localized in the corner of the eye
1.0 Intermittent tickling sensation involving more than the corner of the eye
1.5 Intermittent tickling sensation all over
2.0 Mild continuous itch (can be localized), not requiring rubbing
2.5 Moderate, diffuse, continuous itch that you would like to rub
3.0 Severe itch that you would like to rub
4.0 Incapacitating itch that requires eye rubbing

Hyperemia
0.0 None
1.0 Mild; slightly dilated blood vessels; color of vessels typically pink; can be quadratic
2.0 Moderate; more apparent dilation of blood vessels; vessel color more intense (redder); involves most of the vessel bed
3.0 Severe; numerous and obvious dilated blood vessels; in the absence of chemosis, color is deep red; in the presence of chemosis, leaking interstitial fluid may make the color less red or even pinkish; not quadratic
4.0 Extremely severe; large, numerous, dilated blood vessels characterized by unusually severe deep red color, regardless of grade of chemosis, which involves the entire vessel bed

Chemosis
0.0 None
1.0 Mild; confirmed with slit-lamp evaluation in which the conjunctiva is separated from the episclera
2.0 Moderate; obvious raised conjunctiva without protrusion into the palpebral aperture
3.0 Severe; ballooning of the conjunctiva into the palpebral aperture with exposure of conjunctiva

Advantages of the Conjunctival Allergen Challenge Model

PATHOPHYSIOLOGICAL ADVANTAGES

The CAC model reproduces the signs and symptoms of SAC in a controlled setting. The topical instillation of allergen consistently elicits hyperemia, chemosis, itching, and mucous discharge by activating the innate pathophysiological mechanisms.

PHARMACOLOGICAL ADVANTAGES

Mast cell degranulation after the instillation of allergen has been confirmed with tear assays, thereby providing evidence that the CAC model replicates the natural disease process of SAC. The level of histamine in tears from control subjects was 10.64 ng/mL,[27] whereas that of challenged patients was 107 ng/mL at 3 minutes after challenge,[28] a 10-fold increase. Change in levels of tryptase has also been evaluated in tear samples after topical instillation of allergen.[29] Tryptase is a preformed mediator found exclusively in mast cells. Whereas tear samples from control subjects contained less than detectable levels of tryptase (less than 40 ng/mL), samples collected 10 minutes after challenge contained a mean tryptase level of 362 ng/mL.

REPRODUCIBILITY

The CAC model is highly reproducible because of its controlled, standardized design and its objective evaluation of a drug's efficacy. Each patient's threshold dose is determined and confirmed during the first two visits. This dose is used for all subsequent challenges during the study. Therefore, every patient who qualified for inclusion into the study manifests a minimum of 2+ itching and redness on challenge. Thus, the patients experience a more consistent degree of reaction than that observed in environmental studies. As an internal control, the treated eye can be compared with the naive contralateral eye. In addition, the efficacy of the drug is evaluated by a trained, objective third party according to a preestablished, standardized scale. The data obtained are therefore more reliable and reproducible.

SAFETY

Clinically, the signs of SAC are transient. Redness and chemosis of the conjunctiva and mild lid edema are the only signs of SAC and the CAC model. Itch is the only symptom. The early-phase reaction generally lasts less than 4 hours and is presented in the clinical condition unaccompanied by permanent changes.[35] The CAC model appears therefore safe, and adverse events have not been reported with topical allergen challenge.

PROPHYLACTIC VERSUS THERAPEUTIC EFFECTS

Although this distinction is important in chronic ongoing diseases, SAC is self-limited and lasts only a few hours without any residual pathophysiological alterations. This allergic condition, when it lasts for days or months, is the result of a chain of recurrent episodes of allergen exposure, mast cell degranulation, and receptor binding by mediators and enzymatic termination of the process. Therapies are always prophylactic in this condition, that is, they prevent or diminish the clinical response of the next episode. No lasting effect on tissue requiring therapy occurs, and if future episodes are prevented, the condition will no longer exist.

This having been said, the evaluation of a therapeutic effect defined as increasing the rate of resolution of itching, swelling, and redness, can be performed in the CAC model by administering the drop after antigen challenge. This model can be considered for agents causing vasoconstriction, agents that would rapidly replace histamine at the receptor level, or agents that would degrade any exogenous histamine more rapidly and completely than the endogenous histaminases.

Although the environmental studies can be viewed as prophylactic evaluations designed to diminish the next episode, and at the same time possibly therapeutic in that they increase the rate of sign and symptom resolution of the previous episode, the CAC model can separate and evaluate both these regimens. One must recognize, however, that the prophylactic effect is vastly more prominent in SAC.

USING THE MODEL TO EVALUATE THE EFFECTS OF ONE DROP OR TO DETERMINE THE NECESSARY DOSAGE TO LOAD EFFECTIVELY

The sensitivity of the CAC model allows for the evaluation of the effects of one drop for statistical significance against placebo in a double-masked study as well as the determination of clinical relevance (the change produced that would be noticeable to the patient).

CURRENT USAGE OF THE MODEL

The ability to treat one eye with the drug and the contralateral eye with a comparative drug, placebo, or a different concentration of the same drug has obvious benefits for the pharmaceutical development, regulatory, and marketing processes. The CAC model can determine the number of drops necessary to achieve a therapeutic level by loading before challenge. In addition, the CAC model possesses the ability to determine the exact duration of action, on which one may base the recommended usage. This has proven the case for mast cell stabilizers,[30, 31] antihistamines, vasoconstrictors, steroids, and nonsteroidal anti-inflammatory agents. Data from each of these categories of drug have been submitted to the United States Food and Drug Administration and have been found acceptable from the regulatory perspective for more than 8 years.

EXAMPLES OF ENVIRONMENTAL AND CONJUNCTIVAL ANTIGEN CHALLENGE STUDIES: LEVOCABASTINE/SODIUM CROMOLYN COMPARISONS

The efficacy of levocabastine in alleviating the signs and symptoms of allergic conjunctivitis has been evaluated in both the environmental model[32] and the CAC model.[24, 33] Levocabastine was shown to be active in both models, thus confirming the utility of the CAC model for evaluating new antiallergic agents.

In one environmental study,[32] the investigator's assessment of symptom severity revealed no significant differences between groups treated with levocabastine or sodium cromolyn. At 19 weeks, levocabastine was rated as excellent or good by 54 and 40% of the patients respectively, whereas sodium cromolyn was rated as excellent or good by 56 and 30% of the patients. For the same period, the investigator rated levocabastine as excellent in approximately 45% and good in 65% of the patients. The study therefore determined that both levocabastine and sodium cromolyn possessed comparable, potent anti-inflammatory activity. In another environmental study,[34] levocabastine was significantly more effective than sodium cromolyn in alleviating the signs and symptoms of allergic conjunctivitis, thus conflicting with the results from the Frostad study. Differences in assessing the severity of the allergic response have also been found between investigators and subjects. Although 60 and 35% of the patients rated levocabastine as excellent or good, respectively, in one study, the investigator rated levocabastine as excellent in 40% and good in 35% of the patients, a difference of 20%.[34]

Sixty-three percent of the patients in another study[25] rated the placebo as excellent or good.

In the CAC model, levocabastine was significantly superior to sodium cromolyn in inhibiting the signs and symptoms of allergic conjunctivitis at all time points (3, 5, and 10 minutes after challenge).[33] Mean itching scores for the levocabastine-treated group ranged from approximately 0.25 to 0.5 clinical units, whereas those for the sodium cromolyn–treated group ranged from 1.25 to 1.75 clinical units ($P < .001$). Mean differences for itching ranged from 1.11 to 1.50 clinical units. Mean hyperemia scores for the levocabastine-treated group ranged from approximately 0.5 to 1.25 clinical units, whereas those for the sodium cromolyn–treated group ranged from 1.25 to 2.25 clinical units ($P < .001$). The mean differences for conjunctival, ciliary, and episcleral hyperemia, considered individually, ranged from 0.84 to 1.10 clinical units. The mean differences of the summed scores ranged between 2.63 and 3.14 clinical units. Levocabastine was also significantly superior to sodium cromolyn in preventing chemosis ($P < .001$). Levocabastine maintained its anti-inflammatory activity 4 hours after pretreatment. The CAC model was therefore able to demonstrate objectively that levocabastine was significantly superior to sodium cromolyn in alleviating the signs and symptoms of SAC. Interestingly, sodium cromolyn demonstrated a more variable level of anti-inflammatory activity in the environmental studies than in the CAC study. These studies on levocabastine and sodium cromolyn establish the utility of the CAC model in differentiating among drugs with accepted efficacy in allergic conjunctivitis.

The ability to determine the time of onset, peak effect, and duration of action is a clear benefit of the CAC model not available in environmental studies. This model is part of the development process of most discovery groups in ocular allergy and should not just be accepted but rather required information for a regulatory agency. It is not meant to replace the environmental safety data, but it is a natural extension to allow more precise collection of efficacy data.

REFERENCES

1. Abelson MB, Madiwale NA, Weston JH. Conjunctival eosinophils in allergic ocular disease. Arch Ophthalmol 101:555–556, 1983.
2. Allansmith MR, Baird RS, Kashina K, et al. Mast cells in ocular tissues of normal rats and rats infected with *Nippostrongylus brasiliensis*. Invest Ophthalmol Vis Sci 18:858, 1979.
3. Allansmith K, Greiner J, Baird R. Number of inflammatory cells in the normal conjunctiva. Am J Ophthalmol 86:250, 1978.
4. Levene R. Mast cells and arnines in normal ocular tissues. Invest Ophthalmol 1:531, 1962.
5. Allansmith M. Immunology of the eye. In: The eye and immunology. Allansmith M, ed. St. Louis, CV Mosby, 1982.
6. Prausnitz C, Kustner H. Studien ueber die Ueberemfindlichkeit. Centralbl Bakteriol 86:160, 1921.
7. Kinet J. The high-affinity receptor for immunoglobulin E: structure, function, and role in allergy. In: Inflammation: basic principles and clinical correlates. 2nd ed. Gallin J, Goldstein I, Snyderman R, eds. New York, Raven Press, 1992.
8. Abelson K, Allansmith M. Histamine and the eye. In: Immunology and immunopathology of the eye. Silverstein A, O'Connor G, eds. San Francisco, Masson, 1979.
9. Ash A, Schild H. Receptors mediating some actions of histamine. Br J Pharmacol 27:427, 1966.
10. Black JW, Duncan WA, Durant CJ, et al. Definition and antagonism of histamine 1-12-receptors. Nature 236:385, 1972.
11. Owens DA, Poy E, Woodward DF, et al. Evaluation of the role of histamine H_1 and H_2 receptors in cutaneous inflammation in the guinea pig produced by histamine and mast cell degranulation. Br J Pharmacol 69:615, 1980.
12. Arrange J, Garbarg M, Schwartz J. Autoinhibition of brain histamine release mediated by a novel class (H_3) of histamine receptor. Nature 27:832, 1983.
13. Butrus S, Abelson M, Allansmith M. Ocular allergic disorder. In: Principles of immunology and allergy. Lockey R, Bukantz S, eds. Philadelphia, WB Saunders, 1987.
14. Braquet P. Perspectives in platelet-activating factor research. Agents Actions 15:82, 1987.

15. Spada CS, Woodward DF, Hawley SB, et al. Leukotrienes cause eosinophil emigration into conjunctival tissue. Prostaglandins 31:795, 1986.

16. Schechter NM, Choi JK, Slavin DA, et al. Identification of a chymotrypsin-like proteinase in human mast cells. J Immunol 137:962, 1986.

17. Abelson M, Madiwale N, Weston J. The role of prostaglandin D₂ in allergic ocular disease. In: Advances in immunology and immunopathology of the eye. O'Connor G, Chandler J, eds. New York, Masson, 1984.

18. Tamura N, Agrawal DK, Suliaman FA, et al. Effects of platelet-activating factor on the chemotaxis of normodense eosinophils from normal subjects. Biochem Biophys Res Commun 142:638, 1986.

19. George MA, Smith LM, Berdy GJ, et al. Platelet activating factor induced inflammation following topical ocular challenge. Invest Ophthalmol Vis Sci 31:63, 1990.

20. Kazdan JJ, Crawford JS, et al. Sodium cromoglycate in the treatment of vernal keratoconjunctivitis and allergic conjunctivitis. Can J Ophthalmol 11:300, 1976.

21. Lindsay-Miller A. Group comparative trial of 2% sodium cromoglycate (Opticrom) with placebo in the treatment of seasonal allergic conjunctivitis. Clin Allergy 9:271, 1979.

22. Lindsay-Miller A, Chambers A. Group comparative trial of cromolyn sodium and terfenadine in the treatment of seasonal allergic rhinitis. Ann Allergy 58:28, 1987.

23. Hendrix SG, Patterson R, Zeiss CR, et al. A multi-institutional trial of polymerized whole ragweed for immunotherapy of ragweed allergy. J Allergy Clin Immunol 66:486, 1980.

24. Abelson M, Weintraub D. Levocabastine eye drops: a new approach for the treatment of acute allergic conjunctivitis. Eur J Ophthalmol 4:91, 1994.

25. Davis B, Mullins J. Topical levocabastine is more effective than sodium cromoglycate for the prophylaxis and treatment of seasonal allergic conjunctivitis. Allergy 48:519, 1993.

26. Abelson M, Chambers W, Smith L. Conjunctival allergen challenge: a clinical approach to studying allergic conjunctivitis. Arch Ophthalmol 108:84, 1990.

27. Abelson MB, Leonardi AA, Smith LM, et al. Histaminase activity in patients with vernal keratoconjunctivitis. Ophthalmology 102:1958, 1995.

28. Berdy GJ, Levene RB, Bateman ST, et al. Identification of histaminase activity in human tears after conjunctival antigen challenge (abstract). Invest Ophthalmol Vis Sci 31:65, 1990.

29. Butrus SI, Ochsner KI, Abelson MB, et al. The level of tryptase in human tears: an indicator of conjunctival mast cells. Ophthalmology 97:1678, 1990.

30. Abelson MB, Spitalny L. Combined analysis of two studies using the conjunctival allergen challenge model to evaluate olopatadine hydrochloride; a new ophthalmic antiallergic agent with dual activity. Am J Ophthalmol 125:797, 1998.

31. Abelson MB. Evaluation of olopatadine; a new ophthalmic antiallergic agent with dual activity using the conjunctival allergen challenge model. Ann Allergy Asthma Immunol.

32. Frostad A, Olsen A. A comparison of topical levocabastine and sodium cromoglycate in the treatment of pollen-provoked allergic conjunctivitis. Clin Exp Allergy 23:406, 1993.

33. Abelson M, George M, Smith L. Evaluation of 0.05% levocabastine versus 4% sodium cromolyn in the allergen challenge model. Ophthalmology 102:310, 1995.

34. Odelram H, Bjorksten B, Klercker T, et al. Topical levocabastine versus sodium cromoglycate in allergic conjunctivitis. Allergy 44:432, 1989.

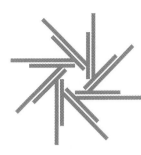

INDEX

Note: Page numbers in *italics* refer to illustrations; page numbers followed by t refer to tables.

ISBN 0-7216-8679-6

90071